DRUG TOXICITY: NEW RESEARCH

DRUG TOXICITY: NEW RESEARCH

CAM E. VELLOTIS
EDITOR

Nova Science Publishers, Inc.
New York

For permission to use material from this book please contact us:
Telephone 631-231-7269; Fax 631-231-8175
Web Site: http://www.novapublishers.com

Library of Congress Cataloging-in-Publication Data

Drug toxicity : new research / Cam E. Vellotis (editor).
p. ; cm.
Includes bibliographical references and index.
ISBN 978-1-60456-320-7 (hardcover)
1. Drugs--Toxicology. I. Vellotis, Cam E.
[DNLM: 1. Drug Toxicity. QV 600 D794 2008]
RA1238.D788 2008
615.9--dc22

2007052696

Published by Nova Science Publishers, Inc. ✢ New York

Contents

Preface

The systemic effects of a drug are related to the overall level of the medication in the bloodstream. Drug toxicity may occur with overdosage of a medication, accumulation of the drug in the body over time or the inability of the patient's body to eliminate the drug. This new book presents recent and important research in the field.

Chapter 1 - Recent high attrition rates have put an immense pressure on pharmaceutical industry which is struggling with even more challenges associated with regulatory hurdles and new products for the pipeline. Poor drug safety profiles have resulted in large fraction of late-stage drug failures. This, in turn, has contributed to a higher cost and lower yield of newer drug innovations. As a result, a greater emphasis has been laid on an earlier detection and verification of drug toxicity in the preclinical phase. Understanding the underlying mechanism of toxicity has become pivotal in the rational designing of research trials involving the drug candidate with superior efficacy.

However, the basic methodology of preclinical evaluation remains unaltered minimally during the last decade and the drug toxicity evaluation still remains an area of great concern. One of the many reasons is that drug toxicity in animal models so far has been evaluated by utilizing chemical, histological and hematological parameters as indicators of the organ damage. The unexpected toxicities encountered after preclinical studies on animal models have been attributed to the failure of adequately mimicking the human in vivo response to drug candidate toxicity. As a result, several newer tools are being developed to expedite the evaluation of toxicity in the drug development process from drug candidate screening to lead optimization. The high-throughput screening (HTS) 'omic' technologies such as genomics, proteomics, metabonomics, transcriptomics as well as in silico filters, molecular imaging, surrogate assays and biomarkers are being utilized in this process. These technologies carry a great potential to their wide spread acceptance in the pharmaceutical industry and would certainly revolutionize the field of drug design.

Moving ahead with this new era of toxicology research would require not only the latest technological innovations but also a multidisciplinary approach to the current safety paradigm involving basic biologists, translational researchers and physician scientists. This will help to deliver higher quality leads with balanced bioactivity and toxicity profile. In this chapter, the authors have reviewed the progress and trends in drug toxicity research and have highlighted a few gaps that need to be filled.

Chapter 2 – The psychotic disorders include schizophrenia, manic phase of bipolar disease, and other psychotic illnesses.

The clinically used agents to treat these disorders are the antipsychotic drugs. They may be classified in typical and atypical following their relative affinity for the antagonism of the dopamine D2 receptors, strong for the typical drugs and discrete or absent for the atypical. The dopamine antagonism is one of the determinants of the clinical effect, but the interaction with other neurotransmitter receptors also is relevant. Secondarily, the antipsychotic drugs may be classified following their chemical structure. Examples of typical antipsychotic drugs are thioridazine, chlorpromazine, fluphenazine, or haloperidol. Examples of atypical antipsychotic drugs are quetiapine, olanzapine, clozapine, or risperidone.

Although the antipsychotics are generally safe drugs, the adverse events profile of these agents is extensive and they are often related to their own pharmacological actions. They include central and autonomic nervous effects (sedation, cholinergic block, both acute and chronic extrapiramidal reactions including the neuroleptic malignant syndrome, and others), cardiovascular events (orthostatic hypotension, electrocardiographic changes and arrhythmias, stroke), endocrine disorders (weight gain, new-onset type 2 diabetes mellitus, and others), haematological disorders (leukocytosis, leukopenia, agranulocytosis, bone marrow suppression), and other adverse events (dermatological reactions, gastrointestinal disorders).

The aims of this chapter are to review several issues of antipsychotics (its supposed mechanism of action, main adverse events related and its habitual management) and to highlight the current research lines of new antipsychotic drugs, focusing on those trying to minimize the adverse event profile.

Chapter 3 – In the last decade, topical corticosteroids have received increasing attention for their sensitizing potential to generate allergic contact dermatitis. Most dermatologists agree that this sensitization is still under-recognized because the anti-inflammatory and immunosuppressive properties of topical glucocorticosteroids make it difficult to suspect the disease and, above all, to perform a correct diagnostic patch test. In fact, the best vehicle, concentration and reading time have not yet been identified. So, despite the growing number of dermatological studies published, the gold standard approach to the management of glucocorticosteroid allergic contact dermatitis has not yet been identified.

In the authors review, we try to provide a comprehensive overview of the clinical and practical aspects of corticosteroids-induced delayed hypersensitivity and its consequences on anti-inflammatory therapeutic choices.

Chapter 4 – Hemodynamic profiles obtained by cardiac catheterization in the context of different clinical scenarios, reflect distinct patho-physiological states enabling clinicians to manage patients in a scientific way. The three most important types of measurements in the cardiac catheterization laboratory are: Pressures, Flows (i.e. cardiac output, systemic blood flow and pulmonary flow etc) resistance indicators and Oxygen Saturations in different chambers.

One should take several general precautions during hemodynamic monitoring. The transducer must be positioned at mid-chest level midway in the frontal and transverse planes close to 4th intercostal space near the sternal margin. This type of leveling assures close proximity of the transducer to the center of the heart, thus excluding the effects of weight of tubing and fluid column. The atmospheric pressure is used as a zero point reference and is therefore, a common need to open the system to air. The tubing should be as short as possible to reflect the accurate timing of pressure tracings. Since air in the system could create grossly erroneous values, adequate and repeated flushing should be performed to ensure an air free system. Fluid to fluid contact should be maintained at all the levels. Intravascular volume status should be closely monitored and adjusted. Etio-pathology of hemodynamic changes should be considered and correlated with the type, severity and duration of each of the valvular and/or pericardial lesions. Influence of pressure and/or volume overload of single or multiple valvular lesions on the volume and pressure profiles of different chambers, arterial and venous vasculature should be considered. Integrity of the pulmonary or hematological system should be taken into account. Correlation with echocardiographic findings should always be considered. Echocardiographic and catheterization findings are always complementary. Intracardiac and extracardiac shunts and anemia have significant influence on pressures, severity of stenoses and insufficiency.

Precise diagnosis of restrictive cardiomyopathy and pericardial diseases using hemodynamic profiles in a busy cardiac catheterization setting is also a challenging task. This is partly due to unavailability of a quick review of case scenarios, equipment selection, methods and interpretation of hemodynamic profiles and key diagnostic points. This review brings together case vignettes, methods and protocols for hemodynamic work up of commonly encountered valvular conditions and pericardial diseases to differentiate them accurately from restrictive cardiomyopathy. Each clinical entity is described with the help of case vignettes, equipment and protocols for hemodynamic work up, methods and interpretation of hemodynamic profiles with emphasis on salient diagnostic features.

Chapter 5 – Artemisinin and its developed derivatives, dihydroartemisinin (DHA), artemether (AM), arteether (AE), artesunate (AS), and artelinate (AL), are highly effective antimalarials with a favorable safety profile. Their pharmacodynamic effects against many stages of the malaria life cycle, from young asexual forms (ring) to early sexual forms (gametocytes), account for their rapid activity, which may protect them from resistance, In the past two decades, toxicity studies have shown a dose-dependent neurotoxic effect in animal species administered intramuscularly or intragastrically with artemisinins, especially with oil-soluble AM and AE. In contrast, few neurotoxic effects are induced by water-soluble AS and AL, which have never produced any CNS side-effects in animal species after intravenous injection. Pharmacokinetic profiles demonstrate that drug exposure time plays a more important role in producing neurotoxicity than drug exposure level, production of the more active metabolite (DHA), or drug location in the CNS system. In addition, it has been demonstrated that at a below human therapeutic dose, injectable AS can cause fetal death due to a build up of high peak concentration of AS during the sensitive period of the early gestation days (GD) in animals. To date, however, the neurotoxicity and reprotoxicity have not been convincingly established in humans treated with any of artemisinins. Fatal neurotoxicity can be avoided by reducing the drug exposure time that varies greatly between the different artemisinin compounds. Also reproductive toxicity can be avoided by limiting the exposure of artemisinins during this sensitive period in fetal development (GD 9–14 in rats and GD 15 to week 6 in humans).

Pharmacokinetic/pharmacodynamic evaluations demonstrate that the rapid efficacy of artemisinins is principally due to the drug peak concentration (Cmax) and their antimalarial potency. Other pharmacokinetic parameters, such as drug exposure level (AUC) and drug exposure time (half-life) tend to be of minor significance. The fundamental and reliable measures of efficacy in cure and mortality rates for uncomplicated and severe malaria show that current artemisinins (AS, AM, and DHA) have great role in artemisinin-based combination therapy (ACT) or monotherapy and provide a clear-cut advantage over other antimalarials currently in use. The artemisinin derivatives in combination with standard antimalarials are now being promoted as the best therapeutic option for treating drug-resistant malaria and retarding the development of resistant. There is clear evidence that combinations improve efficacy without increasing toxicity.

Most recently, a decrease in mortality (34.7%) has been demonstrated in a large study using intravenous AS, as opposed to the standard of care quinine injection. Artemisinins as a group are poorly efficacious at curing malaria as monotherapy. However, this shortfall has been overcome by using ACTs and AS injection in combination or in sequential administration with slower acting antimalarial drugs. When considering the demonstrated rapid parasite killing of parasites and variance between individual patients in both pharmacokinetics and pharmacodynamics, initial monotherapy and larger loading dose of AS injection may be needed to ensure that the maximum effect is obtained in all patients with severe and complicated malaria.

Chapter 6 – Traditional (non-selective) NSAIDs cause nephrotoxicity through inhibition of cyclooxygenase (COX) activity and prostaglandin formation in the kidney. Patients with prostaglandin-dependent disease states are the group at most risk for this adverse effect. It has become apparent that the COX-2 enzyme isoform is constitutively expressed and upregulated in the human kidney during states of renal stress. COX-2 derived prostaglandins importantly modulate renal blood flow and glomerular filtration rate as well as sodium, potassium and water excretion by the kidney. As a result, clinical renal syndromes induced by the selective COX-2 inhibitors are quite similar to those described with the traditional NSAIDs, suggesting that COX-2 derived prostaglandins are important in maintaining normal renal function. Inhibition of prostaglandins causes a reduction in renal blood flow and acute renal failure in patients with predisposing conditions. These include true volume depletion from nausea/vomiting, diarrhea and excessive diuretic therapy. Effective volume depletion from clinical disease states such as heart failure, cirrhosis, and nephrotic syndrome as well as diseases such as chronic kidney disease and renal artery stenosis also portend risk of acute renal failure from prostaglandin inhibition.

Prostaglandins also modulate renal potassium excretion through stimulation of the renin-angiotensin-aldosterone system. Inhibition of prostaglandins can result in hyperkalemia when co-existent conditions such as renal failure, diabetes mellitus and therapy with certain medications (ACE inhibitors, angiotensin receptor blockers, potassium-sparing diuretics) are also present. The classic syndrome of hyporeninemic hypoaldosteronism with a type-4 renal tubular acidosis (RTA) picture (hyperkalemic metabolic acidosis) can be observed when selective COX-2 inhibitor therapy is superimposed. Inhibition of prostaglandins is associated with decreased renal sodium and water excretion and all NSAIDs, including the selective COX-2 inhibitors cause some degree of sodium retention. All patients suffer from this effect, but only patients with certain clinical conditions develop obvious edema, hypertension or heart failure. Patients with underlying hypertension (especially those on antihypertensive medications), heart disease and other salt-retentive disease states (cirrhosis, nephrosis, renal failure) are at highest risk for these complications. Hypertension is a particularly important complication of these drugs as small changes in blood pressure are associated with increased cardiovascular events. Hyponatremia from impaired water excretion also complicates therapy.

Less commonly, acute interstitial nephritis (with or without a glomerulopathy) has been described with these drugs. To reduce adverse renal effects from NSAIDs, including all of available the selective COX-2 inhibitors, identification of patients with renal risk should be undertaken. Defining patient risk profiles based on level of kidney function (stage of chronic kidney disease) as well as on the presence of certain co-morbidities (hypertension, heart failure, diabetes mellitus, liver disease/cirrhosis, electrolyte imbalance, old age, certain medications) is one simple approach that can be taken. Based on the renal risk, recommendations for therapy and monitoring can be utilized in a rational fashion.

Chapter 7 – Ethanol is a small molecule acting on several neurotransmitter systems in the brain. Accumulating evidences suggest that the primary excitatory – i.e. the glutamatergic – neurotransmitter system is a particularly important site of ethanol's action. Several studies showed that ethanol is a potent and selective inhibitor of the N-methyl-D-aspartate (NMDA) receptors and prolonged ethanol exposition leads to a compensatory "up-regulation" of these receptors resulting in enhanced NMDA receptor mediated functions after removal of ethanol. These alterations are supposed to contribute to the development of ethanol tolerance, dependence as well as the acute and delayed signs of ethanol withdrawal. Recently, alterations in subunit composition of NMDA receptors were reported after long-term ethanol exposure. mRNA and/or protein levels of NR2A and NR2B types of subunits were found elevated both by in vivo and in vitro experiments. In primary cultures of rat hippocampal or cortical neurons, especially the NR2B subunit expression and levels of certain NR1 splice variants were increased after 3 days of intermittent ethanol treatment. According to the high calcium permeability, the increased agonist sensitivity and the relatively slow closing kinetics of NMDA ion channels composed of NR1 and NR2B subunits, these changes may underlie the enhanced NMDA receptor activation observed after long-term ethanol exposure. Consequently, novel type of NMDA receptor antagonists - the NR2B subunit selective agents potently inhibited the neurotoxic effect of ethanol withdrawal seen in primary cultures of rat cortical neurons pre-treated with ethanol. Consistent with these observations, enhanced NR2B type of NMDA receptor subunit expression is likely involved in development of alcohol dependence and withdrawal symptoms, therefore this subunit may serve as a possible drug target in pharmacological interventions against alcoholism.

Chapter 8 – Cervical cancer continues to be the major cause of cancer mortality in women in developing countries. Although detection routine screening programs have been implemented since 1975, an increased rate of new cases has also been detected. Some studies have demonstrated a relationship between HPV, cervical intraepithelial neoplasia, and invasive carcinoma of cervix. Additionally, it has been predicted that within 10 years, 66% of all dysplasia -without medical intervention- would progress to carcinoma in situ. It is important to bear these data in mind in order to be able to search new alternatives for cervical cancer treatment.

Cisplatin and its derivatives are important drugs in cervical cancer therapy. However, the administration of cisplatin is associated with serious side effects, including nephrotoxic and neurotoxic events. This issue has motivated the search for new agents or new regimens for cisplatin combinations with the purpose of increasing antitumoral activity and decreasing secondary events.

Among the chemosensitizer drugs, antihormonal agents have been used to modulate the cytotoxic activity of antineoplastic agents, principally in hormone-dependent cancers such as breast and prostate cancers. Although the normal cervix is known to respond to steroid sex hormones, hormonal treatments are not frequently employed in cervical carcinoma therapy. In fact, this carcinoma is traditionally considered not to respond to antihormonal therapy. The authors hypothesize that exposure to antihormonal agents for sensitizer cervical cancer cells to the antineoplastic treatment can be independent of steroid-receptors. The importance of antihormonal agents used to modulate the cytotoxic activity of anticancer drugs in cervical cancer will be explored in this article.

Chapter 9 – It was shown that the scale or direction of correlations between both the several parameters of the lipid composition and the generalized parameters of the phospholipids composition of the murine liver depend on the kinetic characteristics of their lipids (the lipid peroxides content, the capacity of lipids to decompose peroxides). In was found that the combined intraperitoneal administration of the low- toxicity surfactant (Tween 80) and acetone at low doses causes disturbances in the lipid peroxidation regulatory system which manifest themselves in 1 month after the action.

Chapter 10 – D-Serine is nephrotoxic in rats. Intraperitoneal injection of d-serine causes necrosis of the cells in the proximal tubules, resulting in glucosuria, aminoaciduria, proteinuria, and polyuria [1,2]. However, the precise mechanism by which D-serine induces nephrotoxicity is not well understood. D-Amino-acid oxidase (EC 1.4.3.3) is suspected to be involved in the D-serine-induced nephrotoxicity because (a) D-serine is reabsorbed in the straight part (pars recta) of the proximal tubules, where cell damage is observed [1-3], (b) D-amino-acid oxidase is localized in this region [4,5], (c) D-serine is a good substrate for this enzyme [6], and (d) one of the products of the D-amino-acid oxidase reaction, hydrogen peroxide, is a cytotoxin.

However, there are perplexing problems: (a) D-serine is not nephrotoxic in mice, guinea pigs, rabbits, dogs, hamsters, or gerbils that have D-amino-acid oxidase activity comparable to rats [7,8]; (b) D-alanine, which is also a good substrate for D-amino-acid oxidase, is not nephrotoxic in rats [8]. These facts cast doubt on the involvement of this enzyme in d-serine-induced nephrotoxicity.

Thus, D-serine-induced nephrotoxicity is a challenging problem. One example of the induction of the kidney damage by D-serine is described here.

In: Drug Toxicity: New Research
Editor: Cam E. Vellotis, pp.1-28
ISBN 978-1-60456-320-7

Chapter 1

Drug Toxicity Research Trends

Sarabjeet Singh*[*1] and Sanjeev Wasson[2]

[1]Department of Medicine, Chicago Medical School at
Rosalind Franklin University of Medicine and Sciences.
North Chicago, IL-60064
[2]Cleveland Clinic Foundation, Cleveland, OH 44195

Abstract

Recent high attrition rates have put an immense pressure on pharmaceutical industry which is struggling with even more challenges associated with regulatory hurdles and new products for the pipeline. Poor drug safety profiles have resulted in large fraction of late-stage drug failures. This, in turn, has contributed to a higher cost and lower yield of newer drug innovations. As a result, a greater emphasis has been laid on an earlier detection and verification of drug toxicity in the preclinical phase. Understanding the underlying mechanism of toxicity has become pivotal in the rational designing of research trials involving the drug candidate with superior efficacy.

However, the basic methodology of preclinical evaluation remains unaltered minimally during the last decade and the drug toxicity evaluation still remains an area of great concern. One of the many reasons is that drug toxicity in animal models so far has been evaluated by utilizing chemical, histological and hematological parameters as indicators of the organ damage. The unexpected toxicities encountered after preclinical studies on animal models have been attributed to the failure of adequately mimicking the human *in vivo* response to drug candidate toxicity. As a result, several newer tools are being developed to expedite the evaluation of toxicity in the drug development process from drug candidate screening to lead optimization. The high-throughput screening (HTS) 'omic' technologies such as genomics, proteomics, metabonomics, transcriptomics as well as in silico filters, molecular imaging, surrogate assays and biomarkers are being utilized in this process. These technologies carry a great potential to

---

* Address for correspondence: Sarabjeet Singh M.D. Department of Medicine. Chicago Medical School. 3003 Green Bay Road, North Chicago, IL 60064 (USA). Telephone: 773-257-6452. Fax: 209-729-5767. Email: sarabjeetsingh_2000@yahoo.com

their wide spread acceptance in the pharmaceutical industry and would certainly revolutionize the field of drug design.

Moving ahead with this new era of toxicology research would require not only the latest technological innovations but also a multidisciplinary approach to the current safety paradigm involving basic biologists, translational researchers and physician scientists. This will help to deliver higher quality leads with balanced bioactivity and toxicity profile. In this chapter, we have reviewed the progress and trends in drug toxicity research and have highlighted a few gaps that need to be filled.

Keywords: Drug toxicity, Preclinical testing, Animal models, High-throughput screening, 'Omic' technologies.

Abbreviations

ADMET	Absorption, Distribution, Metabolism, Excretion and Toxicology
ADR	Adverse Drug Reaction
ALT	Alanine Transaminase
APD	Action Potential Duration
AST	Aspartate Transaminase
cDNA	Complimentary DNA
CEBS	Chemical Effects in Biological Systems
DNA	Deoxy- ribonucleic Acid
EPA	Environmental Protection Agency
FDA	Food and Drug Administration
hERG	Human Ether-a-go-go
hESC-CM	Human Embryonic Stem Cell Derived Cardiomyocytes
ILSI	International Life Science Institute
MRSD	Maximum recommended safe starting dose
MIAME	Minimum Information About a Microarray Experiment
NCT	National Center for Toxicogenomics
NIEHS	National Institute of Environmental Health Sciences
NOAEL	No observed adverse effect level
NCE	New Chemical Entities
NTP	National Toxicology Program
NIH	National Institute of Health
OSHA	Occupational Safety and Health Administration
PD	Pharmacodynamic
PPAR	Peroxisome Proliferator-Activated Receptor
PLOT	Preclinical Lead Optimization Technologies
QSARs	Quantitative Structure-Activity Relationships
RNA	Ribonucleic acid
SOT	Society of Toxicology
SAR	Structure-Activity Relationship

SIMCA	Soft Independent Modeling of Class Analogy
SGPT	Serum Glutamic Pyruvic Transaminase
SGOT	Serum Glutamic Oxaloacetic Transaminase
SNP	Single Nucleotide Polymorphisms
TI	Toxicity Index

1. Introduction

Despite several years of research, drug toxicity remains a topic of significant concern [1]. Recent drug withdrawals have imposed increased concerns at the time when the pharmaceutical industry yield has leveled [2]. A Food and Drug Administration (FDA) report [3] has suggested that if decreased pipeline production is not delt appropriately, it may create a risk that "the biomedical revolution will not be able to keep up its commitment of providing better health". Moreover, there is an urgent need for applying "omics" technologies, bioinformatics systems, and new imaging modalities to detect safety problems in a timely manner. At the same instance, others have questioned the role of new technologies and their impact on the safety assessment. [4]. To enhance drug safety and better health outcomes, it is essential that we advance our knowledge of mechanisms of drug toxicity, successfully implement new technologies to the practical challenge of predicting drug safety, and improve mechanism-based risk assessment to ensure the safe use of new drugs in mankind.

We offer a perspective on the drug toxicity research trends, its current state and future needs.

2. History

Toxic substances have certainly been used for both offense and defense ever since advent of mankind on this earth. Ancient man likely observed toxic effects in nature partly by accident. He noted the harmful or fatal effect following the causal ingestion of some plant or animal product by one of his fellow tribesmen and possibly used their extracts for hunting or in warfare [5]. Earliest written records were probably the Ebers Papyrus and Hippocrates' description of hemlock as the state poison of the Greeks. [5]. By the time of the Renaissance and the Age of Enlightenment, certain concepts fundamental to toxicology began to take shape. Auroleus Phillipus Theostratus Bombastus von Hohenheim (1493-1541), also known as Paracelsus and widely regarded as the father of modern toxicology, formulated the expression, "All things are poison and nothing is without poison", suggesting that "dose determines the poison". In the late 18th century a Spanish physician, Matthieu Joseph Bonaventure Orfila (1757–1853), working at the University of Paris, first prepared a systematic correlation between the chemical and biological properties of poisons at that time. He demonstrated effects of poisons on specific organs by analyzing autopsy materials and their associated tissue damage. He emphasized that toxicology should be a separate science and chemical analysis must be an integral part of its foundation [5]. He wrote a text, *Traité des Poisons Tirés des Regnes Minéral Végétal et Animal, ou Toxicologie Générale*

Considérée Sous les Rapports de la Pathologie et de Médicine Légale (1814), which went through five editions and was a landmark in not only toxicology but in scientific history [5]. It was Orfila, who introduced qualitative science into toxicology.

Today, it is much easier to define toxicology's coming of age or the transition of toxicology into an academic discipline with journals, textbooks, departments, curricula, societies, annual meetings, certification, etc [6]. Historically, the first step in the transition of toxicology into an academic discipline was the establishment of the Journal of Toxicology and Applied Pharmacology in 1959. The Journal of Toxicology and Applied Pharmacology became the official journal of the Society of Toxicology in 1963. They broadened the scope of this journal to include reviews, editorials, and coverage of contemporary issues in toxicology. During the 1950s many departments of pharmacology began to introduce courses in toxicology into their graduate curriculum and toxicologic materials into the medical school courses. Because there was no textbook for this area of toxicology, DuBois and Geiling wrote and published the first textbook of toxicology in this country in 1959. The formation of the Society of Toxicology (SOT) was the third important event in the history of the transformation of toxicology into an academic discipline. It started in early 1961. In the nearly four decades of SOT's existence, it has exhibited significant progress, its annual meetings have become major scientific events, it has contributed towards the development of toxicology as a science, and transforming it into an academic discipline. During recent years we have seen a virtual explosion in toxicology. Today's toxicology is characterized by sophisticated scientific investigation and evaluation of toxic exposures. The 20th century is marked by an advanced level of understanding of toxicology. During this period, deoxyribonucleic acid (DNA) and various proteins that maintain cellular functions were discovered. Our level of knowledge of toxic effects on organs and cells is now being revealed at the molecular level. Twenty first century has brought the field of toxigenomics. It is recognized that virtually all toxic effects are caused by changes in specific cellular molecules and biochemicals. In September 2000, the National Institute of Environmental Health Sciences developed the National Center for Toxicogenomics (NCT), whose mission is to coordinate a nationwide research effort for the development of a toxicogenomics knowledge base. As stated in their website: http://www.niehs.nih.gov/nct/ there are five goals of the National Center for Toxicogenomics:

1. To facilitate the application of gene and protein expression technology;
2. To understand the relationship between environmental exposures and human disease susceptibility;
3. To identify useful biomarkers of disease and exposure to toxic substances;
4. To improve computational methods for understanding the biological consequences of exposure and responses to exposure; and
5. To create a public database of environmental effects of toxic substances in biological systems.

Because of a diversity of concerns and applications, modern toxicology has developed into three specialized branches: environmental, clinical, and forensic [7]. *Environmental toxicology* is concerned mainly with the harmful effects of chemicals that are encountered by chance because they are in the atmosphere, in the food chain, or are present in occupational environment. *Clinical toxicology*, a subspecialty of medicine, is concerned with the harmful effects of chemicals that are intentionally administered to living organisms for the purpose of achieving a specific effect. The desired effect achieved may be beneficial to the organ, in which case the toxicologist is interested in the adverse or side effects of the agent. *Forensic toxicology* is the division of toxicology that is focused on the medicolegal aspects of the harmful effects of chemicals or poisons [7]. This chapter will review the progress of clinical toxicology by exploring analytical techniques in drug analysis, biological matrices, clinical toxicology, therapeutic drug management, pharmacodynamic monitoring and pharmacogenetics.

3. Background: Safety Assessment

Achieving an acceptable efficacy and safety profile for a new drug molecule is a challenging task, requiring optimization of many variables within a single chemical structure [8]. From a safety perspective, the complexity lies largely in the quality and interpretation of data from a discrete series of experiments and trials that define the preclinical safety assessment paradigm [9].

3.1. Target Validation and Lead Generation

Target validation is defined as the process of allowing the current target object to validate its data before a target change, and to deny change if the data is invalid.

Lead generation is defined as strategies developed to identify compounds which possess a desired but non-optimized biological activity. For novel targets, safety concerns must be inferred from literature on genetic studies in humans and lower organisms or by mining the various pathways involved in a disease process. At the target-to-lead stage, the focus of safety assessment is on anticipated safety problems. In silico analysis of chemical structure and binding to Occupational Safety and Health Administration (OSHA) databases for safety outcomes, such as mutagenicity, are used prior to chemical synthesis [10]. Prototypical small molecules, peptidomimetics or proteins (e.g., antibodies), even if not sufficiently "druglike" for clinical use, can be utilized to investigate safety issues that may emerge during lead optimization. Pharmacodynamic (PD)-based biomarkers of efficacy, such as antibodies that recognize post-translational modifications associated with target modulation; for example, phosphorylation, ubiquitination, and acetylation states of proteins (if these are known), assist link dose-response relationships for target modulation with organ toxicity. If the target in humans has various forms, confirmation of the expression of similar isozymes and selectivity in preclinical animal models is necessary. Mapping the tissue distribution of the drug target is essential to determine if toxicity tracks closely with target expression. In general, multiple approaches are required to unfold the mechanism of target organ toxicity. Having the right tools and an effective risk management strategy are the keys to success.

As toxicities are encountered during the research and development phase, one of the most vital questions to address would be whether the mechanism is related to the intended pharmacology (on-target toxicity) or to the chemical structure itself (off-target toxicity). Distinguishing between these two potential mechanisms is pivotal in designing strategies to enhance safety. Drug development is a high-risk and expensive affair. Thus, appropriate lead candidate selection for preclinical drug development and registration can reduce the high rate of attrition, the cost of which increases with the distance that the failed candidate has proceeded down the pipeline [11].

3.2. Lead Optimization

Lead optimization is categorized into a "synthesis and testing" phase and a "selection" phase. During the former such properties in a compound as potency, selectivity, bioavailability, absorption and metabolism must be assessed. This is achieved by complex functional assays and analytical chemistry. At the same time, lead compounds and their relatives must be synthesized, their molecular structure defined, and their molecular targets constructed. All this is achieved by the use of such advanced techniques including computer assisted drug design and three-dimensional molecular modeling. In the selection phase the pharmacological profile of the compound is completed and chemical and pharmaceutical feasibility evaluated. Increasingly, lead optimization in its selection phase aims to identify and promote only those compounds with an improved realistic chance of completing development. Reducing the rates of attrition during development is a major target for research.

In transition from lead to a drug candidate, the lead is used as a base structure for the synthesis of sometimes hundreds of derivatives in a process known as "Lead Optimization". During this stage, the characteristics of a "good drug" are built into potential clinical candidates [8]. From a safety perspective, the goal is to identify the dose-limiting toxicities, the most sensitive animal species, and set doses for later definitive safety studies. Potential candidates are often screened for safety using pilot repeat dose studies [12]. Toxicity with one molecule can be easily circumvented by testing another, but recurring toxicity within the lead series can be a limiting factor in the development of the drug candidate. However, without understanding the mechanism and relevance to humans, abandoning a novel target or lead series based on toxicity in short-term studies may be premature. However, to proceed further, a strategy to design safer compounds must be thought.

The MOS is defined in preclinical models by the separation between parameters defining the efficacy and safety; in general, they are based on exposure rather than administered dose [13]. Two things are required to widen the MOS during lead optimization: knowledge of mechanism (on- vs off-target) and screening tools to inform the structure-activity relationship (SAR). If the mechanisms cannot be distinguished and a screening method cannot be implemented, finding better compounds may be reduced to empirical screening rather than design of a rational drug. However, if an on- versus off-target mechanism is established, the strategies to increase the MOS will be different. In either case, a mechanism-based screening strategy reduces the time and amount of compound needed to find an optimized drug candidate. Establishing the mechanism and validating the assay are the main goals of mechanistic investigations during lead optimization phase.

3.3. Preclinical Safety Evaluation: From Clinical Candidate to Registration

Once a clinical candidate is identified, the chemical dye is cast, and the biological properties are locked in the structure. The emphasis for preclinical testing shifts from candidate identification to candidate evaluation. Before an application for investigational new drug is submitted, safety is assessed in other species eg. rodents according to requirements of the regulatory committee. [9, 13]. The primary purpose of these safety studies is to identify a maximum recommended safe starting dose (MRSD) [14]. The no observed adverse effect level (NOAEL) is defined as the maximum dose at which adverse effects are not seen preclinically [13]. A human equivalency dose, derived from the NOAEL and divided by a safety factor, establishes the MRSD, the point from where dose escalation begins in the clinic, and main parameter in setting the dose range used to test the clinical hypothesis.

Mechanism-based risk assessment impacts the MRSD and the safety factor used to set the MRSD in multiple ways: (i) understanding mechanisms of species sensitivity, (ii) establishing ways to monitor the risk, and (iii) defining the reversibility of target organ toxicity. In the absence of data on humans, the default position is to estimate the MRSD using the NOAEL from the most sensitive preclinical test species. However, if the mechanism of toxicity in the most sensitive species is not relevant to humans, the interpretation can alter.

In common with any new paradigm shift, the (preclinical lead optimization technologies) PLOT strategy must overcome a number of problems. This is one of the reasons why pharmaceutical drug discovery project teams have made their decisions on compound development based mainly on toxicologic data gathered from short-term, range-finding compound exposures, which provide limited evidence for long-term organ-specific toxicity. This dependence on *in vivo* studies represents a significant obstacle to acceptance of the PLOT strategy, as decisions on a molecule selection/rejection on in vitro PLOT would need to be made before animal testing. Furthermore, since candidate compounds which are chosen for drug development following assessment by PLOT will still need to be assessed in regulatory toxicology studies, it is necessary that the PLOT screens are predictive of the corresponding regulatory test equivalent, if known. This is well illustrated by the use of high throughput mutagenicity-bacterial reporter gene assay (SOS repair system) findings of which correlate well with the regulatory gold-standard Ames assay (Reifferscheid and Heil, 1996). Although it will be difficult to discuss Ames assay in detail but in brief, it was developed by Ames (1971) for short term testing for carcinogenicity subject to the proviso that mutagenicity is equivalent to carcinogenicity and that, since most carcinogens have to undergo metabolism to reveal their carcinogenic action, a preparation of rat liver would provide an activation mechanism similar to that which would occur in human liver. The Ames test is performed on Salmonella typhimurium mutant which does not need amino acid histidine in the medium. If the mutant is exposed to a mutagenic agent it reverts to the original wild strain. This test system is combined with a liver preparation to activate the carcinogen and the test has been further developed with the use of organisms more sensitive to the mutagenic action of chemical agents [15].

There are many reasons for preclinical/clinical drug failure. These include mutagenicity, target organ toxicity and poor bioavailability, the last being due to a number of factors including poor absorption across the gastrointestinal tract, rapid clearance, or metabolism. Finally, unless the correct species is selected for predicting human safety, drug failure may not occur until after preclinical phase. *In vitro* PLOT screening can also help identify the appropriate toxicology non-rodent species in the very early phase of development.

4. *In Silico* Approaches to Drug Safety Evaluation

As the large libraries of compounds are becoming available, recognition of imputed toxicity is needed even before they are synthesized. Thus the utility of predictive toxicology is called for. Quantitative structure-activity relationships (QSARs) exist for a wide range of toxicity endpoints and have been used for the prediction of toxicity of diverse libraries. Fortunately, various expert systems are available for toxicity prediction and most of them cover wide spectrum of toxicity endpoints. Those discussed here include TOPKAT, CASE, DEREK, HazardExpert, OncoLogic and COMPACT. Many examples exist of drug molecules that have had to be withdrawn, because of unacceptable toxicity encountered in clinical studies. This has led to large financial losses. For that reason, in recent years pharmaceutical companies have brought toxicity testing, as well as ADMET (absorption, distribution, metabolism, excretion and toxicology) studies, earlier in the drug development phase.

The modern science of QSAR can be said to date from the seminal 1962 publication of Hansch et al. [16] which established the use of multiple linear regression as an important tool for the correlation of biological activity with descriptors of chemical structure. In order for a QSAR to reflect biological data well, and to be predictive, it is generally acknowledged that all the compounds involved should have the same mechanism of action. Since it is difficult to determine mechanism of action, the compounds involved in a QSAR correlation are usually restricted to a given chemical class in the hope that this will ensure a single mechanism of action. The main reason of developing a QSAR is so that it can be used for predictive purposes. Therefore it is important that the statistics given with the QSAR give an indication of its predictivity. An important point to realize is the utility of a QSAR for toxicity to directly relate to the therapeutic ratio, not toxicity alone. Though the concept of QSAR has been known for a while, but its use has not been that extensive. The main reason for this is the recent advent of combinatorial chemistry in screening diverse libraries, which are not so amenable to classical QSAR analysis. Another reason may be that the pharmaceutical industry is preoccupied with their search for ever-increasing potent drugs. Published drug toxicity QSARs cover numerous end-points, from carcinogenicity to cardiotoxicity to gastric irritancy. It is not feasible to discuss all of them, but it is worthwhile to consider few examples. An example of human drug toxicity was given by King and Moffat [17] in their study, who utilized toxicity index (TI) of barbiturates, the ratio of mortality rates in a given year in United Kingdom in a given year from a specified barbiturate to the number of prescriptions issued for that particular barbiturate. Although the study size was small, the statistics were adequate to reflect the accuracy of the data. In 1987 Hansch et al. [18] proposed their theory of minimal hydrophobicity, which states that 'without convincing evidence to the contrary, drugs should be made as hydrophilic as possible without loss of efficacy'; the reason being that hydrophilic compounds do not accumulate readily in the body, as they are rapidly excreted. On the other hand, the rates of metabolism generally increase with hydrophobicity, as the body tries to eliminate xenobiotics. An example of the above is microsomal demethylation of a group of miscellaneous drugs [19]. As a result, substantial effort has gone into the calculation of octanol-water log P values, and a number of commercial software packages are now available for that reason. Mannhold and Dross [20] published in 1996 a comparative study of 14 such packages; Dearden et al. [18] have recently updated a similar study on commercially available packages for the calculation of aqueous solubility [22]. It should be noted that many pharmaceutical companies have integrated proprietary software algorithms as well.

Expert Systems

An expert system has been defined [23] as 'any formal system, not necessarily computer-based, which enables a user to obtain rational predictions about the toxicity of chemicals. All expert systems for the prediction of toxicity are based on experimental data representing one or more toxic manifestations of chemicals in the database, and/or rules derived from such data'. Expert systems for the prediction of toxicity are broadly divided into four categories: automated QSAR, knowledge-based systems, and automated rule derivation and decision trees. Numerous reviews have been published on the use of expert systems for prediction of toxicity [23-27]. The automated QSAR system is exemplified by TOPKAT. This software uses both continuous and dichotomous measures to predict various toxicity end-points, including carcinogenicity, mutagenicity, teratogenicity, etc. Continuous end-points are modeled using multiple linear regression QSARs, whilst dichotomous measures are modeled using linear discriminant regression. TOPKAT utilizes large, heterogeneous data-bases with selected data while its QSARs usually uses topological, sub-structural and electronic descriptors. TOPKAT can also be used in batch mode from structural data (SD) file input. Enslein et al. [28] reported on the use of TOPKAT in the prediction of carcinogenicity and mutagenicity, whilst Enslein et al. [29] discussed the development of a dermal sensitization module in TOPKAT. The latter was based on a training set of 315 chemicals which yielded a cross-validated specificity between 81 and 91%, and a cross validated sensitivity between 85 and 95%. The CASE technology uses a different mechanism. It creates its own structural alerts. Each molecule is split into multiple fragments which are then categorized statistically as biophobes (not associated with toxicity) or biophores (associated with toxicity). The results are then added into an equation form: CASE units = constant + a (fragment 1) + b(fragment 2) + ... [16]. Cunningham et al. [30] have discussed its role in predicting carcinogenicity; since they reported a cross-validated concordance of 71% between experimental and predicted rat carcinogenicity results for a 745-compound data-set. It may be noted that the CASE technology has been adapted by the United States Food and Drug

Administration (FDA). The new software, known as MCASE QSAR-ES, was designed to enhance the predictability of pharmacological agents for their carcinogenic potential. Another knowledge-based expert system originally designed at Schering, and now developed by LHASA Limited at the University of Leeds, UK is DEREK. This system is similar to other expert systems in that they have similar endpoints like CASE and TOPKAT, including carcinogenicity, mutagenicity, and teratogenicity e.t.c. and, like them, can function in batch mode. Its major benefit is in the prediction of carcinogenicity, mutagenicity and skin sensitization [27]. Lastly, to mention is HazardExpert system. It also offers a similar range of end-points, including carcinogenicity, mutagenicity, teratogenicity, etc.

The user defines the species, route of administration, dose level and period of exposure. Smithing and Darvas [31] have described the rationale behind HazardExpert, and its potential applications. Dearden et al. [23] reported a test of HazardExpert's ability to predict human and animal carcinogenicity; for 192 chemicals evaluated in IARC Monographs, 55% of the chemicals were predicted within ± 1 of the IARC classification when the 'high' exposure condition was chosen, rising to 75% when the 'low' exposure condition was chosen. Brown et al. [32] examined HazardExpert's ability to predict the carcinogenicity of 80 chemicals tested by the National Toxicology Program (NTP) of the US National Institutes of Health; it was found to be good at identifying non-carcinogens (81% correct predictions), but poor at identifying carcinogens (36% correct predictions). It is worthwhile to briefly discuss the toxicity prediction with COMPACT, designed by Lewis and co-workers at the University of Surrey, UK. Although it is inaccessible commercially, but the data needed to utilize it's function is available in publications by Lewis's (for example, [33-35]. COMPACT aids to predict the potential of a drug molecule to act as a substrate for cytochrome P450 system. It depends mainly on two principles, molecular planarity and electronic activation energy. Example of its role to predict mutagenicity was investigated by Lewis et al who found overall concordance to be only 64%. This implies that the predictive ability of expert systems still needs to be improved (36). It is also worthwhile to note that, in general, expert systems are better at predicting toxicity than at predicting lack of toxicity [37, 38]. This might be explained by the fact that positive prediction represents specific information pertaining to a restricted region of the chemical universe; however, characterization of negative toxicity space, lacking any organizing mechanism-based principles, is an inherently more difficult task [38]. Carcinogenicity is the toxicity of great concern in the synthesis of new drug molecules and it would be worthwhile to briefly consider its prediction. Although there is extensive data in relation to prediction of carcinogenicity, unfortunately little is known in reference to drugs. An example of carcinogenicity is Soft Independent Modelling of Class Analogy (SIMCA) approach [39] which has been studied by Dunn and Wold in a series of 4-nitroquinoline 1-oxides. The reduction of 43 descriptors to 4 main components yielded 89% correct predictions for the 18 carcinogens and 70% correct predictions for the 10 non-carcinogens. There is no doubt that carcinogenicity is not one end-point but many, and it would therefore seem highly unlikely that any QSAR modeling could be performed out of the carcinogenic potency of diverse groups of drug candidates. In regard to the enormous financial losses of drug failure secondary to toxicity found in the later phase of the development process, toxicity should be determined as early as possible. This suggests the role of computational prediction of toxicity, and a various approaches to such prediction have been discussed. There is enough of data on existing QSARs for a wide range of toxicity endpoints of drug molecules. But at the same time there is need for further QSAR modeling of toxicity endpoints, provided that adequate experimental data are available to validate the algorithms. At this point there is not much evidence to support that pharmaceutical industry is widely engaged in Insilco toxicity prediction; for example, of the numerous presentations that were made at the 2002 European Symposium on QSAR, only few dealt with the prediction of drug toxicity. Also it would be immensely helpful if pharmaceutical companies share their toxicity data so that development of QSARs could be enhanced.

5. Surrogate Models for Safety Assessment

At the lead optimization stage the lead series narrows to a subset of potential druggable compounds [8]. If unacceptable toxicity is observed e.g., low MOS emerges from initial animal studies, distinguishing between on-target vs off-target mechanism becomes important, but assays that rapidly and reliably estimate SAR are also crucial. Although *In vivo* studies are considered gold standard there exists confusion in comparing the compounds. These results in low throughput and are considered poor SAR tools. Surrogate assays have an edge because of their higher capacity, and that compounds can be compared at equivalent concentrations. But results are only appreciated if can be correlated to pathophysiology *in vivo*. Illustrative examples are outlined below:

5.1. Cell- and Tissue-Based Surrogate Assays

A potentially fatal cardiac arrhythmia, Torsades de Pointes has been diagnosed by linking delayed ventricular repolarization (QT prolongation) detected by batch of surrogate assays. [40]. Electrophysiological recording in cells or tissue explants and screening for binding to the "human ether-a-go-go" (hERG), the potassium channel responsible for repolarization of the cardiomyocyte, are used to screen compounds prior to collecting electrophysiological recordings in conscious animals [38]. Interpreting the liability for Torsade's must be approached on a case-by-case basis; negative results in surrogate assays do not guarantee safety in vivo [37]. Nonetheless, this set of tools has altered our approach from empirical screening to rational drug design and hypothesis testing. Organ slices and primary cell models can be used to address a variety of target organ toxicities. Isolated hepatocytes have been used to screen for hepatotoxicity and drug-drug interactions. Screening for PPARα agonists in isolated hepatocytes has been used. Isolated hepatocytes from rodents, nonrodents, and humans are useful to screen compounds for induction of drug-metabolizing enzymes and drug-drug interactions and to establish human relevance for metabolism [42, 43]. When tissue architecture has to be studied, organ slices serve as useful models, e.g., if toxicity requires interactions between various cell types, and they provide opportunities for species comparisons [44]. Metabolism of many drugs occurs primarily in the liver. This is the main reason for performing n *vitro* studies on drug metabolism using liver preparations. But is also known that other organs, such as lung and kidney also contribute to the drug metabolism. Before a drug is administered to humans, it is obligatory to carry out experiments in the animals to study drug metabolism and toxicity. For this purpose rat and dog are typical surrogates.

Nevertheless, evidence collected from the ongoing research suggests that the differences in metabolic toxic reactions between species can be substantial. These differences in part are secondary to involvement of the various organs in the body in the process of clearance and toxicity. The development of the technique of preparation (Krumdieck et al., 1980) and use of organ slices from liver (Smith et al., 1985), kidney (Ruegget al., 1987) and lung (Stefaniak et al., 1988) caused an increasing use of animal and human liver slices in studies on drug metabolism and toxicity. This technique is generally accepted as a good model to obtain human-specific data (Bach et al., 1996; Olinga et al., 1998a; Parrish et al., 1995; Vickers, 1994). Slices are relatively easy to prepare and they remain viable for at least 24 hours. Recent advances in preservation have increased the viability and drug metabolic capacity of liver slices up to 3±4 days, enabling studies on induction and toxicity (Gokhale et al., 1997; Price et al., 1998). Moreover, human and animal liver slices can be cryopreserved with maintenance of their biotransformation capacity for at least 3 hours after thawing (de Kanter and Koster, 1995; de Kanter et al., 1998).

Although human kidney tissue is used less commonly for drug metabolism studies (Connors et al., 1996; Vickers, 1994), kidney slices have been used extensively for toxicity and uptake studies, (for a review, see McGuinness et al., 1993) . Kidney slices can be prepared from cortex and medulla selectively (Ruegg et al., 1987), enabling the study of regioselective drug metabolism, which is important for the prediction of drug±drug interactions. Also, lung slices have been used successfully in metabolic and toxicity studies (Fisher et al., 1994; Vickers et al., 1997). The preparation of lung slices requires the infusion of low melting agar to solidify the tissue adequately so that it can be sliced easily (Stefaniak et al., 1988). In conclusion, slices play a vital role to study human and organ specific metabolism and toxicity *in vitro.* And the utilization of human organ slices during drug development process could result in a safer administration to mankind and reduction in the number of experimental animals used. Thus, organ slices demonstrate to be an important tool for investigative toxicology studies, particularly for investigating mechanism of injury and repair because of the multicellular and extracellular matrix complexity of the model. Regardless of the assay format used, achievement of the better safety profile will require better understanding of the mechanisms to link results from screening methods with pathophysiology *invivo.*

5.2. Surrogate Animal Models

Lower organisms with shorter life cycles are amenable to higher throughput testing. Developmental and behavioral toxicities are only two examples where disrupting complex interactions among many cell types results in toxicity. The importance of surrogate animal models is being realized; for example, knowledge of apoptosis can be traced to basic mechanisms defined in *Caenorhabditis elegans* [45]. Internationally renowned academic researcher, Mark Fishman, previously the director of the Cardiovascular Research Center at

Massachusetts General Hospital (MGH) who joined Novartis to head its global research operations moved his large-scale zebrafish mutagenesis program through which he has elucidated the genetic pathways of the heart and vascular system. Recent reviews suggest that zebrafish show great promise as surrogate animal models for cardiovascular toxicity [46]. Also *C. elegans* models offer insights into neurotoxicity [47], and amphibian models have contributed to developmental toxicity screening [48]. Both public and private databases, too numerous to reference, offer a wide spectrum of range of genetic, biochemical, and cell biology contents for eukaryotic organisms from yeasts to mice.

6. Application of Stem Cells in Toxicology

Recent advances in stem cells have been the subject of increasing interest because of their use in numerous biomedical applications including potentials to predict drug toxicity *in vitro*. (Figure 1) The striking potential benefits of stem cells, when applied to field of toxicology, result from their unique properties compared to primary human cells; that is, unlimited proliferation ability and more readily available sources of human cells. Particularly, the advances in the technologies in this field and how they could fulfill critical safety issues such as QT prolongation and hepatotoxicity, genotoxicity and reproductive toxicology screens few important causes of failures in preclinical phase of development of new therapeutic agents. For example, the issue of a drug's effect on the QT intervals has been the subject of increasing regulatory review and concern. The QT interval in the electrocardiogram represents the period from the beginning of ventricular depolarization to the end of ventricular repolarization. Prolongation of the QT or QTc interval may be associated with a rare but potentially life-threatening type of ventricular arrhythmia known as torsade de pointes (Morganroth, 1993; Cubeddu, 2003). The present preclinical models of *in vivo* and *in vitro* cardiotoxicity to drug candidates do not precisely predict clinical outcomes and have few limitations. For example, telemetrized animals, which provide insight on the effects of drug on cardiac function, are costly and have suboptimal sensitivity. *In vitro* systems using Purkinje fibers or cloned human ion channels inadequately predict the effect of a drug candidate on human cardiomyocytes. Cultures of human cardiomyocytes provide an excellent in vitro model system (Bird et al., 2003); however, limited availability of tissue from healthy donors restricts the availability of primary cardiomyocytes to be evaluated for high throughput safety. Therefore, the development of novel test systems to screen new chemical entities (NCEs) and predict potential cardiac safety liability in humans is highly desirable. Cardiomyocytes derived from human stem cells is an emerging field to screen NCEs for potential cardiotoxicants and QT interval prolongation and offer a method of minimizing and possibly avoiding undesirable proarrhythmic drug effects. Till now, the source for functional cardiomyocytes has been cultures of human embryonic stem cells (hESC) (He et al., 2003, Lavon and Bevenisty, 2003). These human embryonic stem cell derived cardiomyocytes (hESC-CM) demonstrate the expected morphology and express numerous cardiomyocyte proteins. They also display rhythmic contractions with a longer action potential duration (APD) characteristic feature of cardiomyocytes.

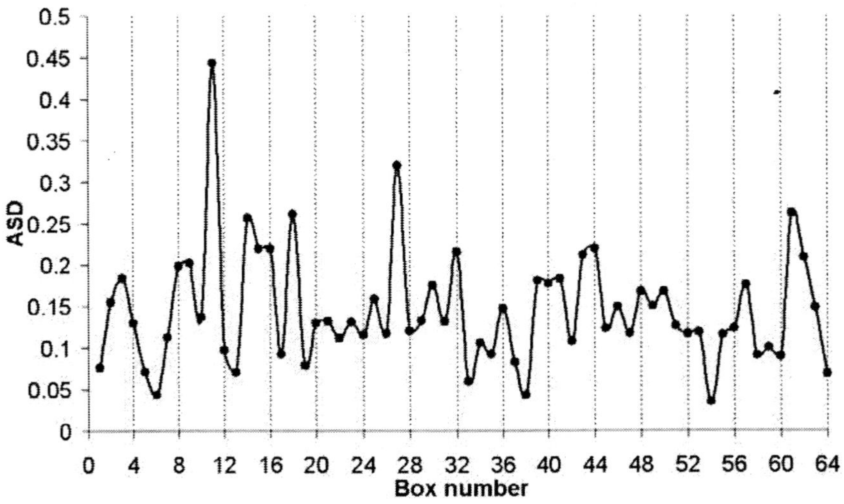

Figure 1. Various Stages of Stem Cell Development and their Potential Use in Drug Toxicity Screening.

Together, these results suggest that hESC-CM is a functional surrogate for primary cardiomyocytes; however, the controversy surrounding the use of hESCs has limited the development of these cells as potential sources of cardiomyocyte progenitors. But there is little controversy using multipotent stem cells compared to pluripotent stem cells requiring blastocysts. Hence, multipotent stem cells (derived from adult tissue; ASCs), such as bone marrow, provide a valuable and more readily acceptable source of cardiomyocyte precursors *in vitro*. These advantages of stem cells will provide essential early mechanistic insight into potential cardiac electrophysiological effects and enhance our decision-making capacity at the discovery and preclinical levels. The information available suggests that stem cell technology has the potential to contribute to the science of toxicology. Extensive research and development is continuing to optimaly use the available resources to establish reproducible *in vitro* assays that will directly address cardiotoxicity, hepatotoxicity, and reproductive toxicology. Moreover, the use of stem cell– derived *in vitro* models will overcome expensive and labor-intensive toxicology studies performed in primary cellular reagents or *in vivo* animal models. Additionally, the advancement in the field of stem cells will generate robust data on human cellular physiology based on the availability of cardiomyocytes and hepatocytes from precursors in the human bone marrow or discarded placentas. It is predicted that in the future, the advent of stem cell technology will possibly yield reagents for assays on other cell type-specific agressors, such as neurotoxins and skin, respiratory, and renal toxicants.

7. Role of Biomarkers

Earlier indications for addressing *in vivo* safety issues can be provided by the preclinical application of biomarkers. Preclinical biomarkers important for mechanism-based risk assessment include PD markers and safety markers. Safety markers can be further divided into premonitory and surrogate markers for injury.

PD biomarkers measure the response of the target and relate drug exposure to target modulation. They also give idea of biological outcome and provide necessary information to differentiate on- vs off-target mechanisms of toxicity. Any measurement tool that monitors a process linked mechanistically to target modulation can be utilized for developing PD biomarkers. Premonitory and surrogate safety biomarkers measure changes that occur prior to, or concurrent with, morphological evidence of pathology, respectively. For example, dogs exhibit focal myocardial necrosis after isoproterenol treatment [49]. Changes in the chronotropic properties of the heart may be premonitory for cardiac injury while rise in cardiac enzymes such as cardiac troponins and/or creatine kinase released coincident with the rupture of cardiomyocytes serve as surrogate markers of cell death. Similarly, the release of ALT/SGPT and AST/SGOT may indicate hepatic injury. Thus, biomarkers might indicate that injury will progress or may accommodate without an increase in severity or collapse of the MOS. Predicting whether or not an early signal is a reversible phenomena or a harbinger of irreversible injury, describes the essence of the predictive toxicology dilemma.

Mechanism-based PD and safety biomarkers permit safety issues to be monitored and species differences to be addressed as a candidate approaches the clinic. Increased research in this field represents an opportunity to improve risk assessment, relate findings in preclinical species to humans, and increase clinical safety profile. Simply associating dose and time dependence with toxicity is inadequate; mechanism-based biomarkers play important role in predicting accurate risk assessment and facilitate clinical monitoring. Additional mechanism-based PD and validated premonitory safety biomarkers are critical to improve preclinical safety assessment, pipeline productivity, and monitoring human safety.

An important issue in this field is species differences. Lack of cross-reactivity for reagents, such as antibodies, is a significant hurdle to applying biomarkers to preclinical safety assessment. Mining the genome and tissue expression profiles are useful for selecting candidate biomarkers, but functional annotation of the rat, dog, and monkey genome, typical rodent and nonrodents species used in preclinical assessment, is inadequate. Species differences in the activity of molecules or proteins targeting important classes of receptors, such as G-protein-coupled receptors create difficulty in interpretation of safety profile and generate uncertainty in assessing on-target safety issues with biologics. Need for biomarkers in necessary to realize to assess preclinical safety. It is also important to streamline the validation criteria. This will require increased understanding between academic, regulatory, and industrial researchers. In addition, a single marker will not be able to predict multiple pathologies in a single organ, e.g., troponins and cardiac death, while combinatorial biomarkers approaches, although more complicated and expensive to develop, provide deeper insight (50) and may be an opportunity for systems toxicology approaches.

8. Application of Genomics in Toxicology

Researchers engaged in toxicogenomic studies (definitions explained in table 1) apply genomic tools to learn how these networks modulate cellular responses to drug exposures

(Figure 2). Microarrays, for example, identify global changes in gene expression of the 30,000 genes comprising our genome associated with specific types of toxic responses. Proteomics- a field with many implications beyond toxicogenomics characterizes the milieu of the gene products the proteins appearing or changing in a cell after a given exposure. Because each gene gives rise to atleast 10 isoforms in the proteome, reflecting splicing and post translational modification this may be more relevant to signaling pathway delineation. And with metabonomics, scientists study broad patterns of chemical metabolites in exposed tissues. The gene, protein, and metabolite profiles that make up toxicogenomics reflect key steps leading from exposure to disease (Figure 2).

By comparing chemically altered genomic profiles to those obtained from nontreated controls, researchers can identify unique biomarkers for disease processes. To give an example, microarray data demonstrates that chemical activates the genes coding for cytochromes P450, a metabolic enzyme found in hepatic cells. If the chemical also leads to hepatic injury, researchers might hypothesize that activated P450 is involved in the toxic response mechanism. The gene expression profile for activated P450 is therefore a potential biomarker for chemically induced injury to the liver. Over 50 % of the population has gene variants in cytochromes P450 (CYP) genotypes with most involving CYP 206, CYP 269 and CYP 2619 that can alter metabolizing almost half of the preclinical drugs. Specifically, preclinical screening models will look for biomarkers to guide the development of safer drugs. Biomarkers that reliably predict certain toxic effects may preclude the need for further testing. Therefore, toxicogenomic tools have the potential to reduce the number of animals used in research. At present, deoxy-ribose nucleic acid (DNA)-based microarrays dominate the field that toxicogenomics is sometimes viewed erroneously as being concerned solely with gene expression. But no laboratories have the ability to assess all the proteins in a biological sample—although new proteomic tools, approaches in multidimensional protein separation and identification by mass spectrometry such as surface-enhanced laser desorption/ionization–time should facilitate this capability within a few years. Others have expressed their opinion that the most effective diagnostic biomarkers will be proteins. This is in part because proteins are more stable molecules and easier to collect in a clinical setting than the ribonucleic acid (RNA) samples used to elucidate gene expression. Over time, proteomics and metabonomics data will become increasingly available for toxicogenomic research, experts say.

The National Institute of Environmental Health Sciences (NIEHS's), National Center for Toxicogenomics (NCT), which was established in December 2000 to combine toxicogenomic information with the knowledge emerging from classical toxicology, has embraced these technologies readily in an institutional setting. This integrated approach of combining all the toxicogenomic biomarkers will aid researchers to develop intricate biochemical/metabolic pathways of drug toxicity. An even better estimate of the human response will emerge from linking toxicogenomic research to studies of inter-individual variation. Researchers are now assembling the gene variants that modulate (increase or decrease) human susceptibility to chemically induced diseases. Among these variants are simple DNA sequence variations called single nucleotide polymorphisms (SNPs). SNPs can influence toxic responses in multiple ways.

Table 1. Definitions commonly used in Toxicogenomics

Term	Definition
Bioinformatics	The science of informatics as applied to biological research. Informatics is the management and analysis of data using networks of computers and databases.
Data mining	Analyzing data to establish relationships and identify patterns in order to satisfy or generate hypothesis
Genomics	The study of structure and function of all genes in an organism based on knowing the organism's entire DNA sequence and extensive reliance on computer technologies. In order to determine how they interact and influence biological pathways, networks, and physiology.
Metabolomics	The study of the total metabolite pool through a wide spectrum of technologies including spectroscopy, chromatography–mass spectrometry, gas chromatography–mass spectrometry, and , and multivariable analysis.
Microarray	A tool for profiling gene and protein expression in cells and tissues.

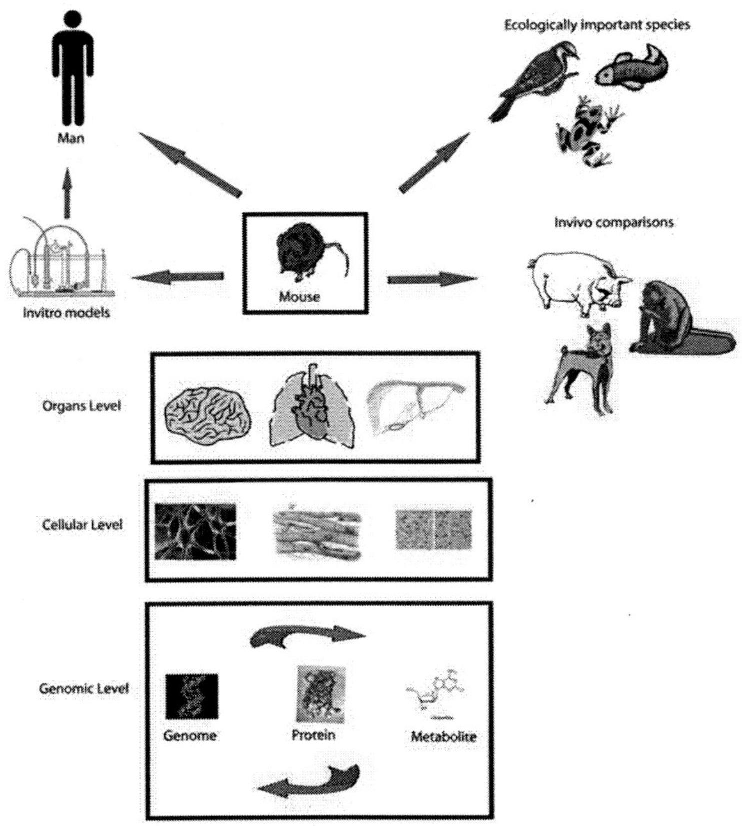

Figure 2. Toxicogenomics: gene, protein, and metabolites pathways can be phenotypically linked to toxicity seen at the cellular and/or tissue level to help us understand the toxic mechanisms.

Enhancement through microarrays experts generally agrees that microarrays enabled the rise of toxicogenomics in the late 1990s. Microarrays are silicon or glass chips coated with thousands of discrete spots of nucleic acids called probes. Each probe corresponds to a specific gene. To use this technology, RNA molecule from a biological sample is "reverse transcribed," or used to synthesize an identical copy of the gene that would normally be produced in a living cell. This complementary DNA (cDNA) is labeled with a radioactive tag and bound to the chip. Ideally, each molecule in the labeled cDNA binds to its complementary probe on the array. Utilizing quantitative imaging techniques that read the radioactivity, researchers assess cDNA binding and thereby identify the genes expressed in the original biological sample and their relative levels of expression. In toxicogenomic studies, the cDNA is obtained from drug exposed animal tissues or cells in culture. At first, the microarrays used in these studies were small and constituted genes for specific pathways such as drug metabolism or DNA repair, Afshari says. These early microarrays and subsequent refinements have enabled researchers to pursue hypothesis-driven studies or trials focused mainly on obtaining additional data about a specific toxicity mechanism. As microarrays evolved, the amount of genes that could be placed on a chip grew up exponentially. Today, investigators can purchase chips containing tens of thousands of genes or even whole genomes for certain species. For example: Affymetrix, the leading manufacturer of chips that represent the entire human and mouse genomes. Scientists who use the larger chips are able to find global gene expression patterns and associated mechanisms resulting from toxic exposures. Gene expression and toxicity involves the ultimate goal of toxicogenomics to link chemically induced gene expression patterns to either detrimental, harmless, or even protective effects. It is also essential to realize that patterns are not necessarily linked to the cause of toxicity and that patterns may be associated with responses that may not have toxicological significance. One way to assess the toxicological significance of the patterns is to "phenotypically anchor" them to standard toxicological indices, such as clinical chemistry or tissue pathology. Such experiments are at present a major activity at the NCT. According to Selkirk, phenotypic anchoring is a technique that couples the unique gene expression patterns induced by chemical exposures to visible evidence of harm. In this manner, the gene expression patterns provide chemical-specific signatures for toxicological pathways and effects. Also according to him the signatures should relate to expression profiles obtained at multiple dose levels. Low-dose signatures, for example, can be correlated with ultrastructural changes in cells or tissues, which are observed only with electron microscopy. In one study [51], it was found that compounds acting through a common mechanism (peroxisome proliferation, a cellular process related to oxidative stress) have similar and collectively distinct gene expression profiles. This means that compounds with similar mechanisms can be arranged together by a common gene signature, which can then be used to predict the chemical class of an unknown compound. Linking signature profiles with toxic effects is the goal of ongoing experiments at the NCT. Some of these experiments are focusing on acetaminophen, a highly studied compound with enormous public exposure. So far, the exposures being considered in all these studies are acute. The reason for this is that acute exposures produce a series of discrete cellular events that researchers can analyze to build confidence in toxicogenomic techniques. Unfortunately, most human exposures are complex in nature. People are generally exposed to many compounds simultaneously, often on a chronic or intermittent basis. Eventually, Tennant says, toxicogenomics will have to address more realistic exposure scenarios. These pathways are much more not simple, he admits. Any evaluation of chronic exposures must contend with the added dimensions of time, adaptive response, and cellular repair. "The signals for each of these processes are masked in the complexity of the response," Tennant says. "With repeat dosing, it all becomes much more intricate." Knowledge and standardization evaluating chronic exposures merely adds to the already overwhelming challenge of managing toxicogenomic data. Just a few years ago, genes involved in a given mechanism were studied one at a time. But with the advent of microarrays, researchers now study gene pathways by the hundreds, or even thousands, for any single exposure. Add multiple doses in varying tissues and species, not to mention proteomic and metabonomics parameters, and the volumes of data generated quickly overpower most analytical capabilities. Data analysis and management for genomics are the realm of the associated field of bioinformatics, which applies computational tools toward the understanding of biology. The goal of bioinformatics is to codify toxicogenomic information in ways that facilitate the rapid extraction of relevant parameters stored in a database to screen biomarkers against signature pathways. Its importance also lies in identifying expressed genes, the degree to which they are expressed, and how those genes are linked to each other. The Chemical Effects in Biological Systems (CEBS) database is being attributed as a "knowledge base" integrating toxicogenomic biomarkers with chemical effects data. Eventually, CEBS data sets will be searchable by compound, structure, toxicity and pathology end point, gene, pathway, and polymorphism, each as a function of dose, time, species, and target tissue. Comparable to the way in which GenBank databases are explored for genome sequences, researchers will explore CEBS to gather information on genes and associated toxicity pathways. If, for example, all that is known about a newly discovered compound is its chemical structure, researchers could explore CEBS using this input to get pathway and toxicity information associated with other, similar compounds. The CEBS output could assist in screening potential effects and new directions for future research on the compound in question. Building such database over time is challenging task—it requires cooperation and data sharing by researchers from various scientific disciplines and cooperation for laying a format for linking toxicogenomic information. The ILSI committee has accomplished the first phase of its research, identifying toxicogenomic parameters for chemicals with hepatotoxic, nephrotoxic, and genotoxic mechanisms. "The idea is to make the data complementary with CEBS and available in a form that can be accessed by others," Pennie says. "The NCT will have continual access, and I hope the data sharing will be reciprocal." According to Pennie, these data are also being gathered to enter into a database managed by the European Bioinformatics Institute, a multinational research organization based in England. The prospect of sharing data across databases and research centers raises a highly challenging issue: the standardization of experimental protocols and data formats. Therefore, a method for ensuring uniform data quality is very important, experts say. However, as in any field, toxicogenomic experiments are unpredictable in terms of approach, outcome, and interpretation. It has also been suggested that researchers should apply standardized methods to minimize this variability. According to Pennie, the ILSI committee dealt this as one of its first priorities. But after discussing this issue for a certain period , he says, committee members concluded that it will be difficult to implement standardized approaches , in part because they felt researchers shouldn't be constrained in method development. "The techniques are still evolving at a rapid pace," he explains. "Furthermore, we want to understand what the sources of variability are." With respect to standardization, he says that they will lean towards the recommendations made by the Microarray Gene Expression Data Society, an international organization working to facilitate the sharing of microarray data. This group has developed a core set of guidelines that is also known as Minimum Information.

About a Microarray Experiment (MIAME). According to the society's website, these guidelines, which apply to microarray gene expression research, will "assist in the development of microarray data repositories and data analysis tools." The guidelines provide a uniform nomenclature for describing toxicogenomic experiments and data.

As said by Waters, "With regards to CEBS, we will follow the recommendations coming from that society in addition to the guidance we obtain from the Toxicogenomics Research Consortium and the NIEHS Microarray Center."The implications of toxicogenomic research ultimately extend far beyond laboratories and clinics, and reach into public and environmental policy. At present policy experts are tackling basic queries about how toxicogenomic information and technology will transform the process of setting standards for chemical hazards. The risk assessment protocols utilized to set these standards have always focused on protecting the most sensitive subgroups of the human population. Usually, these subgroups are defined using equations that relate human responses to lowest-observed-effect levels seen in animal experiments. These low-level effects—usually fairly benign responses such as altered lung function or changes in blood chemistry—are thought to be shared by all members of the population. Therefore, the standards are said to protect against "population-level effects." Today, toxicogenomics is expanding our knowledge of *Low-level effects.* Once the domain of the pathologist, the limits of sensitivity are increasingly being defined according to genetic susceptibility to toxic exposure. Hence, sensitive subgroups are being transformed from an indeterminate entity into a clearly defined genetic subset of individuals within the population. According to Richard Sharp, an assistant professor of medical ethics at the Center for Medical Ethics and Health Policy of the Baylor College of Medicine, the identification of these subpopulations raises some important questions. Most importantly, who bears the cost of protecting these individuals? This issue will probably first come to bear in the workplace, he says. Once sensitive subgroups are identified, employers may refuse applicants on the basis of genetic screens that show them to be sensitive to workplace hazards. "How much discretion should an employer have to make these kinds of decisions?" Sharp asks. Sharp chairs an NCT working group on ethical, legal, and policy issues that is now exploring this and other issues. Regulatory agencies are also tackling with toxicogenomics issues. In June 2002, the U.S. Environmental Protection Agency (EPA) issued its first guidelines for using genomics data for the standard-setting process. In the guidelines, EPA expressed their opinion that toxicogenomics will potentially have an "enormous impact on our ability to assess the risk from exposure to stressors and ultimately to improve our risk assessments." But the guidelines also make clear that "the relationships between changes in gene expression and adverse effects are unclear at this time and may be difficult to evaluate." The EPA's current view point on this subject is that, although informative, toxicogenomic data alone are insufficient for risk assessment. Hence, EPS says that will accept the data but will evaluate them only on a case-by-case basis. The U.S. Food and Drug Administration (FDA) is also closely observing developments in this field. Frank Sistare, director of the Division of Applied Pharmacology Research at the FDA's Center for Drug Evaluation and Research, also previously commented that FDA had completed a series of multistakeholder meetings on the appropriate use of genomic data for drug evaluations. Echoing the concerns of EPA officials, Sistare emphasizes the difficulty of linking microarray results to toxic effects. With respect to submitting toxicogenomic data for drug approval processes, Sistare says, "It's more of a challenge to industry than it is to us right now. I don't think anyone can provide a clear answer on what every signal means on an experiment conducted with microarrays that query thousands of end points at once. This puts industry in the unenviable position of generating all these data that they can't really explain." If data are produced for safety evaluations, they must be submitted to the FDA by law, Sistare adds. Therefore, companies must decide whether the studies are worth the investment, particularly if the outcome data simply immerses them in a drug approval quagmire. Sistare admits the policy might deter drug and biotechnology companies from undertaking toxicogenomic research on developmental compounds. Referring to this particular issue, Sistare adds that viewpoints both within and outside the FDA suggest that companies pursuing toxicogenomic studies for new drug screening (when potential drugs are selected for further research and development) should not be obligated to submit their experimental data. "Either way," he says, "we don't want to inhibit application of the technology to drug development. We think it's a powerful tool, and all of us need to come to resolution on when the data need to be submitted, how the data should be submitted, and how we are going to use them." Clearly, toxicogenomics is a new field brimming with potential benefits. But many hurdles need to be overcome. Scientists are just beginning to explore the complex nature of cellular response mechanisms. But solving the toxicogenomics puzzle will be a challenging task that will need even more advanced tools and decades of research. But the environmental health outcomes are significant: more effective diagnosis and treatment of environmentally related diseases, expedited evaluations of chemicals and new chemical compounds, and better risk assessment. "We have to understand how all the pathways fit together in a systems biology perspective," concludes Samson. "That's the biggest hurdle of all." Charles W. Schmidt Pharmacogenetics (often used interchangeably with pharmacogenomics) investigates the interactions between a patient or animal genome and drug responses [52]. Systems toxicology "represents an analytical approach to the relationships among elements of a system" as applied to toxicology (53). Both require integration of information from multiple sources to describe and predict the behavior of biological systems; summaries of technologies and computational models are available (10, 53-54). Two issues will be discussed in brief, prediction of drug toxicity using 'omic technology and predicting individual patient safety through application of pharmacogenetics data.

Available public and commercial and databases and classification algorithms [53, 54-57] confirm that global transcript and metabolite profiles can be used to classify toxicity from unknown compounds. It is worth appreciating that the classifications appear robust despite the scanty numbers of structurally dissimilar compounds (e.g., ~10 for single pathology) used to train the models [58, 59]. To illustrate, a phospholipidosis classifier was built using 12 model compounds and a signature set of less than 20 genes [60]. This suggests that biological classifiers can be built based on the complexity inherent in the biological data relating to pathogenesis as opposed to an extensive SAR based on similar structures. Although advancement may appear slow compared to expectations, outcomes indicate that the predictive toxicology database can assist in safety predictions and enhance knowledge of the mechanism.

Although genetic polymorphisms may contribute to disease, variability in the phenotype and genotype of the enzymes and transporters involved in the metabolism and disposition of a drug offers promising results with regards to understanding and eliminating toxicity. Although concepts given by Paracelsus are central to toxicological sciences, advancements in the field of pharmacogenetics and epidemiology has increased our understanding that, "The dose determines the poison, but the patient and environment determine the dose that poisons." Because toxicity is directly proportional to exposure, it is not surprising that variation in metabolism and disposition contributes to drug toxicity [52]. Accordingly, differences in metabolism and drug-drug interactions may contribute to ADRs from a wide variety of drugs [61]. Present preclinical safety assessment studies are designed to minimize variability and yield statistically robust outcomes. This experimental necessity underestimates contributions from genetic variability to toxicity. Efforts to understand and apply murine (the Mouse Phenome Project; www.jax.org) and rat (www.physiogenix.com) genetic variability to better understand drug responses may offer opportunities to enhance our knowledge of drug toxicity using preclinical models. In order to establish the importance and implications of genetic diversity in drug responses with preclinical species and human, additional work will be needed. Recent advancement in the tools and application of systems toxicology and pharmacogenetics offer the opportunity to improve preclinical safety testing. Although right utilization of the information and knowledge management apply here as well but are discussed above with regard to in silico applications.

Another area of importance is mechanistic understanding of species differences. Phylogenetics defines the genetic basis for differences among species and relatedness within lineages. The fact that species differences play a key role in preclinical safety assessment calls for a "phylogenetic systems toxicology" approach to safety assessment. Investigation of species differences must progress from descriptive to mechanism-based systems biology approaches. This requires consistent functional annotation of the various genomes and mapping differences in physiology and pathophysiology across species including surrogate animal models. Understanding the genetic concepts of drug toxicity will require systems approaches to integrate a "physiomic" view for preclinical species and humans.

The low incidence of drug toxicity and "curse of dimensionality" are barriers that also confound predicting responses for individual patients [52]. The well-recognized statin-induced rhabdomyolysis incidence is only 3.4 per 100000 and depends on multiple factors [61]. Low frequency of ADRs with complex genetic and environmental etiology may only appear after a drug has been on the market for some time [62]. However, considerable progress is needed to improve pharmacovigilance and streamline phylogenetic systems toxicology approaches to help elucidate the roles of the environment and genetics in mechanisms of ADRs.

Summary: How to Improve Mechanism-Based Risk Evaluation

The preceding discussion provides a perspective and suggestions on future directions for mechanistic research on drug safety as well as practical applications to mechanism-based risk assessment. Toxicology is expected to provide safer drugs to patients at lower cost, but technical and nontechnical challenges must be overcome to realize this vision. Recent advances in understanding the mechanism of metabolic activation of a drug to reactive species [63] and the basic mechanism of cell death [45] offer new insights, but understanding of basic mechanisms of drug-induced target organ toxicity in preclinical animal models and humans is also essential to improve mechanism-based risk assessment for new and existing drugs. Advancement will require both effective translation of basic research to practical applications and a clear focus on the appropriate technical difficulties. A few final comments frame the opportunities and challenges already considered in the preceded discussion.

Improving the accessibility of safety data to fuel public and private collaboration is necessary. The NIH Roadmap and FDA Critical Path documents require more focused utilization of basic science in toxicology. Toxicologists must understand the objective of these documents and make efforts to refine and steer the applications to the most productive results. Regulatory agencies must facilitate the advancement of new technologies and processes by rewarding the pharmaceutical industry to bring forward new safety data. Industry must enter into open collaborations and facilitate the use of relevant compounds and safety data to test novel methods so that existing methods of safety assessment can be improved. All sectors should engage in educating the public to the risk: benefit considerations for any drug [64].

The basic science of toxicology must advance to overcome these hurdles. As noted by Liebler [65], major advances often come from outside the field of toxicology. Changes to study division structure at the NIH has increased the concern in the academic community that the focus of funding for research in toxicology will be diffused across interdisciplinary study divisions. There is always a risk but and change require risk taking. Toxicologists should adapt and compete based on the clinical outcome and application of their research. The high-content nature of systems approaches offers great opportunity and significant barriers that must be understood. They are currently applied often to indicate what "might happen" or what "did happen" but do not predict the probability of an outcome. Risk assessment is neither absolutely qualitative nor a retrospective exercise in nature. Risk assessment, as utilized in pharmaceutical research, attempts to quantify risk (e.g., MOS) in advance to improve risk: benefit decisions regarding therapeutic outcomes and patient safety. Although systems approaches are complex in nature, they must, nonetheless, achieve a level of quantitation and create capabilities for intuitive visualization of outcomes to enhance machine learning to be incorporated into human learning and decision making. Understanding the mechanism is pivotal in defining these relationships. There is no doubt that the future of the toxicological science is promising and will be exciting. However, the future of the art of toxicology may depend on the acceptance by toxicologists that it is integral part of our discipline and is worthy of greater attention.

References

[1] Lasser, K.E., Allen, P.D.,Woolhandler, S.J., Himmelstein, D.U., Wolfe, S.M., and Bor, D.H. (2002).Timing of new black box warnings and withdrawals for prescription medications. *J. Am. Med. Assoc 287* (17), 2215-2220.

[2] Kola, I., Landis, J. (2004). Can the pharmaceutical industry reduce attrition rates? *Nat. Rev. Drug Discovery 3* (8), 711-715.

[3] FDA. (2004). Innovation and Stagnation: Challenges and opportunities on the critical path to new medical products. http://www.fda.gov/oc/initiatives/criticalpath/ whitepaper. html.

[4] Greaves, P., Williams, A., and Eve, M. (2004). First dose of potential new medicines to humans: How animals help. *Nat. Rev. Drug Discovery 3* (3), 226-236.

[5] Fenton, JJ. Toxicology: A Case-Oriented Approach, CRC Press, Boca Raton, FL (2002).

[6] Doull, J. (2001). Toxicology comes of age. Annu. Rev. Pharmacol. Toxicol 41, 1–21.

[7] Poklis, A and Pesce, A. J., Toxicology. In: Lawrence A. Kaplan and Amadeo J. Pesce, Editors, Clinical Chemistry—Theory, Analysis, and Correlation, CV Mosby Company, St. Louis, MO (1984).

[8] Lipinski, C., and Hopkins, A. (2004). Navigating chemical space for biology and medicine. *Nature 432* (7019), 855-861.

[9] Dorato, M. A., and Vodicnik, M. J. (2001). The toxicological assessment of pharmaceutical and biotechnology products. In *Principles and Methods of Toxicology* (Hayes, W. A., Ed.) pp 243-283, Taylor and Francis, Philadelphia.

[10] Ekins, S., Nikolsky, Y., and Nikolskaya, T. (2005). Techniques: Application of systems biology to absorption, distribution, metabolism, excretion and toxicity. *Trends Pharmacol. Sci 26* (4), 202-209.

[11] Stevens, J. L. (2006). Future of toxicology--mechanisms of toxicity and drug safety: where do we go from here? Chem Res Toxicol 19(11),1393-401.

[12] Sasseville, V. G., Lane, J. H., Kadambi, V. J., Bouchard, P., Lee, F. W., Balani, S. K., Miwa, G. T., Smith, P. F., and Alden, C. L. (2004).Testing paradigm for prediction of development-limiting barriers and human drug toxicity. *Chem.-Biol. Interact 150* (1), 9-25.

[13] 1Dorato, M. A., and Engelhardt, J. A. (2005). The no-observed-adverse-effect-level in drug safety evaluations: Use, issues, and definition(s). *Regul. Toxicol. Pharmacol. 42* (3), 265-274.

[14] 14. FDA. (2005). Estimating the maximum safe starting dose in initial clinical trials for therapeutics in adult healthy volunteers. http://www.fda.gov/CDER/ guidance/ 5541fnl.doc.

[15] Ames,B.N. (1971). In: *Chemical Mutagens: Principles and Methods for their Detection*. Ed. A Hollaender. Plenum, New York; pp 267-282.

[16] Hansch, C., Maloney, P.P., Fujita, T. and Muir, R.M. (1962). Correlation of Biological Activity of Phenoxyacetic Acids with Hammett Substituent Constants and Partition Coefficients. *Nature* 194,178.

[17] King, L.A. and Moffat, A.C. (1983). A possible index of fatal drug toxicity in humans. Med Sci Law 23 (3), 193- 198.

[18] 18. Hansch, C., Bjorkroth, J.P. and Leo, A. (1987). Hydrophobicity and central nervous system agents: on the principle of minimal hydrophobicity in drug design. *J. Pharm. Sci.* 76(9):663-87.

[19] Martin, Y.C. and Hansch, C. (1971). Influence of Hydrophobic Character on the Relative Rate of Oxidation of Drugs by Rat Liver Microsomes. *J. Med. Chem.* 14 (9)777.

[20] Mannhold, R. and Dross, K. (1996). Calculations Procedures for Molecular Lipophilicity: A Comparatives Study. *Quantitative structure-activity relationships* 15, 403-409.

[21] Dearden, J.C., Netzeva, T.I. and Bibby, R. (2002). Comparison of a number of commercial software programs for the prediction of aqueous solubility. *J. Pharm. Pharmacol.* 54 (suppl), S-65.

[22] Dearden, J.C., Netzeva, T.I. and Bibby, R. (2002). Comparison of a number of commercial software programs for the prediction of octanol-water partition. *J. Pharm. Pharmacol.* 54 (suppl), S-66.

[23] Dearden, J.C., Barratt, M.D., Benigni, R., Bristol, D.W., Combes, R.D., Cronin, M.T.D., Judson, P.N., Payne, M.P., Richard, A.M., Tichý, M., Worth, A.P. and Yourick, J.J. (1997). Prediction of environmental toxicity and fate using quantitative structure-activity relationships. *ATLA* 25, 223.

[24] Benfenati, E. and Gini, G. (1997). Computational predictive programs (expert systems) in toxicology. *Toxicology*. 119, 213-225.

[25] Richard, A.M. (1999). Application of artificial intelligence and computational methods to predicting toxicity. *Knowledge Eng. Rev.* 14 ,307-317.

[26] Helma, C., Gottmann, E. and Kramer, S. (2000). Knowledge discovery and data mining in toxicology. *Statistical Methods in Medical Research* (9), 329-358.

[27] Greene, N. (2002). Computer systems for the prediction of toxicity: an update. *Adv. Drug Deliv. Rev.* 54 (3), 417-31.17.

[28] Enslein, K., Gombar, V.K. and Blake, B.W. (1994). Use of SAR in computer-assisted prediction of carcinogenicity and mutagenicity of chemicals by the TOPKAT program: Use of SAR for the prediction of rodent carcinogenicity. *Mutation Research* 305, 47-61.

[29] Enslein, K., Gombar, V.K., Blake, B.W., Maibach, H.I., Hostynek, J.J., Sigman, C.C. and Bagheri, D. (1997). A quantitative structure-toxicity relationships model for the dermal sensitization guinea pig maximization assay. *Food Chem. Toxicol.* 35, 1091-8.

[30] Cunningham, A.R., Klopman, G. and Rosenkranz, H.S. (1998). Identification of structural features and associated mechanisms of action for carcinogens in rats. *Mutation Research*. 405, 9-27.

[31] Smithing, M. P., and Darvas, F. (1992). HazardExpert: An expert system for predicting chemical toxicity. In *Food Safety Assessment* (J. W. Finlay, S. F. Robinson, and D. J. Armstrong, Eds., pp. 191–200. American Chemical Society, Washington, DC.

[32] Brown, S.J., Raja, A.A. and Lewis, D.F.V. (1994). A comparison between COMPACT and hazardexpert evaluations for 80 chemicals tested by the NTP/NCI rodent bioassay. *ATLA* 22, 482-500.

[33] Parke, D.V., Ioannides, C. and Lewis, D.F.V. (1990). The safety evaluation of drugs and chemicals by the use of computer optimised molecular parametric analysis of chemical toxicity (COMPACT). *ATLA* 18, 91-102.

[34] Lewis, D.F.V., Ioannides, C. and Parke, D.V. (1998). A combined COMPACT and HazardExpert study of 40 chemicals for which information on mutagenicity and carcinogenicity is known, including the results of human epidemiological studies. *Human and Experimental Toxicology* 17, 577-586.

[35] Lewis, D.F.V. (2001). COMPACT: a structural approach to the modelling of cytochromes P450 and their interactions with xenobiotics. *J. Chem. Tech. Biotech.* 76, 237-244.

[36] Lewis, D.F.V., Ioannides, C. and Parke, D.V. (1993). Validation of a novel molecular orbital approach (COMPACT) for the prospective safety evaluation of chemicals, by comparison with rodent carcinogenicity and Salmonella mutagenicity data evaluated by the U.S. NCI/NTP. *Mut. Res.* 291, 61-67.

[37] Benigni, R. (1995). Predicting chemical carcinogenesis in rodents: the state of the art in light of a comparative exercise. *Mutaion Research* 334, 103-113.

[38] Richard, A.M. and Benigni, R. (2002). AI and SAR approaches for predicting chemical carcinogenicity: survey and status report. *SAR and QSAR in Environmental Research* 13, 1-19.

[39] Dunn, W.J. III and Wold, S. (1978). A structure-carcinogenicity study of 4-nitroquinoline 1-oxides using the SIMCA method of pattern recognition. *W. J. Med. Chem.* 21, 1001-7.

[40] Lawrence, C. L., Pollard, C. E., Hammond, T. G., and Valentin, J. P. (2005) Nonclinical proarrhythmia models: Predicting Torsades de Pointes. *J. Pharmaco. Toxicol. Methods 52* (1), 46-59.

[41] Chiang, A. Y., Holdsworth, D. L., and Leishman, D. J. (2006) A one-step approach to the analysis of the QT interval in conscious telemetrized dogs. *J. Pharmacol. Toxicol. Methods 54* (2), 183-188.

[42] O'Brien, P. J., and Siraki, A. G. (2005). Accelerated cytotoxicity mechanism screening using drug metabolising enzyme modulators. *Cur. Drug Metab 6* (2), 101-109.

[43] Sivaraman, A., Leach, J. K., Townsend, S., Iida, T., Hogan, B. J., Stolz, D. B., Fry, R., Samson, L. D., Tannenbaum, S. R., and Griffith, L. G. (2005). A microscale in vitro physiological model of the liver: Predictive screens for drug metabolism and enzyme induction. *Curr. Drug Metab. 6* (6), 569-591.

[44] Vickers, A. E., and Fisher, R. L. (2005). Precision-cut organ slices to investigate target organ injury. *Exp Opin Drug Metab Toxicol 1* (4), 687-699.

[45] Orrenius, S., and Zhivotovsky, B. (2006).The future of toxicology-does it matter how cells die? *Chem. Res. Toxicol. 19* (6), 729-733.

[46] Zon, L. I., and Peterson, R. T. (2005).In vivo drug discovery in the zebrafish. *Nat Re. Drug Discovery 4* (1), 35-44.

[47] Driscoll, M., and Gerstbrein, B. (2003). Dying for a cause: Invertebrate genetics takes on human neurodegeneration. *Na. Rev. Genet 4* (3), 181-194.

[48] Song, M. O., Fort, D. J., McLaughlin, D. L., Rogers, R. L., Thomas, J. H., Buzzard, B. O., Noll, A. M., and Myers, N. K. (2003).Evaluation of Xenopus tropicalis as an alternative test organism for frog embryo teratogenesis assay-Xenopus (FETAX). *Drug Chem Toxicol 26* (3), 177-189.

[49] Sandusky, G. E., Means, J. R., and Todd, G. C. (1990). Comparative cardiovascular toxicity in dogs given inotropic agents by continuous intravenous infusion. *Toxicol. Pathol. 18* (2), 268-278.

[50] Koop, R. (2005). Combinatorial biomarkers: From early toxicology assays to patient population profiling. *Drug Discovery Today 10* (11), 781-788.

[51] Hamadeh HK, Bushel PR, Jayadev S, Martin K, DiSorbo O, Sieber S, Bennett L, Tennant R, Stoll R, Barrett JC, Blanchard K, Paules RS, Afshari CA. (2002). Gene expression analysis reveals chemical-specific profiles. *Toxicol. Sci.* 67(2), 219-31.

[52] Wilke, R. A., Reif, D. M., and Moore, J. H. (2005). Combinatorial pharmacogenetics. *Na. Rev Drug Discovery 4* (11), 911-918.

[53] Waters, M. D., and Fostel, J. M. (2004). Toxicogenomics and systems toxicology: Aims and prospects. *Na. Rev Genet 5* (12), 936-948.

[54] Fielden, M. R., and Kolaja, K. L. (2006).The state-of-the-art in predictive toxicogenomics. *Curr. Opin. Drug Discovery Dev 9* (1), 84-91.

[55] Fostel, J., Choi, D., Zwickl, C., Morrison, N., Rashid, A., Hasan, A., Bao, W., Richard, A., Tong, W., Bushel, P. R., Brown, R., Bruno, M., Cunningham, M. L., Dix, D., Eastin, W., Frade, C., Garcia, A., Heinloth, A., Irwin, R., Madenspacher, J., Merrick, B. A., Papoian, T., Paules, R., Rocca-Serra, P., Sansone, A. S., Stevens, J., Tomer, K., Yang, C., and Waters, M. (2005). Chemical effects in biological systems-data dictionary (CEBS-DD): A compendium of terms for the capture and integration of biological study design description, conventional phenotypes, and 'omics data. *Toxicol. Sci. 88* (2), 585-601.

[56] Hayes, K. R., and Bradfield, C. A. (2005). Advances in toxicogenomics. *Chem Re. Toxico. 18* (3), 403-414.

[57] Lindon J.C., Holmes, E., Nicholson J. K. (2006). Metabonomics techniques and applications to pharmaceutical research and development. *Pharm. Res. 23* (6), 1075-1088.

[58] Fielden, M. R., and Zacharewski, T. R. (2001). Challenges and limitations of gene expression profiling in mechanistic and predictive toxicology. *Toxico. Sci. 60* (1), 6-10.

[59] Nicholson, J. K., Holmes, E., Lindon, J. C., and Wilson, I. D. (2004). The challenges of modeling mammalian biocomplexity. *Nat. Biotechnol. 22* (10), 1268-1274.

[60] Sawada, H., Takami, K., and Asahi, S. (2005). A toxicogenomic approach to drug-induced phospholipidosis: Analysis of its induction mechanism and establishment of a novel in vitro screening system. *Toxico. Sci 83* (2), 282-292.

[61] Law, M., and Rudnicka, A. R. (2006). Statin safety: A systematic review. *Am. J. Cardiol. 97* (8A), 52C-60C.

[62] Lasser, K. E., Allen, P. D., Woolhandler, S. J., Himmelstein, D. U., Wolfe, S. M., and Bor, D. H. (2002). Timing of new black box warnings and withdrawals for prescription medications. *J. Am. Med. Assoc. 287* (17), 2215-2220.

[63] Baillie, T. A. (2006). Future of toxicology-metabolic activation and drug design: Challenges and opportunities in chemical toxicology. *Chem. Res. Toxicol. 19* (7), 889-893.

[64] Smith, D. A., Johnson, D. E., and Park, B. K. (2006). Editorial overview: Safety of drugs can never be absolute. *Curr. Opin. Drug Discovery Dev. 9* (1), 26-28.

[65] Liebler, D. C. (2006). The poisons within: Application of toxicity mechanisms to fundamental disease processes. *Chem. Res. Toxicol. 19* (5), 610-613.

In: Drug Toxicity: New Research
Editor: Cam E. Vellotis, pp.29-51
ISBN 978-1-60456-320-7

Chapter 2

Antipsychotic Drugs: A Critical Review Focusing on Adverse Event Profile

Francisco José Álvarez*

Health Sciences Research Centre. School of Health Sciences. University of Beira Interior. Covilhã. Portugal. Neurology Department. Pêro da Covilhã Hospital. Colvilhã. Portugal. Infante D. Henrique Av., 6200-506. Covilhã, Portugal

The psychotic disorders include schizophrenia, manic phase of bipolar disease, and other psychotic illnesses.

The clinically used agents to treat these disorders are the antipsychotic drugs. They may be classified in typical and atypical following their relative affinity for the antagonism of the dopamine D2 receptors, strong for the typical drugs and discrete or absent for the atypical. The dopamine antagonism is one of the determinants of the clinical effect, but the interaction with other neurotransmitter receptors also is relevant. Secondarily, the antipsychotic drugs may be classified following their chemical structure. Examples of typical antipsychotic drugs are thioridazine, chlorpromazine, fluphenazine, or haloperidol. Examples of atypical antipsychotic drugs are quetiapine, olanzapine, clozapine, or risperidone.

Although the antipsychotics are generally safe drugs, the adverse events profile of these agents is extensive and they are often related to their own pharmacological actions. They include central and autonomic nervous effects (sedation, cholinergic block, both acute and chronic extrapiramidal reactions including the neuroleptic malignant syndrome, and others), cardiovascular events (orthostatic hypotension, electrocardiographic changes and arrhythmias, stroke), endocrine disorders (weight gain, new-onset type 2 diabetes mellitus, and others), haematological disorders (leukocytosis, leukopenia, agranulocytosis, bone marrow suppression), and other adverse events (dermatological reactions, gastrointestinal disorders).

* 0351-275-329062. franciscoplus@hotmail.com

The aims of this chapter are to review several issues of antipsychotics (its supposed mechanism of action, main adverse events related and its habitual management) and to highlight the current research lines of new antipsychotic drugs, focusing on those trying to minimize the adverse event profile.

Background

Psychotic Disorders

The psychotic disorders are characterized by distortions of thinking and perception and a loss of contact with reality. The patients have beliefs or perceptual experiences not shared by other members of their culture and delusions and hallucinations, or they have a bizarre behaviour. These are the called positive symptoms or psychotic domain. The negative symptoms or the second symptom domain are the blunted or inappropriate affect, anhedonia, apathy, and a reduced quantity and content of speech. Although the consciousness and the intellectual capacity are usually maintained, cognitive deficits may appear in the course of time. Then, the cognitive impairment constitutes the third domain of symptoms. The cognitive impairment affects attention, learning, memory, and different executive functions, like abstract thinking and problem solving [1, 2].

The psychotic disorders include schizophrenia –the most frequent of them-, the manic phase of maniac-depressive illness, the acute psychosis, and other conditions like delusional disorders and severe melancholic depression. Table 1 shows a ICD10-WHO based classification of schizophrenia, schizotypal, and delusional disorders [3, 19].

Table 1.

Schizophrenia:

- Paranoid schizophrenia
- Paraphrenic schizophrenia
- Hebephrenic schizophrenia
- Catatonic schizophrenia
- Undifferentiated schizophrenia
- Post-schizophrenic depression
- Residual schizophrenia
- Simple schizophrenia
- Other schizophrenia
- Schizophrenia, unspecified

Schizotypal disorder.

Persistent delusional disorders:

- Delusional disorder

- Other persistent delusional disorders
- Persistent delusional disorder, unspecified

Acute and transient psychotic disorders:
- Acute polymorphic psychotic disorder without symptoms of schizophrenia
- Acute polymorphic psychotic disorder with symptoms of schizophrenia
- Acute schizophrenia-like psychotic disorder
- Other acute predominantly delusional psychotic disorders
- Other acute and transient psychotic disorders
- Acute and transient psychotic disorder, unspecified

Induced delusional disorder.
Schizoaffective disorders:
- Schizoaffective disorder, manic type
- Schizoaffective disorder, depressive type Schizoaffective disorder, mixed typeOther schizoaffective disorders Schizoaffective disorder, unspecified

Other nonorganic psychotic disorders.

Unspecified nonorganic psychosis.

Etiopathology of Schizophrenia

The etiological basis of schizophrenia remains unknown. Genetic, neurodevelopmental and environmental factors have been proposed. The genetic basis explains the susceptibility in most cases of schizophrenia and the environmental factors may actuate as a trigger and justificate the different clinical presentations of the disease [1, 4-6].

Genetics

The evidence from families, twins, and adoption studies indicates that genetic susceptibility plays a key role in the aetiology of schizophrenia, concluding that the heritability for schizophrenia is around 80%. They are not evidence of Mendelian (monogenic) forms of the disease and it is accepted that multiple susceptibility genes, each of small effect, may act in concert with environmental factors to cause the disease.

The risk of schizophrenia increases 10 fold in the first degree relatives of a patient. The risk is not dependent on the environment, since adoption for a non-schizophrenic parents does not reduces significantly it. Proposed susceptibility genes linked to schizophrenia have been located in short arm of chromosomes 6, 8, 9, and 20 and long arm of chromosome 22.

Neurodevelopmental Disorder

The most prevalent hypothesis for the pathogenesis of schizophrenia posits that the disease is a neurodevelopmental disorder associated with abnormal connectivity resulting from defects in synaptic pruning and migration of neurons. This hypothesis is supported for the presence of premorbid neuropsychological disorders, neuroanatomical and neurohistological changes, and the usual onset of schizophrenia between the ages of 16 and 30 years. Environmental and developmental risk factors for schizophrenia are obstetric complications like perinatal hypoxia, nutritional deficit during first quarter of pregnancy, severe stress during pregnancy, social isolation, and cannabis consumption during adolescence [5, 6]. There is not consistent evidence about the role of viral infections. Experimental evidence and empirical data support that the excessive activation of the hypothalamic pituitary adrenal axis, i.e. for chronic stress, may trigger psychosis.

Different anatomical and cytoarchitectural findings have been reported in these patients, although there are not single anatomic or functional modifications that explain the diversity of findings. Some relevant histologic changes are the modified distribution of interstitial neurons in the white matter underlying the prefrontal cortex (especially dorsolateral areas), hippocampus, and other locations. This may reflect abnormalities in migration of subplate neurons or programmed cell death. Anomalies in cortical and thalamocortical circuitry have been reported.

Classification of Antipsychotic Drugs

The treatment of psychotic disorders is based in the antipsychotic drugs. In the last section of this chapter novel approaches are summarised. As well as psychosis, the antipsychotic drugs are used in the treatment of maniac-depressive illness, severe depression, and severe anxiety.

Classification

The classification of neuroleptic drugs is based on its supposed mechanism of action and its chemical structure [1, 2]. Considering the mechanism of action of antipsychotic drugs they are classified in first generation or typical neuroleptics, and second generation or atypical neuroleptics. A non exhaustive classification is showed in the Table 2.

Table 2. Classification of antipsychotic drugs

First generation or typical antipsychotics:

Phenothiazines:

- Chlorpromazine
- Thioridazine
- Triflupromazine
- Perphenazine
- Trifluoperazine
- Fluphenazine

Mesoridazine

Thioxanthenes:

- Chlorprothixene
- Thiothixene
- Clopenthixol
- Cis-flupentixol
- Piflutixol
- Zuclopentixol

Butirophenones and diphenylbutylpiperidines:

- Haloperidol
- Droperidol
- Penfluridol
- Pimozide
- Dibenzoxazepines:
- Doxapine
- Loxapine
- Clothiapine
- Dihydroindolones:
- Molindone
- Oxypertine

Second generation or atypical antipsychotics:

Benzamides:

- Sulpiride
- Amisulpiride
- Raclopride
- Tiapride

Dibenzodiazepines:

- Clozapine
- Olanzapine

Dibenzotiazepines:

- Quetiapine
- Metiapina

Benzisoxazoles:

- Risperidone

Other:

- Aripiprazole
- Ziprasidone

First Generation or Typical Neuroleptics: History and Mechanism of Action

The phenothiazines were the first drugs synthesized in the late nineteenth century. During the 1930s promethazine was discovered, but its use in psychiatric patients was not successful. Later, chlorpromazine was synthesized by the chemist Paul Charpentier in December 1950, starting the era of neuroleptic drugs. During the same decade, reserpine (an alkaloid derived from the Rauwolfia plant actuating as depletory of monoamines from the terminal nerve vesicles) was used as neuroleptic agent. However, the latency to therapeutic effect and the severity of side effects, relegated it as an antihypertensive and as not as a neuroleptic drug. The psychiatric use of chlorpromazine was introduced in Europe by Jean Delay and Pierre Deniker in 1952 and by Lehmann and Hanrahan in United States in 1954. During the same and next decades, the first thioxanthene and the first butyrophenone and diphenylbutylpiperidine were synthesized by Povl Petersen and Paul Janssen, respectively.

Currently, using receptor binding techniques, it is known that the clinical power of these typical antipsychotics in treating psychotic patients is related to blockade of central D2 dopamine receptors, rather than D1 dopamine. Although this mechanism is related to the clinical benefits of the treatment on positive psychotic symptoms, it is also one of the main determinants of the dose-depending extrapyramidal side effects (EPS) and the exacerbation of negative psychotic symptoms. This is why during the 1970s the first atypical neuroleptics, avoiding the intense blockade of D2 dopamine receptors, were synthesized.

Second Generation or Atypical Neuroleptic: History and Mechanism of Action

The attempt to reduce the EPS conducted the research to synthesize drugs with a more potent 5-HT2A serotonin receptor blocking effect and less intense blockade of D2 dopamine receptors, starting the development of the atypical drugs. The 5-HT2A blockade could reduce the dopamine release from mesolimbic pathway. Other atypical antipsychotics include partial agonists of D2 dopamine receptors. Currently, the only partial D2 agonist antipsychotic approved for clinical use is aripiprazole. Furthermore, this molecule is a 5-HT1A serotonin agonist and 5-HT2A serotonin antagonist.

Some of the approved drugs show a greater overall efficacy than the first-generation antipsychotics and a reduced EPS profile.

Pharmacological Actions and Characteristics of Antipsychotics

Neuroleptic drugs share many pharmacological actions, classified as psychiatric, cognitive, motor, other neurological, endocrine, and vegetative properties. With the aim of determine these effects in humans different experimental animal models and radioligands studies are used. Because the review of these methods is beyond the scope of this chapter the interested reader may find comprehensive information in the additional lectures suggested in the references.

Animal Models

To study behaviour in animals the models used are based on deficits in prepulse inhibition (PPI) observed in rats and mousses. The PPI is a highly conserved phenomenon between vertebrates in which a weak prepulse stimulus attenuates the response to a subsequent startling stimulus. In the human set, PPI is impaired in patients with schizophrenia and other neuropsychiatric disorders. This could reflect the dysfunction of sensorimotor gating mechanisms [8, 9].

The PPI deficit can be induced using pharmacological or developmental methods or genetic models. Pharmacological methods imply the stimulation of D2 dopamine receptors using amphetamine or apomorphine, the stimulation of serotonin receptors using serotonin releasers or direct agonists, and the blockade of N-methyl-D-aspartate receptors using antagonists as phencyclidine. Developmental modifications include long-term consequences of lesions in ventral hippocampus in the neonatal rat, and the isolation rearing. The genetically modified animals have gene or chromosomal deletions or insertions, or induced mutations. An example of genetic model presenting a PPI deficit is the Brattleboro rat. This rat has a mutation in a single pair of autosomal loci that causes a single nucleotide deletion in the second exon. The consequence is the synthesis of non-functional form of vasopresin, resulting in a central diabetes insipidus (similar to disease found in human pathology) and deficits in central nervous system functions, including behaviour, cognition, and drug tolerance [10].

The models used to study extrapiramidal effects in animals include the assessing of catalepsy in rats or dystonia in monkeys for acute effects, and the chewing movements in rats for long term motor effects.

Radioligand Studies

The radioligand studies, using different isotopes with single photon emission computed tomography (SPECT) and positron emission tomography (PET) techniques, allow the visualisation, measurement and characterisation of neurotransmitter pathways at the presynaptic, synaptic, and postsynaptic level, both in normal and pathologic conditions. It also permits the "in vivo" study of pharmacodynamic and pharmacokinetic processes of therapeutic agents, and the estimation of their affinity and distribution for dopamine brain receptors.

The combined use of magnetic resonance imaging (MRI) methods allows reaching a more precise anatomical correlation [7, 11].

Psychiatric and Cognitive Effects

The main psychiatric effect is the antipsychotic effect. It is especially remarkable on positive symptoms of psychosis. Antipsychotic effect characterizes all these drugs and is often used as a synonym of neuroleptic. However, the last term is more complex because includes the antipsychotic effect and other characteristic effects. Considering that the majority of antipsychotics are neuroleptics too, but clozapine, quetiapine, aripiprazole, ziprasidone, and low doses of olanzapine and risperidone are not, the preferred term is antipsychotic, more general.

The concept of neuroleptic was introduced by Delay and was internationally approved in 1955 during the World Congress of Psychiatry. This concept implies a sensory desafferentization, characterised by the suppression of emotional manifestations, lost of interest in the environment, and psychomotor slowing with development of bradykinesia and rigidity. There is a suppression of spontaneous movements and complex behaviours, being the catalepsia the extreme of this effect, when motor immobilization appears. In the psychotic patient positive symptoms like agitation, aggressive behaviour, hallucinations and incoherent thinking are reduced. This effect spares the level of consciousness (although some degree of sedative effect is habitually present, especially when chlorpromazine and other low potency agents are used), the cognitive functions and the motor reflexes [1, 2]. The cognitive symptoms, like attention, verbal memory and executive functions, are usually not improved with dopamine D2 antagonist antipsychotic therapy. Only mixed serotonin 5-HT2a and dopamine D2 antagonist drugs and partial D2 agonists drugs showed some improvement of these symptoms.

The biochemical basis of the antipsychotic effect is the selective blockade of dopamine receptors, both presynaptic and postsynaptic. The blockade of presynaptic receptors increases the liberation of dopamine from the terminal vesicle by suppression of the inhibitory effect of the neurotransmitter when dopamine interacts with it. This results in a continuous depolarisation of the terminal that finally reduces the release of dopamine.

The main dopamine receptor implied in the neuroleptic effect is the D2 subtype, although the D3 and D4 participate too. The percentage of striate D2 receptors occupied to achieve the neuroleptic effect is near 70% and the motor side effects need at least the 80% of occupation of the same receptors. The dopaminergic connections with limbic system and mesocortex may be the more relevant in antipsychotic activity.

The interaction with other receptors also participates in antipsychotic effect. The blockade of serotonin 5-HT2A receptors reduces the mesolimbic release of dopamine. The partial agonist activity on serotonin 5-HT1A receptors reduces the rate of firing in rafe nuclei neurons, reducing the release of dopamine. Antagonism of histamine H1 receptors is related to sedative effect of some antipsychotic drugs, like chlorpromazine [1, 2, 12-15].

Neuroleptics are not related to addiction, although some of physical dependence may be present if the drugs are suddenly discontinued after prolonged use. There is not evidence of reduction of clinical efficacy after long term therapy with antipsychotics. The Table 3 shows the pharmacological profile of different antipsychotic drugs [12-17]. The relative affinity for dopamine and other neurotransmitter receptors are expressed as constant of inhibition (Ki).

Table 3. Pharmacological profile of different antipsychotic drugs. Values express the Ki

	Dopamine D1	Dopamine D2	Dopamine D4	Serotonin 5-HT2A	Cholinergic M1	Adrener-gic Alpha 1	Histamine H1
Typical drugs							
Haloperidol	45	4	10	36	>20.000	6,2	1890
Thioridazine	22	2,3	12	41	10	1,1	16
Chlorpromazine	56	19	12	1,4	60	0,6	9,1
Perphenazine		1,4		5,6	1500	10	
Fluphenazine	15	0,8	9,3	19	2000	9	21
Loxapine	71	-	12	1,69	62	28	5
Pimozide	-	2,5	30	13	-	-	-
Atypical drugs							
Clozapine	38	180	9,6	1,6	7,5	9	2,75
Risperidone	750	3,3	17	0,16	>10.000	2	59
Olanzapine	31	11	9,6	4	1,89	19	7,14
Quetiapine	455	160	1164	294	120	62	11
Ziprasidone	339	4,79	39	0,42	>10.000	10	47
Sulpiride	>1.000	7,4	52	>1.000	>1.000	>1.000	-
Aripiprazole	265	3,4	44	3,4	>10.000	57	61

Adapted from references 12 to 17.

Extrapyramidal Effects

The acute and long term extrapyramidal effects are related to antagonism of dopamine D2 receptors in basal ganglia, both pre and postsynaptic. Then, the dopamine nigrostriate pathway may be the more specifically affected when extrapyramidal effects are considered and the mesocortical and the mesolimbic pathways may be the implied when antipsichotic effects are considered. As it was appointed above, the first consequence of dopamine D2 blockade is the increase in the rate of dopamine production and the increase in the rate of firing in the dopaminergic neurons in the midbrain. Later, the continuous depolarization reduces the presynaptic activity. The role of dopamine D3 and D4 receptors is probably non significant [1, 12, 16, 18].

Neuroendocrine Effects

The dopamine D2 antagonism on lactotropic cells in anterior hypophysis is associated with the increase in prolactine release. In this case, the implied pathway is the tuberoinfundibular tract. This effect is especially intense with older antipsychotics and risperidone and there is no tolerance with years of treatment, although it is rapidly reversible when the responsible drug is withdrawn. Clinically it may be associated to gynecomastia and there is no evidence of increased risk of breast neoplasm. However, these antipsychotic should be avoided in case of carcinoma of breast with known extension. The effect on prolactine is minimum or transient with the use of other atypical drugs.

Other effect reported with antipsychotic drugs is the reduction of the release of gonadotrophins that may be related to amenorrhea in female and sexual dysfunction in male.

The reduction of growth hormone and corticotropin related hormone release has not apparent clinical significance [1, 2, 40, 41].

Autonomic Effects

Autonomic effects are extremely complex because antipsychotics have interactions with peripheral receptor as well as dopaminergic receptors.

The peripheral blockade of cholinergic muscarinic receptors is associated with the reduction in saliva production, constipation, reduction of gastric secretions and motility, acute urinary retention and ejaculation impairment. Anticholinergic effects are especially intense when clozapine, olanzapine or chlorpromazine are used.

The peripheral blockade of alpha adrenergic receptors is strong with chlorpromazine, thioridazhine, and clozapine. It is associated with ortostatic hypotension, due to arterial and venous vasodilatation reducing peripheral resistances, and relaxation of smooth muscle of urinary tract and prostate.

Other autonomic effects are related to the interaction at brain stem level. Most antipsychotics have an antiemetic property related to dopamine antagonism at the chemoreceptor trigger zone in the medulla. The central effect on respiration causes deeper and slower respiratory movements. This effect is extremely slight and the risk of death due to respiratory depression is very low. It is relevant for psychiatric patients, because suicidal attempts with high doses do not depress respiratory centre. The vasomotor reflexes are impaired at central level and ortostatic hypotension is relatively frequent with typical drugs and risperidone. Some old antipsychotics impair the regulation of body temperature, predisposing to hypo or hyperthermia depending on external temperature.

Cardiovascular Effects

Some cardiovascular effects are related to autonomic mediation. Some drugs may have direct heart and vessels activity. Negative ionotropic effect causing prolongation of QT and PR intervals has been related to thioridazine and other phenothiazines, and in less extension to ziprasidone. This effect justified the withdrawal of thioridazine in some countries because cases of sudden death were reported, as it is discussed later.

Pharmacokinetic of Antipsychotic Drugs

The antipsychotics share some general pharmacokinetic properties. The Table 4 shows several pharmacokinetic parameters and habitual initial and maintaining doses of some typical and atypical drugs, respectively [1, 2, 23, 24].

Most antipsychotics have a slow oral absorption, sometimes erratic, with T_{max} values between 2 and 4 hours. The bioavailability is generally about 30% due to hepatic first step effect, but this parameter varies between drugs. As intramuscular administration avoids portal circulation, the bioavailability increases when this route is used.

The percentage of binding of antipsychotics to plasmatic and tissue proteins is high. Habitually more than 90% of the drug is linked to plasma proteins, especially albumin.

Table 4. Summary of pharmacokinetic parameters

	T_{max} (hours)	Bio-availability (%)	Protein binding (%)	Metabolism	$T_{1/2}$ (hours)	Starting dose (mg)	Mean dose (mg)
Typical drugs							
Haloperidol	3-6	40-80	92	CYP2D6	15-30	2,5-5	5-32
Thioridazine	2-4	10-60	99	CYP2D6	10-30	25-100	100-600
Chlorpromazine	2-4	25-65	90-95	CYP2D6	12-36	25-100	200-800
Perphenazine	3-5	60-80	90	CYP2D6	10-20	4-10	8-64
Fluphenazine	2-5	10-50	90-95	CYP2D6	8-32	2,5-5	10-20
Loxapine	1-2	80	91-99	CYP 3A4	4-12	20-50	60-120
Pimozide	4-8	15-25	-	CYP3A4	30-150	1-2	2-10
Atypical drugs							
Clozapine	1-6	40-60	92-95	CYP3A4	12-36	12,5-25	200-600
Risperidone	2	66-82	90	CYP2D6	20-24	1-2	4-16
Olanzapine	5-8	60-80	93	CYP1A2	33	10	5-20
Quetiapine	1-2	9	83	CYP3A4	7	25-100	300-450
Ziprasidone	5	59	99	CYP3A4	7,5	40	40-200
Sulpiride	2-6	15-65	-		6-15	200	800-1600
Aripiprazole	3-5	87	99	CYP3A4	75	2-10	10-30

Adapted from references 1, 2, 14, 23, and 24.

Most drugs are lipophilic and enter through the blood-brain barrier accumulating into the central nervous system. In the case of haloperidol and other drugs the concentration into the brain is 10 times the plasmatic. This is the reason because some antipsychotics are first eliminated from blood and persist later into the brain.

The half life of antipsychotics varies typically between 20 and 40 hours, although exceptions are not uncommon, like ziprasidone, sulpiride, and quetiapine (approximately 7 hours) or pimozide (between 30 and 150 hours).

The main metabolic routes of neuroleptics are hepatic oxidative processes, generally depending on isozymes of cytochrome P-450. Most of the oxidized metabolites are inactive and some drugs may induce their own metabolism. Chlorpromazine, risperidone, ziprasidone and aripiprazole are some examples of neuroleptic drugs having active metabolites that may contribute to clinical effect. The metabolic ability is reduced in the fetus, infant and elderly.

The excretion is performed in urine and feces.

Interactions of Antipsychotics with Other Drugs

Antipsychotics enhance strongly all drugs that depress the central nervous system, like alcohol, sedatives, opioid analgesics, hypnotics, and histamine H1 receptor antagonists. These pharmacodynamic interactions should be considered because the risk of respiratory depression related to opioids and other central depressors may be increased when both class of drugs are combined with antipsychotics [2, 24].

Since the antipsychotics have an antidopaminergic effect, they inhibit the action of levodopa and dopamine agonists, like bromocriptine, lisuride, pergolide, cabergoline, ropirinol, pramipexole, or rotigotine. This interaction is especially relevant in Parkinson disease and Lewy body disease patients. These patients are extremely sensitive to neuroleptics, developing neurological side effects, even low doses are used. If the management of behavioural disorders in these patients requires the use of antipsychotics, clozapine or quetiapine should be preferentially used.

Unpredictable effects have been reported when phenothiazines and antihypertensive drugs are combined. The action of cholinergic and alfa adrenergic agonists may be blocked by antipsychotics. This may enhance anticholinergic side effects and cause ortostatic hypotension, especially in the elderly.

Considering pharmacokinetic interactions, since most antipsychotics are metabolised by cytochromes, inductor drugs like some anticonvulsivants may enhance the metabolism of neuroleptics, and inhibitor drugs like some selective inhibitors of serotonin reuptake antidepressants may increase the plasmatic levels of neuroleptics.

Adverse Effects of Antipsychotic Drugs

Antipsychotics are generally safe drugs with a high therapeutic index and a wide range of doses. Because of the complex pharmacological actions of neuroleptics, the profile of adverse effects is vast[1, 2, 25]. It may be summarised as follows:

- Cardiovascular adverse effects.
- Neurological adverse effects.
- Haematological adverse effects.
- Endocrine adverse effects.
- Dermatological and ocular adverse effects.
- Gastrointestinal and urinary adverse effects.

Cardiovascular Adverse Effects

The most frequent side effect is ortortatic hypotension that may lead to syncope and falls, with the associated risk of secondary damage due to traumatism. This risk is directly related to alpha adrenergic blockade and it is higher in the elderly patient and when phenotiazines and atypical neuroleptics are used.

One of the more important cardiovascular risks is the depression of cardiac repolarization, especially with thioridazine and its active metabolite mesoridazine. The more relevant finding is the prolongation of QT interval, which may lead to ventricular tachycardia ("torsade de pointes" type) and sudden death when corrected QT is higher than 500 msec. The inverted or bicuspid T wave and the presence of U wave have also been reported. This is why the manufacturer of thioridazine discontinued the drug worldwide in June 2005, although it is still available as a generic from other manufacturers. It may be used only as a second line antipsychotic and requires EKG-monitoring and additional white blood cells counts [22, 23].

Isolated cases of myocarditis, pericarditis, and cardiomyopathy have been rarely reported during clozapine therapy. The risk of these cardiac complications ranges from 0.015 to 0.188% and they usually occur within the fist 4 weeks of initiation of drug treatment. The presumed pathophysiology is an IgE mediated acute hypersensitivity because peripheral eosinophilia and eosinophilic myocardial infiltrates have been found. This disorder has a good prognosis with early treatment, based on discontinuation of the neuroleptic and the start of symptomatic treatment. However, it may be fulminant or associated to severe chronic morbidity by development of dilated cardiomyopathy if the diagnosis is delayed.

In our knowledge, 3 isolated cases of myocarditis have been reported with quetiapine [20, 34].

Recently, some atypical antipsychotics have been related to increased risk of ischaemic stroke. This concern emerged from the evaluation of adverse events profile of risperidone, olanzapine, and aripiprazole after clinical trials designed to study the treatment of behavioural disorders in dementia patients. Risperidone duplicates and olanzapine triplicates the risk of cerebrovascular events versus placebo, respectively. The issue is controversial and more information is still necessary. Some retrospective works did not associate the use of atypical antipsychotics with the risk of stroke, because a similar risk was found with the use of typical and atypical drugs. Other analysis explained the increased risk of stroke considering the high vascular risk of the patients population included in these studies [42-46].

In June 2005 the Food and Drug Administration (FDA) issued a warning concerning to the increased mortality risk between elderly demented patients when several atypical antipsychotics, including clozapine, olanzapine, aripiprazole, risperidone, ziprasidone and quetiapine, were used [41]. The conclusion came from the analysis of the data obtained from 17 placebo-controlled trials in elderly demented patients with behavioural disorders. Fifteen studies showed an increased mortality in the active drug groups versus the placebo groups. The risk of mortality was 1.6 to 1.7 times higher in the active drug groups and the rate of death in drug-treated patients was about 4.5%, compared with the rate of 2.6% in the placebo patients. The aetiologies of deaths were primarily due to heart-related events, especially heart failure and sudden death, or pneumonia. As the use of atypical antipsychotic medications for treating behavioural disorders in elderly patients with dementia was associated with increased mortality the FDA requested that manufacturers of these drugs insert a black box warning describing this risk and noting that these drugs are not approved for this off-label indication.

From a clinical point of view, the use of atypical antipsychotics in schizophrenia and mania is not affected by this warning. When demented patients with agitation or psychoses are considered the American Academy of Neurology recommends the use of antipsychotics to treat these symptoms when environmental modifications fail, and suggests that atypical drugs may be better tolerated than typical compounds.

A recently published study of 37.241 elderly patients assessed the 180-days mortality. The authors concluded that the risk of death associated with typical antipsychotic drugs is similar and possibly greater than the risk of death associated with atypical antipsychotics in elderly patients. Then, all antipsychotic drugs should be considered equally risky in this population [47].

Neurological Adverse Effects

The use of antipsychotic therapy is related to different neurological syndromes, which especially affect the extrapyramidal motor system. These adverse events are more intense with the high potency dopamine D2 antagonists and they are less frequent and less severe with aripiprazole, quetiapine, ziprasidone, thioridazine, clozapine and low doses of risperidone and olanzapine.

The extrapyramidal symptoms (EPS) can be classified as acute (acute dystonia, akathisia, parkinsonism, and neuroleptic malignant syndrome) and late (tardive dyskinesia, tardive dystonia, tardive tics, tardive akathisia, and perioral tremor) syndromes. They have a significant impact on tolerability and adherence with antipsychotic therapy [21, 25].

Acute Dystonic Reaction

It is a relatively frequent reaction (2-5%) that commonly occurs during the initiation of antipsychotic therapy, usually between 1 to 5 days, and sometimes hours. The dystonia affects most commonly cranial and axial muscles, causing grimacing, oculogyric crises, torticollis or retrocollis, fixation of the jaw, and contraction of respiratory spinal muscles, phenomenon that may lead to opisthotonos. The limb muscles seem more resistant and they are less frequently implied.

The risk of suffering this side effect is higher in young men and increases with the use of high potency drugs and with the size of dose, whereas the probability of acute dystonia is lower when antipsychotics with stronger anticholinergic effect are used, like thioridazine.

The pathophysiology is unknown, although genetic susceptibility, hypocalcemia, and the excessive activity of the cholinergic system have been suggested.

If this acute reaction is not treated, usually last from seconds to hours and may recur later. If specific therapy is initiated the choice drugs are anticholinergic drugs, like benztropine or diphenhydramine, starting with parenteral dosing and continuing with oral administration 2-3 days.

Akathisia

It is the most common movement disorder related to dopamine antagonists, although it was first described as a manifestation of Parkinson disease. Akathisia is characterised by a subjective restlessness and inability to remain still, and by the movements that satisfy this necessity. The patient feels an anxious distress and discomfort, and the compelling need to be in continuous movements generates a range of activity from distal limb movements to pacing or running movements.

The akathisia induced by antipsychotics is usually acute and generally starts within few days of drug therapy onset. It may appear rarely as a late disorder (tardive akathisia). The development of akathisia is dose dependent and the side effect persists all the time of treatment. The risk of developing akathisia is lower with the use of atypical instead of typical antipsychotics.

To explain the pathophysiology of akathisia the interference of antipsychotic drug with the mesocortical dopaminergic system has been implied. It has been also suggested the participation of setoninergic pathways.

This motor side effect disappears shortly after cessation of the neuroleptic: If the withdrawal is not possible, akathisia may respond to anticholinergics, amantadine, clonazepam or beta-adrenergic antagonists, like propranolol. When a typical antipsychotic is used, another therapeutic option is switching to an atypical drug. The less frequent tardive akathisia is treated as other late effects.

Drug-Induced Parkinsonian Syndrome

This side effect usually develops 2-10 weeks after initiation of treatment in approximately 15% of patients chronically taking antipsychotic drugs. The risk of this EPS increases when the risk of acute complications reduces. The clinical syndrome is similar to idiopathic Parkinson disease (PD). However, when parkinsonian symptoms are related to drugs akinesia is usually the most prominent sign and the disorder tends to be symmetric. The rest tremor, masked facies, reduced arms movements during gait are also present and may be intense like PD.

The risk of developing parkinsonian syndrome depends on the antipsychotic drug used. The risk is low with atypical drugs and lower with clozapine and quetiapine. Both are the elective drugs when it is necessary to treat agitation in PD patients. Currently, there are insufficient data about the use of ziprasidone and aripiprazole.

The parkinsonian manifestations tend to reduce spontaneously after several months despite continuous use of the drug. If symptoms are important, the reduction of dose or substitution by an atypical antipsychotic and the use of antiparkinsonian drugs should be considered. If antiparkinsonian therapy is required, the elective drugs are anticholinergics or amantadine and the continuation of this treatment should be evaluated after 3 months. In most of the cases antiparkinsonian therapy can be withdrawn after this time.

Because the withdrawal of the antipsychotic drug usually causes the suppression of parkinsonian symptoms within weeks, a subclinical PD should be considered in the rare cases of no improvement. Some authors also consider a late side effect called tardive parkinsonism.

Neuroleptic Malignant Syndrome (NMS)

The NMS is an uncommon and serious complication of antipsychotic drug therapy. It was first described in 1967 as “akinetic hypertonic syndrome”. NMS has been reported in the 0.07 to 2.2% of patients receiving neuroleptic medications [27-31].

This motor side effect is unpredictable and it may arise at any time during the treatment. Hwever, it is more common early, especially when high doses of potent drugs are used or when stable doses are quickly increased. This is the reason why NMS may appear with a previously taken drug without side effects. If the same antipsychotic drug is reintroduced later it may not cause the syndrome another time. However, it is recommendable to change to low doses of an atypical antipsychotic if this treatment is still necessary. NMS seems to be more frequent in younger population, especially men, and it has been related to the presence of previous brain disease, dehydration, malnutrition, hyponatremia, and concomitant use of lithium, anticholinergics and some antidepressants.

Two theories have been proposed to explain the pathophysiology of NMS, although remains unknown. The “central theory” explains the NMS by the interference of dopamine antagonists with the thermoregulatory functions of dopamine when central receptors are blocked. The loss of dopamine inhibition allows the stimulation of heat production by serotonin, normally balanced by dopamine activity. The "peripheral theory" implies an excessive muscle contraction induced by dopamine blockade. In vitro investigations have found defects in skeletal muscle activity, usually related to increased calcium release from the sarcoplasmic reticulum. The "peripheral theory" is supported by the existence of similar anatomical findings and mechanisms of disease in cases of malignant hyperthermia.

The NMS is clinically characterised by the presence of extreme rigidity, tremor, dystonia, hyperthermia, signs of autonomic instability (like labile pulse, diaphoresis, variations in blood pressure and respiratory rate), and fluctuating depression of the level of consciousness. Tonic-clonic seizures, opisthotonos, trismus, and mutism are potential manifestations. Frequently, there are analytical alterations like elevation of serum creatine kinase and myoglobinemia (reflecting rhabdomyolysis), leukocytosis, and potential raise of transaminases and acute renal failure secondary to myoglobinuria. Usually, the disorder develops over 24 to 72 hours and can remain 1 to 44 days. Some atypical antipsychotics (clozapine and risperidone) have been related to an atypical form of NMS, characterised by hyperthermia and delirium but without rigidity. However, this concept has been questioned and some authors have suggested that atypical antipsychotics may be related to classical NMS [32].

Different diagnostic criteria have been proposed. However, there is no a general agreement over a determined set of signs, symptoms, and analytical disturbances. The characteristic clinical manifestations in a patient taking antipsychotics, with the expected laboratory findings and the exclusion of other disorders are the basis of diagnosis. Viral encephalitis, malignant hyperthermia, heavy metal poisoning, tetanus, thyrotoxicosis, serotonin syndrome, central anticholinergic syndrome, drugs toxicity (lithium, monoamine oxidase inhibitors), withdrawal states (alcohol, benzodiazepines), and others must be ruled out.

The treatment of NMS is based on the withdrawal of the implied drug and supportive care. The benefits of using specific therapies are controversial. If specific treatment is necessary the currently used drugs are dopaminergic agents (like dopamine, bromocriptine, levodopa, and amantadine) and the peripheral muscle relaxant dantrolene sodium, that inhibits the release of calcium from the sarcoplasmic reticulum. The recommended dose of dantrolene is 2 mg/kg intravenously that may be repeated if necessary reaching 10 mg/kg daily. This drug is only given during the acute phase of disease and hepatic function should be monitored. The recommended dose of bromocriptine is 2.5 to 10 mg up to 4 times daily. The most frequent side effect observed with bromocriptine is hypotension. These drugs may be combined and the treatment should be continued by 2 weeks until symptoms improve.

With early diagnosis and management the recovery often occurs in less than 2 weeks. However, if the therapeutic measures are not initiated the disorder is potentially lethal, with mortality rate between 10% and 30%. The main causes of death are acute renal failure due to rhabdomyolysis, acute respiratory insufficiency due to embolism or pneumonia, disseminated intravascular coagulation, myocardial infarction, and sepsis.

Tardive Dyskinesia

Tardive dyskinesia (TD) is a motor side effect developed after chronic exposure to antipsychotics and it is considered the most common drug related tardive syndrome. Since 1950s, when the first descriptions were reported, different patterns have been outlined. Classical TD refers a syndrome characterised by stereotyped choreic orolingual and masticatory movements, like lip pursing, tongue protrusion and chewing movements. The implication of upper facial, trunk, and limb muscles is less common. If trunk muscles are affected, the patient experiments respiratory dyskinesias and pelvis swinging. When limb muscles are affected the clinical manifestation is a chorea. The movements have 3 main characteristics. First, they tend to be repetitive and stereotypic. Second, usually they do not distress the patient. Third, they may be suppressed moving the affected area and increased moving a different region of the body. This side effect is more frequent in older patients and women. The prevalence is approximately 15-25% of patients treated with older antipsychotics more than 1 year and 50% when the treatment reaches 3 years. The risk of TD is lower with atypical antipsychotics than typical drugs, although risperidone has an intermediate risk.

The presumed pathophysiology of TD is based on the hypersensitivity of striatal dopamine receptors due to chronic denervation. The gabaergic pathways have been also implied in TD.

Even if the causal neuroleptic is withdrawn, TD may remit after months or years in better cases and it may be permanent in many patients. Then, the prevention of the disorder is a especially relevant issue. To prevent this complication, the indication of long term antipsychotic therapy may be reviewed. The preventive treatment with pharmacological doses of vitamin E could be useful, but this measure is not clearly effective. The early diagnosis of TD is basic to minimize the related disability. The first step is the withdrawal of the neuroleptic drug if it is possible. If the disability is minor, pharmacological therapy should not be started because the spontaneous recovery is possible. However, when the disability is more prominent, different drugs, like benzodiazepines, baclofen, or presynaptic dopamine depletors (tetrabenazine or reserpine) may be used. The switch to and atypical antipsychotic may be useful, because these drugs do not worse the TD and even may be used as specific therapy, especially clozapine. However, its long term effect is not well known. The use of antiparkinsonian drugs is not recommended because they may exacerbate the symptoms.

TD should be distinguished of withdrawal-emergent syndrome. This syndrome consists in dyskinesias appeared in schizophrenic patients within 1 month of the sudden cessation of antipsychotic therapy. The characteristic movement is choreiform and usually resolves spontaneously within weeks or few months. One useful approach to minimize the clinical manifestations is the reintroduction of the antipsychotic drug and then to reduce the dose slowly up to definitive withdrawal.

Tardive Dystonia

This motor side effect consists in a focal dystonia. It is usually related to a short course of antipsychotic treatment and often involves the cranial or cervical muscles, being the retrocollis relatively frequent.

As TD, tardive dystonia may persist after the withdrawal of the causal neuroleptic. The therapy of tardive dystonia includes the use of depletors of catecholamines (like reserpine and tetrabenazine), anticholinergics and botulinum toxin.

Other Tardive Syndromes

The tardive tic syndrome is a rare complication that may include motor and vocal tics.

The tardive akathisia syndrome is clinically similar to neuroleptic induced akathisia. It shares with TD the existence of previous long term antipsychotic therapy, the initial and transient worsening when the causal drug is withdrawn, and the improvement with the use of dopamine depletors.

Finally, the perioral tremor or "rabbit syndrome" is a rare tardive syndrome which is handled like TD.

Haematological Adverse Effect

Mild leukocytosis, leukopenia, and peripheral eosinophilia have been reported during treatment with clozapine and low potency phenothiazines, like thioridazine and chlorpromazine. These haematological disorders occur in less than 1 of 10.000 treated patients, habitually within the first 2 months of therapy and they are not clearly related to development of agranulocytosis [24, 33, 48].

Clozapine has been associated with agranulocytosis and bone marrow suppression in approximately 1% of treated patients. This complication occurs usually during the first 3 months of therapy and it is not dependent on the used dose. The onset of the disorder may be sudden and it is obligatory to perform blood counts weekly during the first 6 months of therapy and biweekly thereafter. Agranulocytosis may be reversible when clozapine is withdrawn and it responds to granulocyte-colony-stimulating factor.

Isolated cases of agranulocytosis have been reported during olanzapine or risperidone treatment. It has been suggested the existence of genetic determinants for the development of agranulocytosis. This is one of the determinant mechanisms suggested in a case report of a 19 old year woman who suffered 4 consecutive episodes of neutropenia and agranulocytosis during monotherapy with clozapine, perphenazine, olanzapine and risperidone, respectively.

Endocrine Adverse Effects

The weight gain is a frequent side effect of most antipsychotics. It seems more intense with clozapine and olanzapine and less intense with quetiapine, risperidone, haloperidol, and ziprasidone.

Hyperlipidemia and hyperglycemia, the last as a risk factor for developing type 2 diabetes mellitus, have been related to atypical antipsychotics. The reported relative risk of metabolic disturbances was 4.2 (95% CI 1.5–12.2) for olanzapine and 1.6 (95% CI 0.70-3.8) for risperidone, both compared with typical drugs. Other authors reported an odds ratio of 1.36 (95% CI 1.20-1.53), 1.34, 95% (CI 1.16-1.55), 1.2, and 1.0 for olanzapine, clozapine, quetiapine and risperidone, respectively, versus typical neuroleptics. Globally, the risk of glucose and lipid metabolism disorders seems to be greatest with clozapine and olanzapine, lowest with aripiprazole, risperidone, ziprasidone, haloperidol and other high-potency typical drugs, and intermediate with quetiapine and chlorpromazine and thioridazine [35-40].

The elevation of prolactine level has been related to some atypical and most typical antipsychotics. It has been reported in the 89% of patients treated with risperidone and 24% of patients treated with olanzapine, while it has not been related to clozapine therapy. The supposed mechanism is the blockade of dopamine D2 receptors in the lactotropic cells in anterior hypophysis. Clinically, the elevation of prolactine is related to decrease of libido, menstrual disturbances, galactorrhea, impotence and oligospermia. The same authors reported that side effects due to hyperprolactinemia were present in the 44% and 3% of patients treated with risperidone and olanzapine, respectively. Other authors determined the prolactine levels in patients treated with risperidone, olanzapine, and clozapine. The basal (not related to previous drug administration) levels were increased only in the risperidone group. When levels were determined at 6 hours after the administration of the neuroleptic all the antipsychotics raised the prolactine level transiently, although the increase with olanzapine dose did not reach statistical significance versus baseline. Then, it is probable that risperidone and typical antipsychotics increase persistently both basal and post administration prolactine level and other atypical neuroleptics increase the level of prolactine transiently, related to previous dose of drug .

Dermatological and Ocular Adverse Effects

Chlorpromazine has been related to skin reactions in 5% of patients. The reported disorders are urticaria, dermatitis, photosensitivity, and epithelial keratopathy. Patients may have increased blue greyed pigmentation in sun exposed areas. This phenomenon is related to the accumulation of melanine and it may also appear in cornea and lens. The reaction may be present with other phenothiazines because to cross-sensitivity.

Thioridazine has been related to pigmentary retinopathy, especially when high doses are used. Dermatological and ocular side effects are very uncommon with atypical antipsychotics.

Gastrointestinal and Urinary Adverse Effects

The development of mild jaundice during the first 4 week of treatment with chlorpromazine has been reported in the 0.5% of patients. The supposed mechanism is hypersensitivity, since the disorder is related to peripheral eosinophilia and eosinophilic infiltration of the liver.

The peripheral blockade of cholinergic muscarinic receptors causes reduction in saliva production, reduction of gastric secretions and motility. This may result in a increased predisposition to constipation and urinary retention.

The slowing of gastrointestinal motility may be especially intense when clozapine is used. Isolated cases of severe paralytic ileus have been reported.

Research Lines

The research is guided to developing effective antipsychotic drugs with minimum or absent extrapyramidal effects and lower risk of haematological side effects [1, 49, 53].

Currently, several approaches are investigated. Some of these approaches are summarized attending to the supposed mechanism of action of the drug.

The modulation of NMDA receptor neurotransmission enhancing the NMDA receptor function by acting on the glycine modulatory site is one of the studied approaches to improving cognitive function and reducing negative symptoms. It has been reported that high-dose glycine, D-serine, or the partial agonista D-cycloserine improve negative symptoms, cognitive dysfunction, and depression of schizophrenic patients, but an antipsychotic drug may be used to treat effectively positive psychotic symptoms [50, 51].

The blockade of 5-HT2A receptors is related to the decrease of dopamine in the mesolimbic pathway. This mechanism may reduce the necessity of intense dopamine D2 blockade. Then, serotonin 5-HT2A antagonists were explored as a selective target for developing antipsychotic drugs. The highly selective 5-HT2A receptor antagonist M100907 was discontinued after several studies showing an efficacy similar to placebo or inferior to haloperidol. The phase 2 study of eplivanserin (SR46349B) also showed antipsychotic efficacy intermediate between haloperidol and placebo [53].

The role of these agents in the clinical management of psychosis is unclear, since they are less effective than haloperidol and present important side effectse,. Then, mixed dopamine D2 and 5-HT2A serotonin receptors antagonists, like asenapine, clothiapine, iloperidone, or terguride are under development [52].

Dopamine D4 receptor antagonist antagonists have not shown effectiveness in the treatment of psychosis. Two drugs, L-745,870 and sonepiprazole, were compared with placebo and active comparator (olanzapine), respectively, showing a worsening of patients treated with the drug under research [54].

The mechanism of action of partial D2 dopamine agonists like roxindole or bipefrenox is similar to aripiprazole, modulating the receptor without the development of hypersensitivity and the associated late effects.

The development of mixed D2 dopamine antagonists and muscarinic modulation and D3 dopamine receptor antagonists are other approaches currently under research.

Other therapeutic options are under research. For examples, antagonists of neurokinin 3 NK3 receptors (modest efficacy, probably between haloperidol and placebo), antagonists of neurotensin NTS1 (the study performed with SR48692 showed that this drugs was ineffective), antagonists of cannabinoid CB1 receptors (the trial with rimonabant showed its ineffectiveness), agonists of alpha 7 nicotinic receptors (3–2, 4 dimethoxy benylidene), AMPA potentiators, serotonin 5-HT2A inverse agonist, and other [1, 49, 53].

References

[1] Baldessarini RJ, Tarazi F. Pharmacotherapy of psychosis and mania. In, Goodman and Gilman's. *The pharmacological basis of therapeutics* (Brunton LL, Lazo JS, Parker, KL, eds.). McGraw-Hill, New York, 2006, pp. 461-500.

[2] Florez J. Fármacos antipsicóticos neurolépticos. In, *Farmacología humana* (Flórez J, Armijo JA, Mediavilla A, eds.). Masson, Barcelona, 2004, pp. 563-577.

[3] Mental and behavioural disorders. Schizophrenia, schizotypal and delusional disorders (World Health Organization – ICD versión 2007). Available at: http://www.who.int/classifications/apps/icd/icd10online/ accessed 26 March 2007).

[4] Lee PE, Gill SS, Freedman M, et al. Atypical antipsychotic drugs in the treatment of behavioural and psychological symptoms of dementia: systematic review. *BMJ* 2004;329: 75-79.

[5] Selemon LD. Regionally diverse cortical pathology in schizophrenia: clues to the etiology of the disease. *Schizophrenia Bulletin* 2001; 27: 349-377.

[6] Corcoran C, Walker E, Huot R, et al. The stress cascade and schizophrenia: etiology and onset. *Schizophrenia Bulletin*, 2003; 29: 671-692.

[7] Catafau AM, Dogan AS. PET and SPECT of cerebral neurotransmission. *Rev. Esp. Med. Nuclear* 2003; 22: 109-121.

[8] Geyer MA, McIlwain KL, Paylor R. Mouse genetic models for prepulse inhibition: an early review. *Molecular Psychiatry* 2002; 7: 1039–1053.

[9] Geyer MA, Krebs-Thomson K, Braff DL. Pharmacological studies of prepulse inhibition models of sensorimotor gating deficits in schizophrenia: a decade in review. *Psychopharmacology* (Berl). 2001; 156:117-54.

[10] Bohus B, de Wied D.The vasopressin deficient Brattleboro rats: a natural knockout model used in the search for CNS effects of vasopressin. *Prog. Brain Res.* 1998;119:555-73.

[11] Lammertsma AA. Radioligand studies: imaging and quantitative analysis. *Eur. Neuropsychopharmacol.* 2002; 12:513-6.

[12] Wadenberg ML, Soliman A, VanderSpek S. Dopamine D2 receptor occupancy is a common mechanism underlying animal models of antipsychotics and their clinical effects. *Neuropsychopharmacology* 2001; 25: 655- 641.

[13] Bymaster FP, Calligaro DO, Falcone JF, et al. Radioreceptor binding profile of the atypical antipsychotic olanzapine. *Neuropsychopharmacology*. 1996 Feb;14:87-96.

[14] Schotte A, Janssen PF, Gommeren W, et al. Risperidone compared with new and reference antipsychotic drugs: in vitro and in vivo receptor binding. *Psychopharmacology* (Berl). 1996 Mar;124: 57-73.

[15] Lawler CP, Prioleau C, Lewis MM, et al. Interactions of the novel antipsychotic aripiprazole (OPC-14597) with dopamine and serotonin receptor subtypes. *Neuropsychopharmacology*. 1999 Jun; 20: 612-27.

[16] Arnt J, Skarsfeldt T. Do novel antipsychotics have similar pharmacological characteristics? A review of the evidence. *Neuropsychopharmacology* 1998; 18: 63-101.

[17] Farde L., Nordström A.-L., Wiesel F.A., et al. Positron emission tomographic analysis of central D_ and D_ dopamine receptor occupancy in patients treated with classical neuroleptics and clozapine. *Arch. Gen. Psychiat.* 1992; 49: 538–544.

[18] Ossowska K. Neuronal basis of neuroleptic-induced extrapyramidal side effects. *Pol. J. Pharmacol.*, 2002, 54, 299–312.

[19] Peralta V, Cuesta MJ. The nosology of psychotic disorders: a comparison among competing classification systems. *Schizophrenia Bulletin*, 29(3):413- 425,2003.

[20] Roesch-Ely A, Van Einsielder R, Kathöfer S, et al. Myocarditis With Quetiapine. *Am. J. Psychiatry* 2002; 159: 1607-1608.
[21] Riley DE, Lang AE. Movement disorders. Drug-induced movement disorders. In, *Neurology in clinical practice* (Bradley WG, Daroff RB, Fenichel GM, Marsden CD, eds.). Butterworth-Heinemann, Boston, 2000, pp. 1921-1924.
[22] Alderman J. Coadministration of sertraline with cisapride or pimozide: an open-label, nonrandomized examination of pharmacokinetics and corrected QT intervals in healthy adult volunteers. *Clin. Ther.* 2005; 27:1050-63.
[23] Daniel DG. Tolerability of ziprasidone: an expanding perspective. *J. Clin. Psychiatry* 2003; 64 (suppl 19): 40-49.
[24] Olesen OV, Linnet K. Identification of the human cytochrome P450 isoforms mediating *in vitro N*-dealkylation of perphenazine. *British Journal of Clinical Pharmacology* 2000; 50: 563–571.
[25] Casey DE. Side effects profiles of new antipsychotic agents. *J. Clin. Psychiatry* 1996; 57 (suppl 11): 40-45.
[26] Hasan S, Buckley P. Novel Antipsychotics and the Neuroleptic Malignant Syndrome: A Review and Critique. *Am. J. Psychiatry* 1998; 155:1113–1116.
[27] Chandran GJ, Mikler JR, Keegan DL. Neuroleptic malignant syndrome: case report and discussion. *CMAJ* 2003; 169: 439-442.
[28] Adnet P, Lestavel P, Krivosic-Horber R. Neuroleptic malignant syndrome. *Br. J. Anaesth* 2000; 85: 129-135.
[29] Caroff SN. The neuroleptic malignant syndrome. *J. Clin. Psychiatry* 1980; 41: 79-83.
[30] Henderson VW, Wooten GF. Neuroleptic malignant syndrome: pathogenetic role for dopamine receptor blockade? *Neurology* 1981; 31: 132-137.
[31] Pelonero AL, Levenson JL, Pandurangi AK. Neuroleptic malignant syndrome: a review. *Psychiatr. Serv.* 1998; 49: 1163-1172.
[32] Hasan S, Buckley P. Novel antipsychotics and the neuroleptic malignant syndrome: a review and critique. *Am. J. Psychiatry* 1998; 155:1113–1116.
[33] Hong X, Wang X. Agranulocytosis and neutropenia with typical and atypical neuroleptics. *Am. J. Psychiatry* 2001; 158: 1736-1737.
[34] Merrill DB, Ahmari SE, Bradford JM, et al. Myocarditis during clozapine treatment. *Am. J. Psychiatry* 2006; 163: 204-208.
[35] Gardner DM, Baldessarini RJ, Waraich P. Modern antipsychotic drugs: a critical overview. *CMAJ* 2005;172:1703-1711.
[36] Koro CE, Fedder DO, L'Italien GJ, et al. Assessment of independent effect of olanzapine and risperidone on risk of diabetes among patients with schizophrenia: population based nested casecontrol study. *BMJ* 2002;325:243-7.
[37] Lambert BL, Chou CH, Chang KY, et al. Antipsychotic exposure and type 2 diabetes among patients with schizophrenia: a matched case-control study of California Medicaid claims. *Pharmacoepidemiol Drug Saf* 2005; 14: 417-425.
[38] Cohen D. Atypical antipsychotics and new onset diabetes mellitus. An overview of the literature. *Pharmacopsychiatry* 2004; 37: 1-11.
[39] Turrone P, Kapur S, Seeman MV, et al. Elevation of prolactin levels by atypical antipsychotics. *Am. J. Psychiatry* 2002; 159:133–135.

[40] Melkersson K. Differences in prolactin elevation and related symptoms of atypical antipsychotics in schizophrenic patients. *J. Clin. Psychiatry* 2005; 66: 761-7.

[41] FDA issues public health advisory for antipsychotic drugs used for treatment of behavioral disorders in elderly patients [FDA Talk Paper]. Rockville (MD): US Food and Drug Administration; 2005. Available: www.fda.gov/ bbs/topics/ ANSWERS/2005/ANS01350.html (accessed 2007 May 1).

[42] Gill SS, Rochon PA, Herrmann N, et al. Atypical antipsychotic drugs and risk of ischaemic stroke: population based retrospective cohort study. BMJ 2005;330;445-450.

[43] Herrmann N, Mamdani M, Lanctôt KL. Atypical antipsychotics and risk of cerebrovascular accidents. *Am. J. Psychiatry* 2004; 161:1113–1115.

[44] Layton D, Harris S, Wilton LV, et al. Comparison of incidence rates of cerebrovascular accidents and transient ischaemic attacks in observational cohort studies of patients prescribed risperidone, quetiapine or olanzapine in general practice in England including patients with dementia. *J. Psychopharmacol.* 2005; 19:473-482.

[45] Herrmann N, Lanctot KL. Do atypical antipsychotics cause stroke? *CNS Drugs*. 2005;19:91-103.

[46] Lenzer J. FDA warns about using antipsychotic drugs for dementia. *BMJ* 2005;330:922.

[47] Schneeweiss S, Setoguchi S, Brookhart A, et al. Risk of death associated with the use of conventional versus atypical antipsychotic drugs among elderly patients. *CMAJ* 2007; 176: 627-632.

[48] Alvir JM, Lieberman JA, Safferman AZ, et al. Clozapine-induced agranulocytosis. Incidence and risk factors in the United States. *N. Engl. J. Med.* 1993; 329: 162-167.

[49] Marek G, Merchant K. Developing therapeutics for schizophrenia and other psychotic disorders. *NeuroRx* 2005; 2: 579-589.

[50] Coyle JT, Tsai G. The NMDA receptor glycine modulatory site: a therapeutic target for improving cognition and reducing negative symptoms, *Psychopharmacology* 2004; 174: 32–38.

[51] Coyle JT, Tsai G, Goff DC. Ionotropic glutamate receptors as therapeutic targets in schizophrenia. *Curr. Drug Target CNS Neurol. Disord.* 2002;1: 183–189.

[52] Marder SR. Limitations of dopamine-D2 antagonists and the search for novel antipsychotic strategies. *Neuropsychopharmacology* 1999; 21 [Suppl 6]:S117.

[53] Meltzer HY, Arvanitis L, Bauer D, et al. Meta-Trial Study Group. Placebo-controlled evaluation of four novel compounds for the treatment of schizophrenia and schizoaffective disorders. *Am. J. Psychiatry* 2004; 161: 975–984.

[54] Kramer MS, Last B, Getson A, Reines SA; D4 Dopamine Antagonist Group. The effects of a selective D4 dopamine receptor antagonist (L-745,870) in acutely psychotic inpatients with schizophrenia. *Arch. Gen. Psychiatry* 1997; 54:567–572.

In: Drug Toxicity: New Research
Editor: Cam E. Vellotis, pp.53-72

ISBN 978-1-60456-320-7

Chapter 3

A Critical Approach to an Allergic Paradox: Allergic and Allergic-Like Reactions to Glucocorticoids. Delayed Hypersensitivity Mechanisms

M. T. Ventura**, G. F. Calogiuri, R. Buquicchio, R. A. Tummolo and M. Digregorio

Department of Internal Medicine, Immunology and Infectious Diseases (MIDIM),
University of Bari Medical School, Policlinico, Bari, Italy
4th Division Pneumologic Hospital A,
Galateo - San Cesario di Lecce (Lecce, Italy)

Abstract

In the last decade, topical corticosteroids have received increasing attention for their sensitizing potential to generate allergic contact dermatitis. Most dermatologists agree that this sensitization is still under-recognized because the anti-inflammatory and immunosuppressive properties of topical glucocorticosteroids make it difficult to suspect the disease and, above all, to perform a correct diagnostic patch test. In fact, the best vehicle, concentration and reading time have not yet been identified. So, despite the growing number of dermatological studies published, the gold standard approach to the management of glucocorticosteroid allergic contact dermatitis has not yet been identified.

In our review, we try to provide a comprehensive overview of the clinical and practical aspects of corticosteroids-induced delayed hypersensitivity and its consequences on anti-inflammatory therapeutic choices.

* Correspondence to: M.T. Ventura, M.D., Department of Internal Medicine, Immunology and Infectious Diseases, University of Bari, Policlinico, Piazza G. Cesare n° 11, 70124 Bari (Italy). E-mail: mt.ventura@allergy.uniba.it

Introduction

In 1952, Glucocorticosteroids (GCs) were introduced in clinical practice as topical formulations (creams, ointments, lotions). Nowadays, they are widely used in the therapy of allergic and autoimmune dermatological diseases for their anti-inflammatory, immunosuppressive and antiproliferative properties.

Although the rationale of employment of topical GCs was that of reducing their systemic absorption and severe side effects, their use could favour some cutaneous alterations ranging from steroidal acne, atrophy, the appearance of telangiectasis and hypertrichosis, to the appearance of the so-called "steroidal skin" characterized by thinning and cutaneous atrophy, and of telangiectasis and purpura.

The first cases of allergic contact dermatitis to Hydrocortisone (HC) were described in literature in 1959 [1]; nevertheless, the possibility that topical GCs could cause allergic contact dermatitis (ACD) seems a remote and exceptional eventuality, in view of the greater risk of the allergic sensitisation to the preservatives (paraben, lanolin, ethylenediamine, etc...) contained in the topical HC preparations.

In 1960 Church reported that contact sensitisation to HC acetate was caused by a precursor contaminating some compounds for topical use. This precursor (HC $_{21}$-diol-acetate) represented the true sensitising agent, being responsible for a more intense patch test positivity in comparison with HC [2].

Pharmaceutical chemical research has changed the basic formula of HC (Figure 1) by introducing halogenations of the carbonic rings and the esterification of ring D in position C_{17} and/or C_{21}. These changes cause an increased immunosuppressive and anti-inflammatory activity by enhancing the lipophilicity and favouring a good penetration of the topical steroid into the cutaneous hydrolipidic mantle [3].

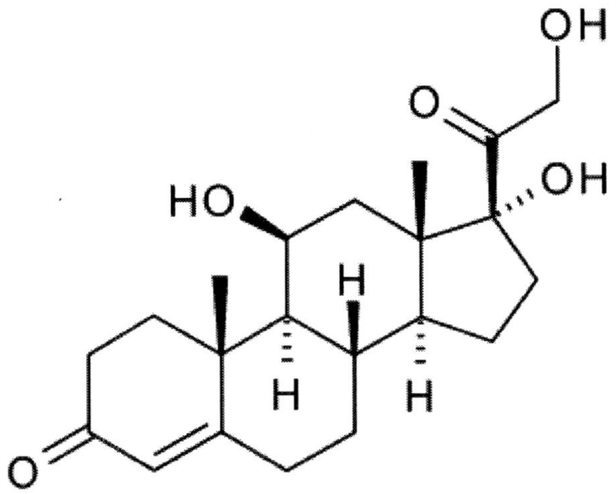

Figure 1. Molecular structure of cortisol.

Nevertheless, it appears evident to dermatologists that HC represents a potential hapten [4] and that allergic sensitisation to this or derived molecules, rather than being a remote and paradoxical eventuality, is in fact an underhand clinical entity, underestimated and difficult to diagnose [5]due to the anti-inflammatory activities of topical GCs [6].

Therefore, with the new topical GC preparations [7], the frequency and incidence of ACD to GCs appears to have increased.

Clinical Aspects of Allergic Contact Dermatitis to Topical GCs

GCs for local use are not responsible for eczematous dermatitis, but rather for sub-acute or chronic eczema, which is aggravated by the application of topical steroids [8].

The site of application of topical GCs can also influence the clinical picture of the ACD. In fact, after the local application of prednicarbate [9], intense genital edema has been described, with erythema and vesicles located on the penis and on the scrotum, while the classic erythematous-eczematous reactions accompanied by mucositis have been reported [10], with itching and vesicles located on the face and the wings of the nose, after the use of budesonide by the inhalation route [11].

Exceptionally, a case of sensitisation far from the site of application was described [12], while only one report of photodermatitis to HC [13] has yet been reported.

It has been demonstrated that mononuclear cells withdrawn from patients with ACD in response to HC can proliferate in culture in the presence of HC (after the removal of the inhibitory activity of the free cortisol [14], as in presence of an immunological stimulus. This condition has alerted dermatologists to the possibility that the administration of systemic GCs might be able to induce allergic generalized dermatitis in these patients.

In the literature, many allergic cutaneous reactions to GCs have been reported after administration by oral, intramuscular, intravenous or inhalator route.

Intra-articular administration has provoked local and/or systemic border-line dermatitis involving the skin at the level of the treated joint, with activation and migration of lymphocytes in the synovial fluid [15]. In the case of retro-bulbar injection of methylprednisolone acetate [16, 17] eczematous dermatitis has been described, with edema and inflammation of the surrounding soft tissue.

The cutaneous adverse reactions correlated to the administration of systemic GCs induce more complex and variegated clinical-morphological syndromes in comparison to the local preparations. Many authors have described eczematous generalized dermatitis, maculo-papular exanthemas [20, 21], sometimes with exfoliative aspects [22] and diffuse erythematous eruptions [23, 24], after the inhalation of high dosages of budesonide [18, 19].

Some cases of dermatitis with erythrodermal [25, 26], erythema multiforme-like [27, 28], urticarioid [29, 30] and eczematous-urticarioid [31] aspects have been reported in the literature after the administration of triamcinolone acetonide, that induced fixed drug erythema in one case [32].

In two reports [33, 34] an acute generalized exanthematous pustolosis has been described, provoked by dexamethasone and methylprednisolone. In a patient in daily therapy with 90 mgs of deflazacort [35], after 3 weeks polymorphous erythema [36, 37], Stevens-Johnson syndrome [38] and toxic epidermal necrolysis (TEN) occurred.

All these reactions share a common immediate [33] or delayed [22, 29] onset of the manifestations.

Some professional categories such as doctors, chemists and nurses can develop sensitisation after manipulating corticosteroid preparations [39], including pills [36].

In patients with immediate allergic reactions such as bronchospasm, urticaria, angioedema or anaphylaxis induced by systemic GCs, an ACD to topical GCs [8, 40] has been hypothesized. However, patch tests to confirm the diagnosis have rarely been performed [30, 41].

Recently, specific Ig-E for HC and methylprednisolone have been isolated from the serum of patients with a clinical history of type I allergic reactions to systemic GCs [42, 43, 44], showing that adverse reactions to GCs are common in clinical practice.

In a group of 7 patients with ACD to HC [45], the presence in the same patient of humoral and cells-mediated sensitisation suggests that type I and type IV response mechanisms may be simultaneously present.

The trans-cutaneous absorption of topical compounds [46, 47] can also be responsible for anaphylactic reactions if GCs are applied on a large skin area [48].

Pathogenetic Mechanisms and Risk Factors in Contact Sensitisations to Topical GCs

Cortisol is a hapten of around 400 Daltons molecular weight, whose structure consists of a steroid ring, formed by the condensation of three rings of hexane (conventionally denominated A, B and C), with a ring of pentane called D (figure 1) which, for its dimensions and liposolubility, may penetrate into the cutaneous layer, thus representing a perfect contact allergen [49].

In subjects sensitised to topical HC, after making a punch-biopsy of skin submitted to patch tests to HC, Lauerma found that the perivascular inflammatory infiltrate consisted of lymphomonocytes and the derma presented exocytosis and spongiosis, occurs in subjects with ACD to nickel [50].

Subsequently, Wilkinson performed immunohistochemical examinations on samples of derma withdrawn with the same method in subjects with positive epicutaneous tests to Thixocortol Pivalate (TP) and to nickel sulphate. The presence of interleukin-1 (IL-1) and tumour necrosis factor-alpha (TNF-α) receptors was revealed, and an increased expression of ICAM-1 and ELAM-1 on keratinocytes and on endothelial cells, with immunological activation and migration of lymphocytes in the dermis.

The examination confirmed that there were no qualitative differences between ACD induced by GCs and by nickel [51].

According to Church [2], contact allergy to HC could be provoked by a precursor or a degradation product of cortisol. This suggestion was supported by Bungaard [52]. He studied, in aqueous solution, C_{21} degradation of the HC molecule in a glioxal steroid-, so allowing a covalent bond to develop with the guanidyl groups of arginine and the lateral chains on C_{17}. The transformation of a steroidal hapten into a complete antigen permits the presentation of the steroidal molecule carbonic rings to immunocompetent cells (figure 2); the immunogenicity is correlated to the bond stability of the steroidal hapten with the cutaneous proteins [52]. The affinity of HC and topical preparations to arginine is a key factor in the development of an allergic delayed sensitisation to topical GCs [53]. The alkaline pH seems to favour the oxidation and degradation of cortisol [53] determining a great accumulation of glioxal steroid, that binds to the arginine. The cutaneous pH is usually equal to 5.5, but in the underarm and perineal sites, these values are equal to 7.2-8 due to the greater perspiration [53].

Other conditions that favour a rise in the cutaneous pH are bacterial infections, occlusions, eczematous lesions, allergic and irritant contact dermatitis [53]. This could explain the association between ACD to topical GCs and stasis dermatitis, varicose ulcers of the legs and perineal dermatitis [54,55]. By contrast, all chronic dermatosis forms like dyshydrosis, genital lichen simplex, seborrhoic dermatitis, atopic and contact eczemas, represent risk factors for an allergic contact sensitisation to GCs [56].

Reitamo and coll. [57] have identified as risk factors the presence of 2 or more positive patch tests to other topical drugs like neomycin, anesthetics or topical disinfectants. Other researchers have confirmed that patients with clinical delayed hypersensitivity to drugs have a greater probability of developing allergic reactions to topical GCs [5].

Glioxal steroid is a degradation product of cortisol which contains an alpha-ketoaldehyde on C_{21}. The aldehydes are extremely toxic and unstable metabolites.

In the case of drug allergy reactions, Knowles and Uetrecht have proposed the "Hapten Theory" and the "Danger" of Matzinger's theory [58]. According to this theory, to activate the immune system a drug or its metabolite must be able to bind with a high affinity to the proteins of the organism, and must possess a certain toxicity [58]. In particular, the cellular stress produced during necrosis, and the release of proteins or chemokines, has been shown to be able to activate the immune system [58].

Aldehydes and GCs are degraded by an aldolase (aldehyde-dehydrogenases), which metabolises the alcohol and the derived aldehydes [59], for this reason the frequency of positive patch tests to ethanol is high in patients with contact allergy to GCs [60,61].

A deficit of the aldolase activity, due to impaired liver function or chronic hepatic disease, but also to genetic diseases, could be responsible for an accumulation of the aldehydes or the glioxal steroid-, increasing the risk of allergic sensitisation to systemic GCs. In addition, since the skin metabolic activity includes a variety of enzymes like cytochrome P450, N-acetyl-transferase, glutathione-S-transferase and also aldolase [62], a genetic deficiency of this enzymatic activity could be responsible for the accumulation of toxic metabolites of topical drugs, leading to the activation and recruitment of the immunocompetent cells.

Children with atopic eczema could therefore be another group at risk for delayed type sensitisation to topical GCs, due both to chronic dermatological diseases and to the immaturity of enzymatic pathway [63]; in addition due to their smaller skin surface, they have a greater percutaneous absorption of topical GCS than adults [46].

According to Lauerma, in vitro sensitisation to topical GCs occurs through HLA-associated *cognate interaction,* since the presence of Langerhans cells such as Antigen Presenting Cell (APC) is required to introduce the steroidal hapten to the T effector lymphocytes [64]. Some researchers have investigated the association between contact sensitisation to HC and a particular Major Histocompatibility Complex (MHC) haplotype. The Authors postulated that HLA B8 (MHC-I) and DR3 (MHC-II) haplotypes, associated to the development of many autoimmune diseases (SLE, celiac disease, Sjogren syndrome, etc…), represents a protective factor for contact dermatitis to HC, but the results obtained did not confirm this hypothesis. A multicentric study carried out in 10 European countries by the EECDRG (European Environmental Contact Dermatitis Research Group) [66] highlighted that the incidence of ACD to topical GCs is almost double in the female sex. In fact, among 189 patients with ACD to topical GCs, 67 were men and 122 were women [66]. Likely this difference is due to cyclical progesterone fluctuations, that seem to make the female sex more susceptible to contact sensitisation to topical GCs [67]. In patients with ACD to HC and to other topical GCs, the lack of correlation reported between ACD and autoimmune dermatitis to progesterone, demonstrated with patch tests performed with progesterone and its precursors, is probably due to the limited number of patients enrolled (19 subjects).

Nevertheless, the formation of a glioxal is not the only way for a steroidal molecule to bind firmly to cutaneous proteins and become a complete antigen. Thixocortol pivalate (TP) is a GC for topical and inhalator use with a thioester on C_{21} (figure 3), that is able to establish sufficiently stable disulphuric bridges (-S-S-) with cutaneous amino acids such as methionine. TP resulted a powerful sensitising hapten for guinea-pigs, and an intradermal injection of 4-5 mgs of TP on Freund adjuvant sensitised all animals by day 23 [68]. For this reason many Authors consider TP to be a sensitive and specific marker for ACD to HC, employed at the concentration of 1% in vaseline [69, 70].

Non fluorinated GCs, in more recent formulations [7], can bind to arginine, measured as an equal or greater absorption, as compared to HC (table 1); for this reason non fluorinated GCs have a higher sensitising activity than halogenated GCs.

Table 1. Degree of binding capability of some GCs to arginine (measured as absorption)

Budesonide	7.65
Hydrocortisone and Thixocortol pivalate	6.95
Hydrocortisone-17-butyrate	6.13
Betamethasone valerate	1.03
Clobetasol propionate	0

The halogenations on C_9 confer to halogenated GCs a great affinity for the specific target cells receptor [71] and prevent binding to arginine and the consequent haptenation process, making these halogenated GCs less allergenic.

The Problem of Allergic Cross-Reactivity in Topical GCs

Although in the early '70s Alani and Alani [72] hypothesized a possible allergic cross-reactivity (CRA) among topical GCs, from a clinical point of view it was difficult to distinguish a concomitant sensitisation from cross-reactivity. At the same time, the previous use of different topical GCs, and the development of chronic dermatitis led to the prescription of more powerful topical GCs.

Nevertheless, the possibility of an allergic cross-reactivity was confirmed by some epidemiological studies of the incidence of ACD to GCs in patients with positive patch tests to never commercialised GCs [73], which had therefore never had the opportunity to induce sensitisation.

In 1989 Coopman and Dooms-Goossens, after having analysed literature data and submitted a group of 19 patients to patch tests with various topical GCs, identified 4 classes of CRA, denominated classes A, B, C and D. The Authors demonstrated that within every class, positive results of patch tests are 6-7 times more frequent than to GCs of different classes [74]. The 4 classes of topical GCs are shown in table 2.

The researchers identified the D ring as the key that permits discrimination among the different GCs. Subsequently, the authors confirmed the validity of their classification, showing the existence, through computerized conformational analysis of topical GC molecules, of a precise spatial steroidal structure, that is representative in the form, volume and distribution of the charges for groups A, B and D (Figure 2), but not C.

Moreover, these studies underlined that budesonide has two isomeric conformations: D-budesonide, that resembles GCs of the B group and L-budesonide, that mimics the ester class that seems to belong to group D [75].

This structural anomaly had already been described by a Japanese group [76]. These authors hypothesized that, in view of the propyl substitute's ability to freely rotate at the c-terminal of 16α, 17α –butyldene dioxy portion, budesonide could exhibit conformational variants, besides D and L-budesonide, as well as the raceme variant, that is extremely unstable. These variants have not yet been correctly characterized, as in the Coopman and Dooms-Goossens classification.

Table 2. Classes of allergenic cross-reactivity among topical corticosteroids (Coopman and Dooms-Goossens, 1989)

Class A	(HC type with no change of ring D or of C_{20}-C_{21} or the presence of esters with a brief chain on C_{20}-C_{21}): HC, Prednisolone and Methylprednisolone and their ester acetates, sodium-phosphates and succinate, Cortisone, Prednisone, Thixocortol pivalate;
Class B	(Triamcinolone acetonide type with C_{16}, C_{17}-cis-ketal or -diol changes): Triamcinolone acetonide, Fluocinolone acetonide, Halcinonide, Dexonide, Fluocinonide, Halcinonide, Budesonide, Amcinonide, Flunisolide, etc
Class C	(Betamethasone type with methylation $-CH_3$ on C_{16}, but without esterifications on C_{17}-C_{21}): Betamethasone, Dexamethasone, Paramethasone, Desoxymethasone, Fluocortolone.
Class D	(Clobetasone type or HC esterification with a long chain at C_{17} and/or C_{21} and with or without a methylic group at C_{16}): Clobetasone-17-butyrate, Clobetasol-17-propionate, HC-17-propionate, HC-17-butyrate, Beclomethasone dipropionate, Betamethasone valerate, Betamethasone dipropionate, Methylprednisolone aceponate, Fluocortolone caproate, Prednicarbate, etc...

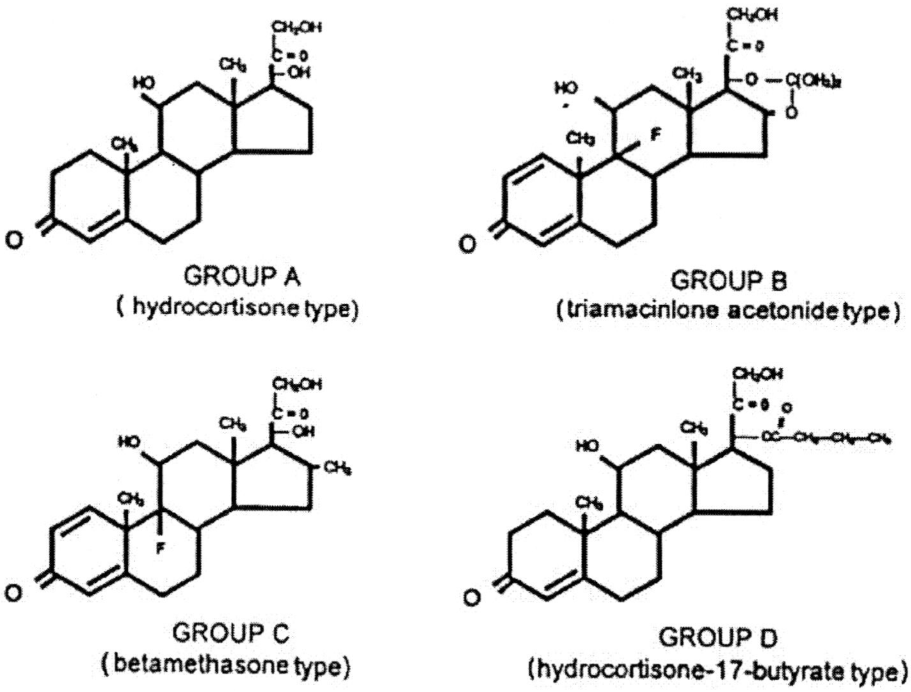

Figure 2. The patterns of corticosteroid cross-reactivity according to Coopman and Doom-Goossens.

Isomeric variations are capable of influencing the immunogenicity of Budesonide and, in addition, for conferring a different affinity for the receptor and a different clinical effectiveness [77]. Although Coopman and Dooms-Goossens' classification in 4 classes of CRA seems very simple and efficacious in its application in comparison to other classifications [78], some objections have been raised by other Authors.

Wilkinson proposed that the immunogenicity of cortisol was attributable to the whole structure of the steroid ring [79]. In a study in 96 patients with ACD to HC, the author found through mathematical analysis that the correlation between the changes operated on the carbonic rings and patch test positivity declined, in order, with the substitutions effected on C_6, on C_9 and on C_6 and C_9. Therefore, the B ring could represent another site of the GC molecule that could affect CRA [80].

It is conceivable that the presence of a halogen atom like chlorine or fluorine on C_9, determining an electron-attractive effect on C_{11} [81], besides causing a refolding of the GC molecule, confers a notable conformational stability. This is indirectly verifiable since a fluorinated GC such as Fluticasone Propionate (FP) introduces only one isomer while budesonide exhibits three variations. In addition, halogenated GCs (C group), do not have a three-dimensional representation [75].

In another study, 46 subjects with positive results to budesonide were submitted to patch tests with 17 different topical GCs. The Author hypothesized that the changes operated on C_{21} favouredbinding with cutaneous proteins, without any immunological influence [82]; in fact, keratinocytes possess an esterase responsible for rapid hydrolysis of the esters present on C_{21} [83]. The enzymatic hydrolysis can thus modify the class of affiliation of a topical GC, above all for group D; Prednicarbate (a GC of group D) is a product of Prednisolone, that has an ethylcarbonate on C_{17} and a propionate group on C_{21}. It is quickly hydrolysed after its cutaneous absorption into prednisolone-17-ethylcarbonate, that again belongs to group D, and subsequently to prednisone (group A). [84].

Therefore it is possible, with GCs of group D, to develop a concomitant sensitisation to GCs of group A (not halogenated) and C (halogenated). For this reason, Dooms-Goossens modified the classification, dividing group D GCs into two subgroups: D1 (with fluorination on C_9, methylation on C_{16} and a lateral esterified chain on C_{17}, that can cross-react with group C GCs or cause co-sensitisation to these latter, as in the case of Clobetasol propionate) and D2 (no halogenations on the carbonic rings, no methylic group on C_{16}, foreign???? on C_{17} as in Methylprednisolone aceponate, the possibility of cross-reactions or co-sensitisations for the GCs of group A) [85].

Frequently, other Authors [86] have reported patch test cross-reactivity between HC (group A) and HC -17-butyrate (group D). However, not all the GCs for topical or systemic use can be classified according to Coopman-Dooms-Goossens; molecules like Deflazacort, FP, Momethasone Furoate (MF), in view of their peculiar formulation (an oxazolinic ring on C_{16}/C_{17} in deflazacort, esterifications with short lateral chains on C_{17}, the presence of a halogen on C_{21} and C_{17} as in FP and MF) are difficult to include in one of the 4 groups of CRA [87].

The particular structure of FP and MF could justify the lower risk of allergic contact sensitisation reported by some authors [87,88]. For this reason these molecules could be a good alternative molecule in patients with contact sensitisation to 2 or more allergenic classes of topical GCs [89].

Recently, Wilkinson also revised the importance of changes on C_6/C_9 in the influence of CRA of topical GCs. In fact, he proposed that the immunodominant sites capable of influencing the immunogenicity of the basic HC molecule and consequently allergic cross-reactions, were positions C_6/C_9 of the B ring and positions C_{16}/C_{17} of the D ring (figure 3) [90], thus finally admitting the importance of the D ring.

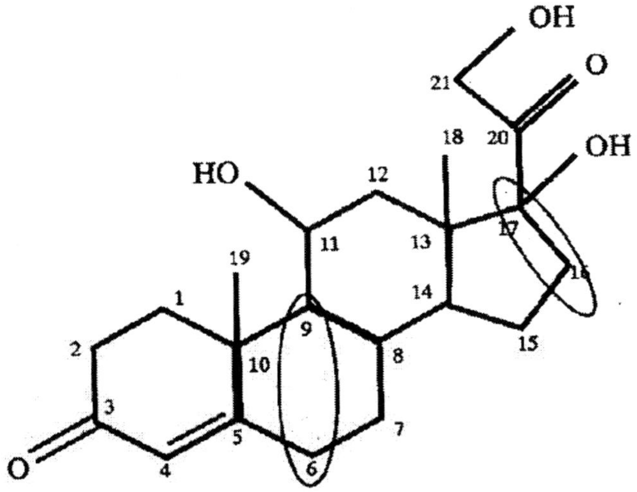

Figure 3. Site modifications influencing corticosteroid cross-reactivity according to Wilkinson.

On the basis of the results of our study of 10 patients, we agree with Wilkinson that it is possible to identify an alternative molecule in the case of immediate adverse reactions to systemic GCs [91].

Diagnostic Allergy Tests in Contact Allergy to GCs: Methods, Validity and Limits

In the case of ACD to topical GCs, it is necessary to confirm the diagnosis with specific allergic tests to identify the GCs responsible, in order to avoid the use of this drug and to find an alternative GC [91].

PTs are the tests of choice in patients with ACD and their use has also been proposed by the European Academy of Allergy and Clinical Immunology (EAACI) [92] and the International Contact Dermatitis Research Group (ICDRG) [93] in the diagnosis of cutaneous adverse reactions to drugs.

The anti-inflammatory and vasoconstrictor effects of GCs may hide an allergic sensitisation after the removal of the patch test, and some authors have advised further readings at 48 and 96 hours, and up to day 7 [94].

Another problem is represented by the bioavailability of GCs: the high concentration of GCs in PT favours a good cutaneous penetration, but on the other hand it inhibits the skin reaction in virtue of its immunosuppressive capacity. Although a low concentration of some commercial GCs can determine the onset of contact allergy on damaged skin, PTs to the same concentration can false negative results when performed on the healthy skin of the back. This phenomenon, known as the "paradox of the parabens" can also occur with GCs [95].

The "edge effect" at the PT reading, usually considered an irritant effect of the same test, should be taken into account when it appears after the removal of epicutaneous tests with topical GCs. Usually, at the first reading, infiltration and erythema are present on the edge of the patch test only, while the site of application of the hapten becomes eczematous later on. The effect has been attributed to the anti-inflammatory property of GCs and disappears with higher concentrations of the GC, causing a suppression of cell-mediated reactions, although these still appear on the edge, where the GC quantity is reduced, and hence also its anti-inflammatory activity [96].

The possibility that PTs with GC could suppress the adjacent skin reactions has been excluded since it was observed that PT with Clobethasol propionate 1% in ethanol, that has a high anti-inflammatory activity, had no influence on skin reactions in a group of patients allergic to Nickel [97].

The identification of an optimal diluent is another problem when performing epicutaneous tests: according to some Authors, at the same concentration (the concentration of 1% seems to be optimal for PTs with GCs) [98], ethanol is a better vehicle than vaseline; in fact, using vaseline, PTs were previously negative [99].

Even so vaseline seems to be a good vehicle for hydrosoluble GCs. By contrast, for lyposoluble GCs ethanol at the dilution of 1% is a better diluent [99, 100].

Nevertheless, ethanol causes other problems, such as irritant dermatitis. This effect is correlated to the presence of degradation products and impurities, identified by chromatography [98].

The evaporation of ethanol provokes PTs deterioration: in fact, Isaksson showed that GCs in ethanol were stable for six months or one year at -18° C, whereas the same preparations in vaseline were stable for at least one year, regardless of the temperature [101].

Since ethanol could also be responsible for ACD when it is utilized as a diluent [60, 61, 103], due to the presence of aldehydes and acetaldehydes [103] it is necessary to carry out control PTs also with the hydroalcohol solution alone.

Boffa et al. showed that PTs with 6 different topical GCs diluted in ethanol or vaseline identified 91.3% of patients with ACD to GCs [104]. Even so, another study outlined that the optimal dilution of budesonide was 0.002% [105].

In addition, although PTs with TP and Budesonide 1% in ethanol seem to confirm the diagnosis in all allergic patients to HC and budesonide, in the case of other GCs, the use of ethanol is not always able to identify false positive and false negative reactions. In particular, PTs with HC-17-butyrate at 1% in ethanol did not confirm the diagnosis in 30% of the examined patients; intradermal delayed tests (reading at 48 hours) had to be carried out with 1 mg of GC diluted 1:1 in physiological solution [106].

Previously, intradermal reactions with HC hemisuccinate 1 mg/ml in physiological solution confirmed the validity of PTs with TP as a reliable diagnostic marker in the case of HC dermatitis, therefore their extensive employment has been suggested in the diagnosis of ACD to GCs [107].

Nevertheless, this method exposes patients to a risk of adverse reactions during its execution [25, 30] and it is practicable only for GCs that have commercially available hydrosoluble formulations: succinate or sodium phosphate salts. On the other hand, for most topical steroid molecules, due to their poor hydrosolubility, the dilutions should be performed with a hydrosoluble solution, but this itself has an irritant effect if injected in the derma.

By contrast, Freeman proposed the diagnosis of GCs-induced ACD using PTs with the same GCs commercial preparation employed by the patient [108], (better in cream than in ointment), rather than utilizing the diluted active principle in 1% ethanol or vaseline. However, using the commercial preparation there is the risk of allergic sensitisation caused by the excipients.

The main preservatives present in the topical GCs preparations responsible for ACD are shown in table 3.

Other preservatives in topical GCs which have never been associated with ACD include : Triethanolamine 5% vas., Isopropyl myristate 5% vas., Disodium edetate 1% acq., Carboxyvinyl-polymer as such.

The risk that patients can develop a "compound allergy" suggests that PT should ne carried out with commercial preparations. A “compound allergy” is a contact allergy that can appear after the use of commercial preparations, but, when epicutaneous tests are performed with the single hapten contained in it (active principle, preservative, etc...), the skin test results negative. Some rare cases of “compound allergy "to topical GCs have been reported in the literature [121]. The possible causes of this phenomenon are shown in table 4.

Table 3. Principal preservatives in GC topical preparations responsible for allergic contact sensitisation, and their commercial patch test concentrations (Firm F.I.R.M.A. – Florence)

Ethyl alcohol (102) 5% aq. and as such	Sorbitan-sequiolate (115) 20% vas.
Benzyl alcohol (109) 5% vas	1,2,6- hexanetriol (116) % vas. *
Isopropyl palmitate (109) 5% vas.	Lanoline (117) 30% vas.
Paraben (110) 3% vas.	Cetostearyl alcohol (117) 30% vas.
Chlorocresol (111) 1% vas.	Ethylenediamine hydrochlorate (118) 1% vas.
Propylene glycol (111) 10% acq.	Propylgallate (119) 0,1% vas.
Sodium bisulphite (112) 5% vas.	Sodium lauryl sulphate 0,1% acq.(120)
Dioctyl sodium sulfosuccinate (113) 1% acq.*	Mystril γ picolinium chlorure (16) 0.1% vas*
Polysorbate 60 (114) 5% vas.	

N.B.: vas.: vaseline - aq.: aqueous - *Concentration used by the author, not included in the F.I.R.M.A. catalogue (F.I.R.M.A. Inc.- Florence – Italy).

Table 4. Possible causes of "compound allergy"[122]

(1) Commercial preparations of GCs permit a greater cutaneous penetration of the hapten than with the patch test;
(2) Injured skin favours penetration more than healthy skin;
(3) The allergen responsible is a degradation product in the commercial preparation, lost when the preparation is decomposed;
(4) The allergen is a tertiary product derived from the combination, or interaction, of 2 substances present in the commercial product;
(5) The allergen derives from oxidation of the product container (for example the Zn^{++} ions or the plastic polymers in the tube where the preparation is manufactured).

For this reason, the use of the ROAT (Repeated Open Application Test) [108] has been advised. This consists in the application of a small quantity of topical GCs twice a day for seven days, as commercial preparations diluted at 1% in ethanol or vaseline, on the forearm surface, with readings up to day 7, and sometimes day 15 [12] in doubtful cases [12,108] with multiple sensitisation to various molecules GCs [123]. This method would be surer, risk-free and deontologically correct in comparison to exposure/challenge tests with oral GCs [124,125] or inhalator tests [126].

Epidemiological Importance of Topical GCs ACD

In the early '70s Alani and Alani submitted 1830 patients to PT with HC 25% in vaseline to investigate the incidence of ACD to topical GCs. They observed these patients for 14 months, identifying 6 patients with unexpected skin positivity, thus yielding an annual incidence equal to 0.3%. An extension of the investigation to all patients examined during the previous 8 years found 17 new suspicious cases of delayed hypersensitivity to GCs.

Conclusions

Although the problem of allergic sensitisation to GCs has not been completely studied, it is important to emphasize the following data:

(1) allergic contact sensitization to GCs must be suspected when in patients with dermatitis or eczema the repeated use of topical GCs does not improve the clinical findings;
(2) dermatological diseases are risk factors for the development of GCs sensitization;
(3) in vivo allergological tests, like patch tests and intradermal reactions, should be carried out and read by specialists, due to their difficulty of interpretation;
(4) it is necessary to effect several readings after removing the patch tests;
(5) it may be useful to perform patch tests for the excipients contained in GC topical preparations, both to identify associated contact sensitization and to exclude any possible responsibility of the preservatives contained;
(6) the Coopman-Dooms-Goossens classification is easy to apply and helps to avoid the administration of other topical or systemic GCs similar to those implicated in the allergic sensitisation.

In conclusion, immunologists, dermatologists and clinical pharmacologists should be informed about the risks of allergic topical sensitisation of GCs. In fact, due to their frequent assumption of topic GCs, atopic subjects can develop allergic dermatitis and other adverse reactions after therapy with, or the manipulation of GCs.

References

[1] Kooji, R., Hypersensitivity to hydrocortisone, *Brit. J. Dermatol.*, 1959,71: 392-4.
[2] Church, R., Sensitivity to hydrocortisone acetate ointment, *Brit. J. Dermatol.*, 1960,72: 341-3.
[3] Shroot, B., Caron, J.C., Ponec, M., Glucocorticoid specific binding: structure-activity relationship, *Brit. J. Dermatol.*, 1982,107: 30-4.

[4] Wilkinson, S.M., Cartwright, P.H., English JSC. Hydrocortisone: an important cutaneous allergen, *Lancet*, 1991,337:761-2.

[5] Dooms-Goossens, A., Degreef, H., Marien, K.J., Coopman, S.A., Contact allergy to corticosteroids: a frequently missed diagnosis?, *J. Am. Acad. Dermatol.*, 1989,21: 538-43.

[6] Crijns, M.B., Nater, J.P., van Oosten, F., van der Walk, P.G., Vasoconstrictor and the anti-inflammatory effects of seven corticosteroids, *Contact Dermatitis*, 1994,11: 108-11.

[7] Degreef, H., Dooms-Goossens, A., The newer corticosteroids: are they effective and safe?, *Dermatol. Clin.*, 1993,11: 155-60.

[8] Dooms-Goossens, A., Degreef, H., Clinical aspects of contact allergy to corticosteroids, *Dermatology*, 1994,189: 54-5.

[9] Miranda-Romero, A., Sanchez-Sambucety, P., Bajo, C., Martinez, M., Garcia-Munoz, M. Genital oedema from contact allergy to prednicarbate, *Contact Dermatitis*, 1998,38 : 228-9.

[10] Iglesias-Cadarso, A., Diaz, C., Laguna, J.J., Hernandez-Weigand, P., Allergic contact dermatomucositis to budesonide, *J. Allergy Clin. Immunol.*, 1994,94: 559-60.

[11] Sastre, J., Ibanez, M.D., Contact allergy to budesonide contained in a nasal spray, *Allergy*, 1992,47: 661-2.

[12] Weber, F., Barbaud, A., Reichert-Penetrat, S., Danchin, A., Shmutz, JL., Unusual clinical presentation in a case of contact dermatitis due to corticosteroids diagnosed by ROAT. *Contact Dermatitis*, 2001,44: 105-6.

[13] Rietschel, RL., Photocontact dermatitis to hydrocortisone, *Contact Dermatitis*, 1978,4: 334-7.

[14] Wilkinson, SM., English JSC., Mattey DL., In vitro evidence of delayed-type hypersensitivity to hydrocortisone, *Contact Dermatitis*, 1993,29: 241-5.

[15] Konttinen, YT., Friman, C., Tolvanen, E., Reimamo, S., Johansson, E., Local skin rash after intra-articular methylprednisolone acetate injection in a patient with rheumatoid arthritis,*Arthritis Rheumat.*, 1983,26: 231-3.

[16] Mathias, C.G., Robertson, D.B., Delayed hypersensitivity to corticosteroid suspension containing methylprednisolone. Two cases of conjuntival inflammation after retrobulbar injection, *Arch Dermatol.*, 1985,121: 258-61.

[17] Lyon, C.C., Beck, M.H., Allergic contact dermatitis to corticosteroids in periorbital inflammation and conjunctivitis, *Eye*, 1998,12: 148-9.

[18] Poon, E., Fewings, M., Generalized eczematous reaction to budesonide with cross-reactivity to triamcinolone., *Austr. J. Dermatol.*, 2001,42: 36-7.

[19] Holmes, P., Spongiotic (eczematous-type) dermatitis after inhaled budesonide, *Austr. N. Zel. J. Med.*, 1992,22: 511.

[20] Bircher, A.J., Levy, F., Langauer, S., Lepoittevin, J.P., Contact allergy to topical corticosteroids and systemic contact dermatitis from prednisolone with tolerance of triamcinolone, *Acta Dermatol. Venereol.*, 1995,75: 490-5.

[21] McKenna, D.B., Murphy, G.M., Contact allergy to topical corticosteroids and systemic allergy to prednisolone, *Contact Dermatitis*, 1998,38: 121-2.

[22] Reinhold, K., Schneider, L., Hunzelmann, N., Krieg, T., Scharfetter-Kochanek, K., Delayed-type allergy to systemic corticosteroids, *Allergy*, 2000,55: 1095-6.

[23] Fernandez de Corres, L., Bernaola, G., Urrutia, I., Munoz, D., Allergic dermatitis from systemic treatment with corticosteroids, *Contact Dermatitis*, 1990,22: 104-5.

[24] Whitemore, S.L., Dexamethasone injection induced generalized dermatitis, *Brit J Dermatol.*, 1994,131: 296-7.

[25] Wilkinson, S.M., Smith, A.G., English JSC., Erythroderma following the intradermal injection of the corticosteroid budesonide, *Contact Dermatitis*, 1992,27: 121-2.

[26] Fernandez de Corres, L., Urrutia, I., Audicana, M., Echechippa, S., Gastaminza, G., Erythroderma after intravenous injection of methylprednisolone, *Contact Dermatitis*, 1991,25: 68-70.

[27] Stingeni, L.,Caraffini, S., Assalve, D., Lapomarda, V.,Lisi, P., Erythema multiforme-like contact dermatitis from budesonide, *Contact Dermatitis*, 1996,34: 154-5.

[28] Valsecchi, R., Resenguetti, A., Leghista, P., Cologni, L., Cortinovis, R., Erythema multiforme-like lesions from triamcinolone acetonide, *Contact Dermatitis*, 1998,38:362-3.

[29] Scala, E., Giani, M., Pastore, S., Pallotta, S., Guerra, E.C., Pirrotta, L. Locanto, M.L., Frezzolini, A., DePità, O., Puddu, P.,Distinct delayed T-cell response to betamethasone and penicillinn G in the same patient, *Allergy,* 2003,58: 439-44.

[30] Pollock, B., Wilkinson, S.M., McDonald-Hull, S.P., Chronic urticaria associated with intra-articular methylprednisolone, *Brit. J. Dermatol.*, 2001,144: 1228-30.

[31] Ijsselmuiden, O.E., Knegt-Junk, K.J., van WijK, R., van Joost, T., Cutaneous adverse reaction after intra-articular injection of triamcinolone acetonide, *Acta Dermatol. Venereol.*, 1995,75: 57-8.

[32] Sener, O., Caliskaner, Z., Yazicioglu, K., Karaayvaz, M., Ozanguc, N., Non pigmenting solitary fixed drug eruption after skin testing and intrarticular injection of triamcinolone acetonide, *Ann. Allergy Asthma Immunol.*, 2001,86: 335-6.

[33] Demitsu, T., Kosuge, A., Yamada, T., Usui, K., Katayama, H., Yaoita, H., Acute generalized exanthematous pustolosis induced by dexamethasone injection, *Dermatology* 1996,193: 53-8.

[34] Mussot-Chia, C., Flechet, M.L.,Napolitano M., Hersan, S., Frances, C.; Chosidow, O., Pustolose exanthematiqué aigué generalisée à la methylprednisolone, *Ann. Dermatol. Venereol.*, 2001,128: 241-3.

[35] Navarro-Llanos, A., Elizalde Eguinoa, J., Boto de los Buyes, A., Puyol de la Llave E., Necrolisis epidermica toxica en una paciente en tratamento con altas dosis de deflazacort, *Med. Clin.*, 1996,106: 599.

[36] Garcia-Bravo, B., Reciso, J.B., Camacho, F., Systemic contact dermatiti sto deflazacort,*Contact Dematitis*, 2000,43: 359-60.

[37] Lew, D.B., Higgins, G.C., Skinner, R.B., Snider, M.D., Myers, L.K., Adverse reaction to prednisone in a patient with systemic lupus erythematous, *Pediatric Dermatol.*, 1999,16:146-50.

[38] Femiano, F., Cozzolino, F., Belnome, G., De Luca, P., Stevens-Johnson syndrome. Description of an unusual clinical case due to glucocorticoid therapy for oral lichen planus. *Minerva Stomatol.*, 1999,48: 277-82.

[39] Lauerma, A.I., Occupational contact sensitization to corticosteroids, *Contact Dermatitis*, 1998,39: 328-9.

[40] Ventura, M.T., Muratore, L., Calogiuri, G.F., Dagnello, M., Buquicchio, R., Nicoletti, A., Altamura, M., Sabbà, C., Tursi, A., Allergic and pseudoallergic reactions induced by glucocorticoids: a review. *Current pharmaceutical design*, 2003,9: 1956-64.

[41] Gomez, C.M., Higuero, N.C., Moral de Gregorio, A., Quiles, M.H., Nunez-Aceves, A.B., Lara, M.J., Sanchez, C.S., Urticaria–angioedema by deflazacort, *Allergy*, 2002,57: 370-1.

[42] Burgdorff, T., Venemalm, L., Vogt, T., Landhaler, M., Stolz, W., IgE-mediated anaphylactic reaction induced by succinare ester of methilprednisolone, *Ann. Allergy Asthma Immunol.*, 2002,89: 425-8.

[43] Rasanen, L., Tarvainen, K., Makinen-Kiljunen, S., Urticaria to hydrocortisone, *Allergy*, 2001,56: 352-3.

[44] Nakamura, H., Matsuse, H., Obase, Y., Mitsuta, K., Tomari, S., Saeki, S., Kawano, T., Kondo, Y., Machida, I., Shimoda, T., Asai, S., Kohno, S., Clinical evalutation of anaphylactic reactions to intravenous corticosteroids in adult asthmatic, *Respiration*, 2002,69: 309-13.

[45] Wilkinson, S.M., Mattey, D.L., Beck, M.H., IgG antibodies and early intradermal reactions to hydrocortisone in patients with cutaneous delayed-type hypersensitivity to hydrocortisone, *Brit. J. Dermatol.*, 1994,131: 495-8.

[46] Patel, L., Clayton, P.E., Addison, G.M., Price, D.A., David, T.J., Adrenal function following topical steroid treatment in children with atopic dermatitis, *Brit. J. Dermatol.*, 1995,32: 950-5.

[47] Keckes, A., Jahn, P., Mathes, H., Kulhmann, R.K., Lange, L., Systemic effects of topically applied methylprednisolone aceponate in healthy volunteers, *J. Am. Acad. Dermatol.*, 1993,28: 798-802.

[48] Pippen, R., Anaphylactoid reaction after chymacort ointment, *Brit. Med. J.,* 1966,5496: 1172.

[49] Bos, J.D., Meinerdi, M.M., The 500 Dalton rule for the skin penetration of chemical compounds and drugs, *Exp. Dermatol.*, 2000,9: 165-9.

[50] Lauerma, A.I., Visa, K., Pekonen, M., Forstrom, L., Reitamo, S., Cellular kinetics of delayed hypersensitivity test reactions to topical glucocorticosteroids, *Arch. Dermatol. Res.*, 1987,279: 379-84.

[51] Wilkinson, S.M., Andrew, S.M., Maseruka, H., Beck, M.H., Immunohistochemical appearance of corticosteroid contact hypersensitivity reactions, *Contact Dermatitis*, 1994,31: 304-7.

[52] Bundgaard, H., The possible implication of steroid-glyoxal degradation products in allergic reactions to corticosteroids, *Arch. Pharm. Chem., Science Ed.*, 1980,8: 83-90.

[53] Wilkinson, S.M., Jones, M.F., Corticosteroid usage and binding to arginine: determinants of corticosteroids hypersensitivity, *Brit. J. Dermatol.,* 1996,135: 225-30.

[54] Wilkinson, S.M., English, J.S.C., Hydrocortisone sensitivity: clinical features of 59 cases. *J. Amer. Acad. Dermatol.* 1992,27: 683-7.

[55] Wilkinson, S.M., Cartwright, P.H., English J.S.C., The significance of tixocortol pivalate positive patch tests in leg ulcer patients, *Contact Dermatitis*, 1990,23:120-1.

[56] Corazza, M., Mantovani, L., Maraini, C., Bacileri, S., Virgili, A., Contact sensitisation to corticosteroids: an increased risk in long term dermatosis, *Eur. J. Dermatol.* 2000,10: 533-5.

[57] Reitamo, S., Lauerma, A.I., Stubb, S., Kayhko, K., Visa, K., Forstrom, L., Delayed hypersensitivity to topical corticosteroids, *J. Am. Acad. Dermatol.*, 1986,14: 585-9.

[58] Knowles, S.R., Uetrecht, J., Shear, N.H., Idiosyncratic drug reactions: the reactive metabolite syndromes, *Lancet*, 2000,356: 1587-91.

[59] Leanza, W.J., Combere, J.P., Rogers, E.F., Pfister, K., Aldehydes derived from cortisone and hydrocortisone, *J. Am. Chem. Soc.*, 1953,76: 1691-4.

[60] Dooms-Goossens, A., Is there a relation between contact allergy to alcohols and contact allergy to corticosteroids?, *Eur. J. Dermatol.*, 1993,3: 713.

[61] Dooms-Goossens, A., Lepoittevin, J.P., Vigand, M., (Oct, 1994), Simultaneous positive patch test reactions to ethanol and/or aldehydes and corticosteroids, Proceedings of the 2nd Congress of European Society of Contact Dermatitis, pg. 14-6.

[62] Merk, H.F., Jugert, F.K., Frankenberg, S., (1996), Biotrasfomation in skin, In: *Dermatotoxicology*, 5th Ed, Marzulli F.N., Maibach H.I., Eds. Taylor and Francis Ed: Washington DC, 61.

[63] Morren, M.A., Dooms-Goossens, A., Corticosteroid allergy in children: a potential complication of atopic eczema, *Eur. J. Dermatol.* 1994,4: 106-9.

[64] Lauerma, A.I., Rasanen, L., Reunala, T., Reitamo, S., Langerhans cells but not monocytes are capable of antigen presentation in vitro in corticosteroid contact hypersensitivity, *Brit. J. Dermatol.* 1990,123: 699-705.

[65] Wilkinson, S.M., Morrey, K., Hollowood, K., Heagerty, A.H., English, J.S.C., HLA-A, B and DR antigens in hydrocortisone hypersensitivity, *Contact Dermatitis*, 1993,28:295-7.

[66] Dooms-Goossens, A., Andersen, K.E., Brandao, F.M., Bruynzeel, D., Burrows, D., Camarsa, J., Ducombs, G., Frosch, P., Hannuksela, Lachapelle, J.M., Lahti, A., Menné, T., Wahlberg, J.E., Wilkinson, J.D., Corticosteroid contact allergy: an EECDRG multicentre study, *Contact Dermatitis*, 1996,35: 40-4.

[67] Schoenmakers, A., Vermorken, A., Degreef, H., Dooms-Gossens, A., Corticosteroids or steroids allergy?, *Contact Dermatitis*, 1992,26: 159-62.

[68] Hausen, B.M., Fossereau, J., The sensitising capacity of tixocortol pivalate, *Contact Dermatitis,* 1988,18: 63-4.

[69] Wilkinson, S.M., English, J.C.S., Hydrocortisone sensitivity: a prospective study of the value of tixocortol pivalate and hydrocortisone acetate as patch test markers, *Contact Dermatitis*, 1991,25: 132-5.

[70] Dooms-Goossens, A., Identification of undected corticosteroid allergy, *Contact Dermatitis*, 1988,18: 124-5.

[71] Wolf, M.E., Baxter, J.D., Kollmann, P.A., Lee, D.L., Kuntz, I.D., Bloom, E., Matulich, D.T., Morris, J., Nature of steroid-glucocorticoid receptor interactions: thermodynamic analysis of the binding reaction, *Biochemistry*, 1978,17: 3201-8.

[72] Alani, M.D., Alani, S.D., Allergic contact dermatitis to corticosteroids, *Ann. Allergy*, 1972,30: 181-5.

[73] Dooms-Goossens, A., Morren, M., Results of routine patch testing with corticosteroid series in 2073 patients, *Contact Dermatitis*, 1992,26: 182-91.

[74] Coopman, S., Degreef, H., Dooms-Goossens, A., Identification of cross-reaction patterns in allergic contact dermatitis to topical corticosteroids, *Brit. J. Dermatol.*, 1989,121: 27-34.

[75] Lepoittevin, J.P., Drieghe, J., Dooms-Goossens, A., Studies in patient with corticosteroid contact allergy. Understanding cross-reactivity, *Arch. Dermatol.*, 1995,131: 31-7.

[76] Noda, H., Matsunaga, K., Noda, T., Abe, M., Ohtani, T., Shimizu, Y., Ashi, K., Noriyasu, T., Masutani, M., Ueda, H., Contact sensitivity and cross-reactiviy of budesonide, *Contact Dermatitis,* 1993,28: 212-5.

[77] Dahlberg, E., Thalen, A., Brattsand, R., Gustaffson JA, Johansson U, Roempke K, Saatok T., Correlation between chemical structure, receptor binding and biological activity of some novel highly active 16–17 (acetal-substituted) glucocorticoids, *Mol. Pharmacol.* 1984, 25: 70-8.

[78] Oh-I, T., Contact dermatitis due to topical steroids with conceivable cross-reactions between topical steroid preparations, *J. Dermatol.*, 1996,23: 200-208.

[79] Wilkinson, S.M., English, J.S.C., Hydrocortisone sensitivity. An investigation into the nature of the allergen, *Contact Dermatitis*, 1991,25: 178-81.

[80] Wilkinson, S.M., Hollis, S., Beck, M.H., Reactions to other corticosteroids in patients with allergic contact dermatitis from hydrocortisone, *Brit. J. Dermatol.*, 1995,132: 766-71.

[81] Haynes, R.C. jr. (1985). Inhibitors of adrenocortical steroids biosynthesis. In: *Goodman-Gillman Eds. The Pharmacological Basis of Theurapeutics, Adrenocorticotropic hormone: Adrenocortical steroids and their synthetic analogs.* McMillan Publishing Company, p.1459-89, New York.

[82] Wilkinson, S.M., Hollis, S., Beck, M., Reactions to other corticosteroids in patients with positive patch test reactions to budesonide, *J. Am. Acad. Dermatol.*, 1995,33:963-8.

[83] Kitano, Y., Hydrolisis of hydrocortisone-17-butyrrate-21-propionate by cultured human keratinocytes, *Acta Dermatol. Venereol.*, 1986,66: 98-102.

[84] Stingeni, L., Lisi, P., Contact allergy to prednicarbate: frequency of positive reactions in consecutively patch tested patients, *Contact Dermatitis*, 1999,40:286-7.

[85] Goossens, A., Matura, M., Degreef, H., Reactions to corticosteroids: some new aspects regarding cross-sensitivty, *Cutis*, 2000,65: 43-5.

[86] Lauerma, A.I., Screening for corticosteroid contact hypersensitivity: comparison of tixocortol pivalate, hydrocortisone-17-butyrate and hydrocortisone, *Contact Dermatitis*, 1991,24: 123-30.

[87] Goossens, A., Huygens, S., Matura, M., Degreef, H., Fluticasone propionate: a rare contact sensitizer, *Eur. J. Dermatol.*, 2001,11: 29-34.

[88] Wilkinson, S.M., Beck, M.H., Fluticasone propionate and mometasone furoate have a low risk of contact sensitization, *Contact Dermatitis*, 1996,34: 365-6.

[89] Grandolfo, M., Vena, G.A., Angelini, G., Bianchi, B., Mometasone furoate versus betamethasone vale rate in the treatment of allergic contact dermatisis, *J. Eur. Acad. Dermatol. Venereol.,* 1999,12 :78.

[90] Wilkinson, S.M., Corticosteroid cross-reactions: an alternative view, Contact Dermatitis, 2000,42: 59-63.

[91] Ventura, M.T., Calogiuri, G.F., Matino, M.G., Dagnello, M., Buquicchio, R., Foti, C., Di Corato, R., Alternative glucocorticoids for use in case of adverse reaction to systemic glucocorticoids: a study on 10 patients, *Brit. J. Dermatol.*, 2003,148: 139-41.

[92] Brockow, K., Romano, A., Blanca, M., Ring, J., Pichler, W.J., Demoly, P., General consideration for skin test procedures in the diagnosis of drug hypersensitivity. *Allergy*, 2002,57: 45-51.

[93] Calnan, C.D., Fregert, S., Magnusson, B., The International Contact Dermatitis Research Group, *Cutis*, 1976,18: 708.

[94] Dooms-Goossens, A., Corticosteroid contact allergy: a challenge to patch testing, Am. *J. Contact Dermatitis*, 1993,4: 120-6.

[95] Dooms-Goossens, A., Verschaeve, H., Degreef, H., van Berendrocks, J., Contact allergy to hydrocortisone and tixocortol pivalate: problems in detection of corticosteroid sensitivity, *Contact Dermatitis*, 1986,14: 94-102.

[96] Bjornasson, B., Flosadottir, E., Fischer, T., Reactivity at edges of corticosteroid patch tests may be an indicator of a strong positive test response, *Dermatology*, 1999,199: 138-44.

[97] Bruze, M., Isaksson, M., Dooms-Goossens, A., The influence of patch tests with clobetasol propionate on adjacent patch test reactions, *Contact Dermatitis*, 1995,32: 167-70.

[98] Forstrom, L., Lassus, A., Salde, L., Nierni, K.M., Allergic contact eczema from topical steroids, *Contact Dermatitis*, 1988,19: 128-33.

[99] Reitamo, S., Lauerma, A.I., Forstrom, L., Detection of contact hypersensitivity to topical corticosteroid with hydrocortisone 17-butyrate, *Contact Dermatitis*, 1989,21: 159-65.

[100] Wilkinson, S.M., Beck, H.M., Corticosteroid contact hypersensitivity: what vehicle and concentration?, *Contact Dermatitis*, 1996,34: 305-8.

[101] Isaksson, M., Gruvberger, B., Parsson, L., Stability of corticosteroid patch test preparations, *Contact Dermatitis*, 2000,42:144-7.

[102] Barbaud, A., Trechort, P., Reichert-Penetrart, S., Schmutz, J.L., Eczema de contact à l'alcool ethylique: comment realiser le tests?, *Ann. Dermatol. Venereol.*, 2001,127: 484-7.

[103] Matura, M., Leipottevin, J.P., Arbez-Gindrè, C., Goossens, A., Testing with corticosteroid aldheydes in corticosteroid sensitive patients (preliminary results), *Contact Dermatitis*, 1998,36:106-8.

[104] Boffa, M., Wilkinson, S.M., Beck, M.H., Screening for corticosteroid contact hypersensitivity, *Contact Dermatitis*, 1995,33: 149-51.

[105] Isaksson, M., Bruze, M., Goossens, A., Leipottevin, J.P., Patch testing with budesonide in serial dilutions: the significance of dose, occlusion time and reaig time, *Contact Dermatitis*, 1999,40: 24-31.

[106] Seukeran, D.C., Wilkinson, S.M., Beck, M.H., Patch testing to detect corticosteroid allergy: is it adequate?, *Contact Dermatitis*, 1997,36:127-30.

[107] Wilkinson, S.M., Heagerty, A.H., English, J.S.C., A prospective study into the value of patch and intradermal tests in identifying topical corticosteroids allergy, *Brit. J. Dermatol.*, 1992,27: 22-5.

[108] Freeman, S., Corticosteroids allergy, *Contact Dermatitis*, 1995,33: 240-5.

[109] Lazzarini, S., Contact allergy to benzyl alcohol and isopropyl-palmitate, ingredients of topical corticosteroids, *Contact dermatitis*, 1982,8: 342.

[110] Fischer, A., Cortaid cream dermatitis and the paraben paradox, *J. Am. Acad. Dermatol.*, 1982,6: 116-7.

[111] Oleffe, J.A., Blonded, A., De Conich, A., Allergy to chlorocresol and propylene glycol in a steroid cream, *Contact Dermatitis*, 1975,5: 53.

[112] Heshmati, S., Maibach, H.I., Active sensitization to sodium metabisulfite in hydrocortisone cream, *Contact Dermatitis*, 1999,41:166.

[113] Lee, A.Y., Lee, K.H., Allergic contact dermatitis from dioctylsodium-sulfosuccinate in a topical corticosteroid, *Contact Dermatitis*, 1998,38: 355.

[114] Maibach, H.I., Conant, M., Contact urticaria to a corticosteroid cream: Polysorbate 60, *Contact Dermatitis*, 1977,3:350.

[115] Green, C., Kenicer, K.J., A case of "contact allergy to corticosteroid", *Contact Dermatitis*, 1993,28: 39-40.

[116] Miura, Y., Allergic contact dermatitis from 1,2,6 hexanentriol in fluocinonide, *Contact Dermatitis*, 1999,41:118.

[117] Marston, S., Contact dermatitis from cetostearyl alcohol in hydrocortisone butyrate lipocream and from lanolin, *Contact Dermatitis*, 1991,24: 372.

[118] De Groot, A.C., Contact allergy to EDTA in a topical corticosteroid preparation, *Contact Dermatitis*, 1986,15: 250-2.

[119] Hernandez, N., Assier-Bonnet, M., Terki, N., Revuz, J., Allergic contact dermatitis from propylgallate in desonide cream (Locapred), *Contact Dermatitis*, 1997,36:111.

[120] Coksey, R.J., Bryan, H.G., Contact dermatitis to methylprednisolone, *JAMA*, 1967,199:136.

[121] Corazza, M., Mantovani, L., Romani, I., Bettoli, V., Virgili, A., Compound allergy to topical budesonide, *Contact Dermatitis*, 1994,30: 246-7.

[122] Kellet, J.K., King, C.M., Beck, M.H., Compound allergy to medicaments, *Contact Dermatitis*, 1986,14: 45-8.

[123] Chang, Y.C., Clarke, G.F., Maibach, H.I., The provocative use test (PUT) ROAT (Repeated Open Application Test) in topical corticosteroid allergic contact dermatitis, *Contact Dermatitis*, 1997, 37:309-10.

[124] Lauerma, A.I., Reitamo, S., Maibach, H., Systemic hydrocortisone/cortisol induces allergic skin reactions in presensitized subjects, *J. Am. Acad. Dermatol.*, 1991, 24:182-5.

[125] Rasanen, L., Tuomi, M.L., Yilitalo, L., Reactivity of tixocortol pivalate-positive patient in intradermal and oral provocation tests, *Brit. J. Dermatol.*, 1996,135:931-4.

[126] Isaksson, M., Bruze, M., Allergic contact dermatitis in response to budesonide reactivated by inhalation of the allergen, *J. Am. Acad. Dermatol.*, 2002, 46: 880-5.

In: Drug Toxicity: New Research
Editor: Cam E. Vellotis, pp.73-88
ISBN 978-1-60456-320-7

Chapter 4

Hemodynamic Profiles in Clinical Cardiology: Diagnosis of Valvular, Myocardial and Pericardial Heart Diseases by Coupling Hemodynamics with Clinical Picture

Sanjeev Wasson [*1] ***and Hanumanth K. Reddy*** [2]
[1]Department of Cardiology/Cardiac Electrophysiology,
Cleveland Clinic Foundation
[2]Medical Center of South Arkansas

Keywords: clinical hemodynamic, hemodynamic profiles, valvular heart disease, constrictive pericarditis, cardiac tamponade, restrictive cardiomyopathy.

Introduction

Hemodynamic profiles obtained by cardiac catheterization in the context of different clinical scenarios, reflect distinct patho-physiological states enabling clinicians to manage patients in a scientific way [1]. The three most important types of measurements in the cardiac catheterization laboratory are: Pressures, Flows (i.e. cardiac output, systemic blood flow and pulmonary flow etc) resistance indicators and Oxygen Saturations in different chambers.

One should take several general precautions during hemodynamic monitoring. The transducer must be positioned at mid-chest level midway in the frontal and transverse planes close to 4th intercostal space near the sternal margin. This type of leveling assures close

* Address for correspondence and reprints: Sanjeev Wasson, M.D. Department of Cardiology/Cardiac Electrophysiology; Cleveland Clinic Foundation; 9500 Euclid Avenue, Desk F-15; Cleveland, OH 44195; E-mail: wassons@health.missouri.edu

proximity of the transducer to the center of the heart, thus excluding the effects of weight of tubing and fluid column. The atmospheric pressure is used as a zero point reference and is therefore, a common need to open the system to air. The tubing should be as short as possible to reflect the accurate timing of pressure tracings. Since air in the system could create grossly erroneous values, adequate and repeated flushing should be performed to ensure an air free system. Fluid to fluid contact should be maintained at all the levels. Intravascular volume status should be closely monitored and adjusted. Etio-pathology of hemodynamic changes should be considered and correlated with the type, severity and duration of each of the valvular and/or pericardial lesions. Influence of pressure and/or volume overload of single or multiple valvular lesions on the volume and pressure profiles of different chambers, arterial and venous vasculature should be considered. Integrity of the pulmonary or hematological system should be taken into account. Correlation with echocardiographic findings should always be considered. Echocardiographic and catheterization findings are always complementary. Intracardiac and extracardiac shunts and anemia have significant influence on pressures, severity of stenoses and insufficiency.

Precise diagnosis of restrictive cardiomyopathy and pericardial diseases using hemodynamic profiles in a busy cardiac catheterization setting is also a challenging task. This is partly due to unavailability of a quick review of case scenarios, equipment selection, methods and interpretation of hemodynamic profiles and key diagnostic points. This review brings together case vignettes, methods and protocols for hemodynamic work up of commonly encountered valvular conditions and pericardial diseases to differentiate them accurately from restrictive cardiomyopathy. Each clinical entity is described with the help of case vignettes, equipment and protocols for hemodynamic work up, methods and interpretation of hemodynamic profiles with emphasis on salient diagnostic features.

Aortic Stenosis

Case Vignette: A 79 year old gentleman farmer, very active in his family farming, presents with lightheadedness and exertional chest pressure. His family physician heard a severe grade IV crescendo-decrescendo, systolic ejection murmur and muffled 2nd heart sound. There were no signs of congestive heart failure. EKG showed left ventricular hypertrophy. An echocardiogram performed at a local hospital reportedly showed aortic stenosis (AS) with a peak trans-aortic pressure gradient of 36 mmHg. The aortic valve area was calculated as 1.2 cm^2 by continuity equation. Because of the discrepancy between the clinical assessment and echocardiographic measurements, the patient was referred for cardiac catheterization. Indications and equipment for right and left heart catheterization in cases of aortic stenosis are summarized in Table I [2], Table II and Table III respectively. A particular set of protocol should be followed during performance of catheterization in these cases (Table IV).

Table I. Indications of heart catheterization aortic stenosis [2]

Most Common Indications

(1) To ascertain coronary anatomy in patients with suspected coronary artery atherosclerosis (CAD) and known severe aortic stenosis by clinical and echocardiographic assessment.
(2) To delineate coronary anatomy and determine aortic valve area in patients with discordance between clinical and echocardiographic evaluation of the valve area
(3) To exclude pulmonary hypertension, other valvular or congenital heart diseases when suspected

Less Common Indications

(1) In patients with significant symptoms of chest pain, syncopal or pre-syncopal sensation and heart failure with clinical and echocardiographic evidence of non-critical stenosis.
(2) To evaluate aortic valve area in patients with low trans-aortic pressure gradient and low cardiac output. Valve area is calculated using cardiac output and pressure gradient measurements at baseline and following physiological and pharmacologic stress such as dobutamine stress.

Table II. Equipment for right heart catheterization in cases of aortic stenosis

(1) 7 French venous sheath
(2) 7 French Swan-Ganz catheter
(3) 10 blood gas syringes for estimation of oxygen saturation
(4) A separate manifold attached to pressure transducer
(5) Thermodilution cardiac output machine
(6) Oxygen saturation analyzer
(7) 0.025 wire to guide Swan-Ganz catheter to superior vena cava and/or pulmonary artery (PA) if needed

Table III. Equipment for left heart catheterization in cases of aortic stenosis

(1) A standard left sided manifold attached to a separate transducer
(2) 6 French arterial sheath
(3) A dual port 6 French pig tail catheter with left ventricle (LV) side holes and aortic side holes (Cordis) or alternatively, a 90 cm 7 French Mullin's Sheath to record ascending aortic pressure simultaneously with 5 French pigtail catheter in the left ventricle.
(4) A 5 French angled pigtail catheter and 0.038 straight-tipped safety guide wire. Alternative catheters in case of difficulty with crossing the aortic valve include right Judkin's catheter (J), right and left amplatz catheters, multipurpose catheters. Transseptal approach is rarely needed.
(5) A 0.035 exchange length 260cm guide wire.
(6) Standard coronary catheters, JL4, 3D RC (Williams) or JR4

Table IV. Protocol for right and left heart catheterization in cases of aortic stenosis

(1) Compulsive measures for baseline and repeated calibration and flushing of the right and left sided transducers and catheters to ensure air free and thrombus free systems is extremely important.
(2) Routine right heart catheterization with screening oximetry to exclude concomitant congenital heart diseases.
(3) 5000 units of heparin and frequent flushing of sheaths.
(4) Baseline recording of short or long arterial sheath pressure before the introduction of pig tail catheter.
(5) Crossing the aortic valve with pig tail catheter with frequent flushing and recording of simultaneous aortic and ventricular pressures and simultaneous ventricular and pulmonary artery wedge pressures and thermodilution estimation of cardiac output soon after the recording of trans-aortic pressure gradient.

Discussion

Hemodynamic findings in aortic stenosis are characterized by an increase in transvalvular pressure gradient. Transvalvular gradient is measured by simultaneous measurement of the left ventricular pressure (by a catheter in the left ventricle advanced retrogradely via aorta or via transseptal approach), and central aortic pressure (by a pigtail catheter in the aorta just above the aortic valve). Femoral arterial pressure obtained from the side arm of the arterial sheath is most commonly utilized along with LV pressure. However, because of time delay of about 40-50 msecs between femoral artery pressure and LV pressure, the upstrokes of femoral artery and left ventricular pressures should be matched. Also, the usually higher femoral artery pressure relative to ascending aortic pressure should be considered in the valve area calculation. Aortic pressure tracing shows very slow upstroke and delayed rate of pressure rise, while the LV tracing depicts high left ventricular systolic and diastolic pressures. Pulmonary artery wedge pressure (PCWP) tracing demonstrates large "a" waves due to hypertrophied left atrium and a noncompliant left ventricle causing elevated left ventricular end diastolic pressure (LVEDP). Aortic valve area (AVA) can be calculated (Table-V) using Gorlin's Formula [3]:

$$AVA\ (cm^2) = (SV \div SEP) \div (44.3 \times [\text{sq rt}\ \Delta P])$$

where SV = stroke volume (mL per beat), SEP = systolic ejection period (sec per beat), and ΔP = mean systolic pressure gradient between the left ventricle and aorta (mmHg).

Alternatively, AVA could be calculated by Hakki's formula [4] which is a simplified version of Gorlin's equation. This formula is based on finding of the product of heart rate, SEP or DFP and Gorlin's equation constant being 1 in all patients at a resting state.

AVA (cm^2) = *Cardiac output (liters/ minute)*

√ Trans-aortic peak to peak pressure gradient

Table V. Aortic valve area calculations

Location	Pressure mmHg Systolic	Diastolic	Mean	Oximetry O_2 saturation
Right Atrium	9	6	5	63%
Right Ventricle	43	0		60%
Pulmonary Artery	43	16	29	64%
Pulmonary Artery Wedge	18	18	14	
Central Aortic	117	86	102	96%
Left ventricle	179	20		

Peak to Peak Trans-Aortic Pressure Gradient 62 mmHg
Cardiac output 4.42 l/min
Mean Trans-Aortic Pressure Gradient 54
Systolic Ejection Period 0.39 sec
Trans-Aortic Blood Flow per second 182.7
Gorlin's Formula 182.7/ 1.0x44.3x √54
Calculated Aortic Valve Area by Gorlin Formula 0.56 cm^2
Calculated Aortic Valve Area by Hakki Formula 0.57 cm^2

However, several pitfalls of Gorlin's formula have been described. Gorlin's formula being flow-dependent usually underestimates the valve area in low output states (below 3 L/min) [5, 6]. Symptomatic low gradient AS patients with a small transvalvular gradient (<30 mmHg), low cardiac output, and a calculated valve area of ≤0.7 cm2 [7] present a diagnostic and therapeutic dilemma. Using maneuvers to increase cardiac output as with dobutamine or nitroprusside, which increase calculated valve area, except in severe AS, further facilitates surgical decision making in regard to calculation of aortic valve area [8].

Severe AS is suspected when there is mean trans-aortic pressure gradient of greater than 40 mm Hg in the setting of normal cardiac output [9]. The mean trans-aortic pressure gradient is approximately 80 and 90% of peak to peak gradient in moderate and severe AS respectively. Approximately 10mmHg pressure gradient caused by the catheter across the aortic valve is considered clinically insignificant. In atrial fibrillation or any irregular rhythm, at least 10 cardiac cycles should be measured for average pressure gradient. In cases of severe AS with low cardiac output, dobutamine administration may assist in sorting out true severe AS (gradient same or increases) from less severe AS (gradient decreases).

Aortic Insufficiency

Case Vignette: A 68 year old lady with a history of obesity, severe hypertension, hyperlipidemia, family history of coronary artery disease, idiopathic aortic dilatation and severe aortic insufficiency (AI) and previously known LV dilatation (left ventricular end-diastolic dimension (LVEDD) 6.5cm and end-systolic dimension 5.3 cm) and normal ejection fraction of 70%. Prior to her most recent hospitalization, the patient has gained about 30 pounds of weight over a period of 6 months, pedal edema and increasing dyspnea despite therapy with ACE inhibitors, calcium channel blockers and diuretics. A repeat echocardiogram showed poorly defined LV endocardium with an ejection fraction of 45%. Therefore, a complete cardiac catheterization was performed. Table VI summarizes the common indications of cardiac catheterization in cases of aortic insufficiency [9].

Table VI. Common Indications of Cardiac Catheterization in Cases of Aortic Insufficiency [9]

(1)	In acute aortic insufficiency due to aortic dissection where aortography and coronary angiography are needed.
(2)	In patients with symptomatic aortic insufficiency and indeterminate echocardiographic assessment of severity of insufficiency and left ventricular systolic function
(3)	To study coronary anatomy in patients with suspected coronary artery disease and severe aortic insufficiency prior to surgery.
(4)	Exercise right heart catheterization may provide useful information in some patients with severe AI, LV dilatation approaching the cut-off criteria, and borderline or normal systolic function.

Discussion

The regurgitant fraction (RF) during each cardiac cycle is the difference between the LV stroke volume measured angiographically (A) and the stroke volume measured by the Fick method (F).

RF = [stroke volume (A) - stroke volume (F)]/stroke volume (A)

In chronic compensated severe AI, the right heart pressures and left ventricular end diastolic pressure may be normal or mildly elevated. In advanced cases of severe AI, the hemodynamic profile shows wide pulse pressure because of systolic volume overloading and diastolic emptying of peripheral arterial system with a high stroke volume that dissipates rapidly into the left ventricle with aortic insufficiency. Because of this rapid transmission of a large volume and pressure from a high pressure aorta to the left ventricle with exhausted compliance, there is a rapid rise of LV diastolic pressure. The higher augmentation of femoral arterial pressure relative to LV pressure is due to a brisk, high volume LV output into peripheral arteries with reflected waves that augment femoral arterial systolic pressure. Aortic pressure tracing shows a rapid upstroke, an increased systolic pressure, a rapid fall and wide pulse pressure. The aortic and LV pressures become equal near the end of diastole. Due to increased LV compliance, LV pressure tracings reveal normal LVEDP despite of increased end diastolic volume (EDV). Left atrial (LA) pressure waveforms are normal in the absence of left ventricular hypertrophy (LVH).

In cases of acute AI, right and left heart catheterization shows severe elevations of LVEDP and PCWP due to sudden volume overloading of normal sized left ventricle. LVEDP is often much higher than PCWP because of an early closure of mitral valve. However, florid pulmonary edema is not uncommon and these patients need intravenous vasodilators, diuretics and ventilatory support. Due to lack of time for adaptation and impaired compliance, LV pressure tracing shows a rapid rise in diastolic pressure, marked elevation in LVEDP and narrow pulse pressure due to decreased aortic systolic pressure from reduced forward stroke volume. LA pressure tracing shows elevated LA pressure with a small "a" and "v" wave, with small nadir of the "x" and "y" descents. Hill's sign signifies the difference in femoral artery systolic pressure (i.e., 25-70 mm Hg) above aortic pressure that most likely indicates chronic and severe AI. In acute severe aortic insufficiency, the patho-physiology that brings about Hill's sign has not had time to develop and this sign is not present. With acute insufficiency, these patients have low stroke volume and cardiac output despite compensatory tachycardia and are often in cardiogenic shock with excessive mortality and morbidity. They need early surgical intervention and use of an intra-aortic balloon pump is contraindicated.

Mitral Stenosis

Case Vignette: A 45 year old morbidly obese woman presents with gradually worsening dyspnea on exertion, paroxysmal nocturnal dyspnea (PND) and hemoptysis. No fever or any signs of pulmonary infection were noted. Physical examination showed morbid obesity, no discernible jugular venous pressure (JVP), distant heart sounds, a hardly detectable mid-diastolic murmur, bibasilar lung crackles and severe lower extremity edema. Echocardiogram showed calcified mitral valve that appeared to be ballooning out during diastole, which was not clearly visualized. Common indications [2] and equipments for left heart catheterization in cases of mitral stenosis are described in Table VII and VIII respectively. Equipment and protocol for right heart catheterization in mitral stenosis are same as those for aortic stenosis. Essentially the same precautions as for routine right and left heart catheterization except that oximetry as described above and an accurate pulmonary artery wedge pressure to reflect left atrial pressure should be obtained. The following guidelines should be followed: Confirm the wedge position of Swan Ganz catheter PA port by watching the balloon move with movements of lungs with respiration. While the balloon is inflated, check the saturation of PA port blood to be above 95%. The mean wedge pressure is always lower than the mean pulmonary artery pressure.

Discussion

Similar to AS, mitral valve area (in cm2) to assess the severity of mitral stenosis is calculated by Gorlin formula [3] (Table IX) and can be graded into different grades of severity (Table X).

$$MVA = (SV \div DFP) \div (37.7 \times [\text{sq rt } \Delta P])$$

where SV = stroke volume (mL per beat), DFP = diastolic filling period (sec per beat), and ΔP = mean diastolic pressure gradient between the left atrium and left ventricle (mmHg).

Table VII. Indications of heart catheterization in mitral stenosis [2]

Most Common Indications

(1) Discrepancy between the hemodynamics data from echocardiography and the clinical symptoms.

(2) Elevated pulmonary artery pressure out of proportion to mean trans-mitral pressure gradient and valve area.

(3) To evaluate severity of suspected mitral insufficiency in association with mitral stenosis (MS).

(4) To delineate coronary anatomy in patients with suspected coronary atherosclerosis.

Less Common Indications

(1) Discrepancy between symptoms and hemodynamic data-exercise hemodynamic assessment in severely symptomatic patients with resting hemodynamics not indicating moderate to severe MS.

(2) Patients younger than 40 years with pure mitral stenosis without any co-existent valvular pathologies and any angina.

Table VIII. Equipment for left heart catheterization in cases of mitral stenosis

Equipment for left heart catheterization

(1) A standard left sided manifold attached to a separate transducer

(2) 5 French arterial sheath

(3) 5 French pig tail catheter, standard coronary catheters, JL4, JR4 or 3DRC catheters.

(4) A 0.035 regular length J-tipped wire.

Table IX. Mitral valve area calculations

Location	Pressure mmHg Systolic	Diastolic	Mean	Oximetry O_2 saturation
Right Atrium	7	4	5	61%
Right Ventricle	80	10		62%
Pulmonary Artery	80	32	51	64%
Pulmonary Artery Wedge	36	32	22	
Central Aortic	138	77	102	94%
Left ventricle	120	0	7(LVEDP)	
Cardiac output	3.4 l/min			
Heart Rate	75 beats/min			
	Pre-Valvotomy			Post-valvotomy
Mean Diastolic Pressure Gradient	15 mmHg			4.55 mm Hg
Diastolic Filling Period	0.36 sec			0.32 sec
Trans-Mitral Blood Flow per second	125.9			137.2
Gorlin's Formula	$125.9/\ 0.85 \times 44.3 \times \sqrt{15}$			$145.8/\ 0.85 \times 44.3 \times \sqrt{4.55}$
Calculated Mitral Valve Area by Gorlin Formula	$0.87\ cm^2$			$1.82 cm^2$

Table X. Valve area and gradient criteria used for grading severity of various stages of mitral and aortic stenosis

	MITRAL VALVE		AORTIC VALVE AREA (cm^2)
	AREA (cm^2)	GRADIENT(mm Hg)	
NORMAL	4 - 6	0	2.5-4.0
MILD STENOSIS	>1.5	5	>1.5
MODERATE STENOSIS	1.0-1.5	5-10	1.1-1.5
SEVERE STENOSIS	1.0	>10	<1.0
CRITICAL STENOSIS	<1.0		<0.75

Transvalvular gradient is measured by the simultaneous measurement of the left ventricular pressure (by a catheter in the left ventricle retrogradely via aorta), and the left atrial pressure (by a transseptal approach or indirectly with PCWP) during diastole. Hemodynamic PCWP tracings demonstrates gradual "y" descent and a prominent "a" wave [10]. Since PCWP is delayed compared to LVEDP, phase shifting of "v" waves to LV pressure down slope is important before the diastolic pressure gradient is calculated.

Various factors like abnormal heart rate or rhythm or LV function, and coexistent valvular disorders, would affect the Gorlin's formula. Since a small difference in mitral gradient may make a large valve area difference, multiple cycles i.e. at least 10 cycles should be used for pressure gradient measurement in any irregular rhythm. Tachycardia increases transvalvular gradient because of the reduced diastolic filling period. Mean of valve gradients over 10 cardiac cycles is taken for valve area computation in atrial fibrillation [11]. PCWP and direct left atrial pressure measurement by transseptal catheter may not correlate in conditions like cor-tritriatum or chronic pulmonary venous disease. In patients with both MS and mitral insufficiency (MI), the Gorlin formula is not as accurate as 2-D-echocardiography in regard to the MVA. In patients with both MS and MI, the Gorlin formula tends to underestimate the MVA.

Mitral Insufficiency

Case Vignette: A 58 year lady with previously known moderately severe MI due to mitral valve prolapse presents with increasing dyspnea despite optimal medical therapy. A repeat echocardiogram showed mild LV dilatation (LVEDD of 6.0 cm) and a normal ejection fraction of 75%. Because of this discrepancy between clinical presentation and echocardiographic findings, a complete cardiac catheterization was performed. Table XI summarizes the common indications of cardiac catheterization in cases of mitral insufficiency [2].

Table XI. Indications of cardiac catheterization in cases of mitral insufficiency [2]

(1)	Discrepancy between clinical and echocardiographic findings.
(2)	To assess severity of mitral insufficiency prior to valve repair or replacement.
(3)	To exclude coronary artery disease in patients with risk factors for CAD or in patients with mitral insufficiency of ischemic origin.
(4)	To assess LV size, function and severity of mitral insufficiency in patients in whom echocardiographic assessment is indeterminate.

Discussion

Similar to the situation in acute aortic insufficiency, in patients with acute mitral insufficiency due to rupture of papillary muscle or chordae tendinae in bacterial endocarditis or acute ischemic syndrome, right and left heart catheterization show severe elevations of pulmonary artery wedge pressure and left ventricular end-diastolic pressure due to sudden volume overloading of normal sized left ventricle. Due to lack of time for adaptation and low compliance, the LA pressure tracings show a very tall "v" wave. The amplitude of the "v" wave and that of LV systole becomes equal by the end of systole. Florid pulmonary edema is common and these patients need intravenous vasodilators, diuretics and ventilatory support. These patients have low stroke volume and cardiac output despite compensatory tachycardia and are often in cardiogenic shock with excessive mortality and morbidity. They need early surgical intervention and balloon pump is indicated.

In chronic compensated mitral insufficiency, the right sided pressures and left ventricular end diastolic pressure may be normal or mildly elevated. In advanced cases, the hemodynamic profile is characterized by the elevated left ventricular end-diastolic pressure and pulmonary artery wedge pressure with prominent *'v'* waves. The magnitude of 'v' waves is dependent on left atrial size, loading conditions and acuity of mitral insufficiency. One should keep in mind that the "v" wave height may not accurately indicate the actual degree of MI. It is well known that "v" wave height may be increased in MS as well as in patients with VSD. Pulmonary hypertension and low cardiac output may be expected. A rapid y descent with rapid emptying of high left atrial volume into left ventricle happens when mitral valve opens. A small transmitral early diastolic pressure gradient is not uncommon.

The regurgitant fraction (RF) during each cardiac cycle is the difference between the LV stroke volume measured angiographically (A) and the stroke volume measured by the Fick method (F).

RF = [stroke volume (A) - stroke volume (F)]/stroke volume (A)

LA Pressure tracings show a tall "v" wave or "c-v" wave, which are sensitive but not specific for MI. Such waves are also seen in ventricular septal defect (VSD) [12]. Due to a very compliant left atrium, the amplitude of "v" wave is lower than that of left ventricular systole. Due to increased LV compliance and the forward stroke volume being normal in chronic MI, the LV pressure waveforms in systole and diastole are normal.

Cardiac Tamponade

Case Vignette: A 72 yr old woman had sharp pleuritic chest pain with acute hypotension following difficulty with manipulation of a ventricular lead during permanent pacemaker placement. An emergent echocardiogram showed moderate amount of pericardial fluid with signs of cardiac tamponade. Common indications for cardiac catheterization in cardiac tamponade are described in Table XII. The same equipment are required for right and left heart catheterization as described in paper1 for valvular heart diseases. Three transducers are utilized to record simultaneous pressures of right heart, left heart and pericardial cavity. High quality pressure tracings may be obtained at a higher gain, fast paper speed and coupled with respiratory cycle as well as EKG. Diastolic equalization of right heart, left heart and pericardial pressures is diagnostic of cardiac tamponade. Pulmonary artery wedge pressure in the absence of severe mitral insufficiency may be used to represent left ventricular end-diastolic pressure thus obviating left heart catheterization.

Table XII. Indications for cardiac catheterization in cardiac tamponade

Most common indications

(1) To identify cardiac tamponade as a cardiac emergency in cases of equivocal clinical and echocardiographic findings especially in post cardiac surgery cardiac tamponade.

(2) To evaluate the efficacy of pericardiocentesis procedure

(3) To differentiate pseudotamponade due to right ventricular failure from true tamponade physiology.

Less Common Indications

(1) Hemodynamically stable patients with the evidence of moderate to severe pericardial effusion of known etiology on non-invasive monitoring.

Discussion

Hemodynamic Findings are characterized by the elevation of central venous pressure (CVP) with blunted Y descent producing pulsus paradoxus [13]. There is an absence of dip and plateau on right ventricle (RV) pressure tracings. Equalization of right heart, left ventricular diastolic and pericardial pressures is diagnostic of cardiac tamponade. This diastolic equalization of pressures will no longer be seen after pericardiocentesis. Cardiac tamponade is suggested by a dominant x descent. Patients with pseudotamponade due to RV failure after mitral valve replacement usually have arterial hypotension, elevated cardiac filling pressures and elevated CVP. This entity is differentiated from true tamponade by predominant diastolic y descents on venous waveforms, which is attenuated in true tamponade.

Constrictive Pericarditis

Case Vignette: A 57 year old insurance executive underwent coronary artery bypass surgery 8 weeks prior to his presentation with increasing dyspnea and fatigue. Physical examination showed a moderately built individual with tachycardia and borderline low blood pressure, moderately elevated jugular venous pressure with positive Kussmaul's sign and quiet precordium. Echocardiogram showed low normal LV systolic function and thickened pericardium with a small pericardial effusion. Table XIII describes the common indications for catheterization in this clinical entity. Essential equipment for right and left catheterization are 5F arterial sheath, a 5 F angled pig tail catheter, 7 F venous sheath, Swan Ganz catheter, and two pressure transducer systems to obtain simultaneous pressure measurements. Careful, simultaneous, high gain recording of right atrial (RA)/ LV, RA/PCWP, RV/LV pressures should be performed. If diastolic equalization of the above described pressure is not apparent then all the pressures should be repeated after administering one liter of normal saline over 10 minutes.

Table XIII. Indications of cardiac catheterization in constrictive pericarditis

(1)	To differentiate right ventricular infarction from pericardial constriction.
(2)	To differentiate constrictive and restrictive physiology
(3)	Co-existent atrial fibrillation may make interpretation of hemodynamics difficult in pericardial constriction and right ventricular infarction.
(4)	To study effects of various respiratory changes on constrictive and restrictive cardiomyopathy including Kussmaul's sign.

Discussion

Constrictive pericarditis is suggested by a dominant y descent. Hemodynamic CVP tracings show exaggeration of all components including a, c, v waves, as well as x and y descents. RA pressure is elevated during inspiration in constrictive pericarditis producing W or M configuration, which is known as Kussmaul's sign [14]. RV infarction mimics constrictive pericarditis unless there is coexisting RA infarction, which produces decreased a, c waves and x descent. Atrial fibrillation associated with constrictive pericarditis and RV infarction causes absent a wave, attenuated x descent and dominant y descent. LV pressure tracings show a very rapid upstroke immediately after LVEDP (=0 mmHg) and then, followed by sharp attenuation. LV and RV diastolic pressures are elevated, equal and exactly superimposed producing classic square root (or dip and plateau) wave pattern during diastole in both ventricles. The square root sign noted on right and left heart diastolic wave forms is most commonly seen with pericardial constriction; however, may occasionally be noted in patients with cardiac tamponade. Similarly, RA and LV diastolic pressure patterns also superimposed with increased RA y-descent. Early y-descent and rapid drop in LV diastolic pressure to zero mmHg differentiate constrictive from restrictive hemodynamics. PA tracings show triphasic response with low flow pattern and pulmonary artery diastolic pressure

(PADP) almost equal to LVEDP. PCWP tracings almost superimposes on RA pressure tracings. RA a wave occurs at nadir of diastolic nadir of PA pressure due to pressure time delay.

Effusive constrictive pericarditis [15], usually seen in tuberculous pericarditis, is characterized by pulsus paradoxus (rare in classical constrictive pericarditis because of the absence of transmission of the inspiratory decline in pressure to the right heart chambers), less prominent y descent and absent Kussmaul's sign. During pericardiocentesis in such patients, pericardial pressure is lowered to normal, but RA pressure remains elevated, y-descent becomes predominant and respiratory variation is impaired.

Restrictive Cardiomyopathy

Case vignette: A 72 year gentleman with a long standing hypertension presented to the hospital with 6 month history of gradually worsening dyspnea and lower extremity edema. Physical examination showed moderately elevated jugular venous pressure, soft first and second heart sounds, grade 2 tricuspid insufficiency murmur 3+ lower extremity edema. EKG showed small R wave voltage, poor precordial R wave progression. Echocardiogram showed normal sized left ventricle with an ejection fraction of 50% and echo-reflective thick LV and RV walls and a small pericardial effusion. Cardiac catheterization was requested to make an accurate diagnosis of etiology of heart failure. Cardiac catheterization is indicated in only specific circumstances in cases of suspected restrictive cardiomyopathy (Table XIV). Equipments and protocols are same as that used for constrictive pericardium. Additionally, a 54 cm bioptome is utilized to obtain endomyocardial biopsy via right internal jugular vein under echocardiographic guidance to avoid myocardial puncture and injury to the tricuspid apparatus.

Table XIV. Indications of cardiac catheterization in restrictive cardiomyopathy

(1)	To make diagnosis of etiology of new onset heart failure
(2)	To obtain the hemodynamic profile of heart failure patients for effective management
(3)	To exclude common causes of heart failure such as coronary artery disease and valve disease before performing echo-guided endomyocardial biopsy via the right internal jugular vein.

Discussion

Hemodynamic pressure tracings would show rapid x and y descents dip and plateau known as square root sign. LVEDP exceeds right ventricular end diastolic pressure (RVEDP) with concordance of RV and LV pressures during respiration (as opposed to discordance seen in constrictive physiology) [16].

Summary

Appropriate correlation of the hemodynamic spectrum with the clinical presentation could be a challenging task to an unwary clinician. While obtaining hemodynamic data in the cardiac catheterization laboratory, great attention should be paid to the details and all the variables must be correlated with the patient's clinical picture. When appropriately obtained, hemodynamic profiles serve to broaden the horizons of clinical diagnosis, confirm clinical diagnosis already made and clinch the diagnosis in a confounding clinical situation. Hemodynamic profiles and clinical manifestations of constrictive pericardium and restrictive cardiomyopathy are quite similar and therefore could pose a diagnostic dilemma to a busy clinician (Table XV).

Table XV. Pathophysiological profiles of constrictive pericardium and restrictive cardiomyopathy

	Constrictive pericardium	Restrictive cardiomyopathy
Causes	Abnormal scarring of the pericardium preventing normal LV diastolic function	Intramyocardial accumulation of foreign material leading to wall stiffening and inelasticity leading to restrictive type of impaired LV diastolic function
Historical clues	Previous history of heart or chest surgery or trauma or radiation or connective tissue disease	History of amyloidosis, hemochromatosis, glycogen storage disease and other infiltrative diseases. Endomyocardial biopsy might show eosinophilic endomyocardial disease or endocardial fibroelastosis
Hemodynamic distinction	Narrowed right ventricular pulse pressure because of heightened diastolic pressure in the presence of normal systolic pressure Near equalization of diastolic pressures in all 4 chambers Square root-like or Dip-plateau type of right ventricular pressure wave form represents initial rapid ventricular filling followed by a brisk rise of diastolic pressure to a flattened state	A greater elevation of more than 5mmHG on left side compared to right side. Square root sign in restrictive cardiomyopathy is very similar to that of constrictive pericardium.
Variation of ventricular pressures with respiration	Right ventricular peak systolic pressure rises while the left ventricular pressure falls out of phase in a discordant manner during respiration	Right ventricular and left ventricular pressures vary with respiration in a concordant manner

The clinical context of constrictive pericardium is quite distinct from that of restrictive cardiomyopathy. The hemodynamic profiles of the two conditions are quite similar albeit there are some clues to favor on or the other condition. Remembering that in patients with restrictive physiology and pathology, the LVEDP will be higher than the RVEDP, may assist in sorting out restriction vs. constriction. The distinction between the constrictive pericardium and restrictive cardiomyopathy mainly rests on the unique clinical courses and a host of noninvasive tests including an echocardiogram (Figure 1). Endomyocardial biopsy may clinch the diagnosis of restrictive cardiomyopathy and therefore should be considered whenever there is continued uncertainty about the diagnosis.

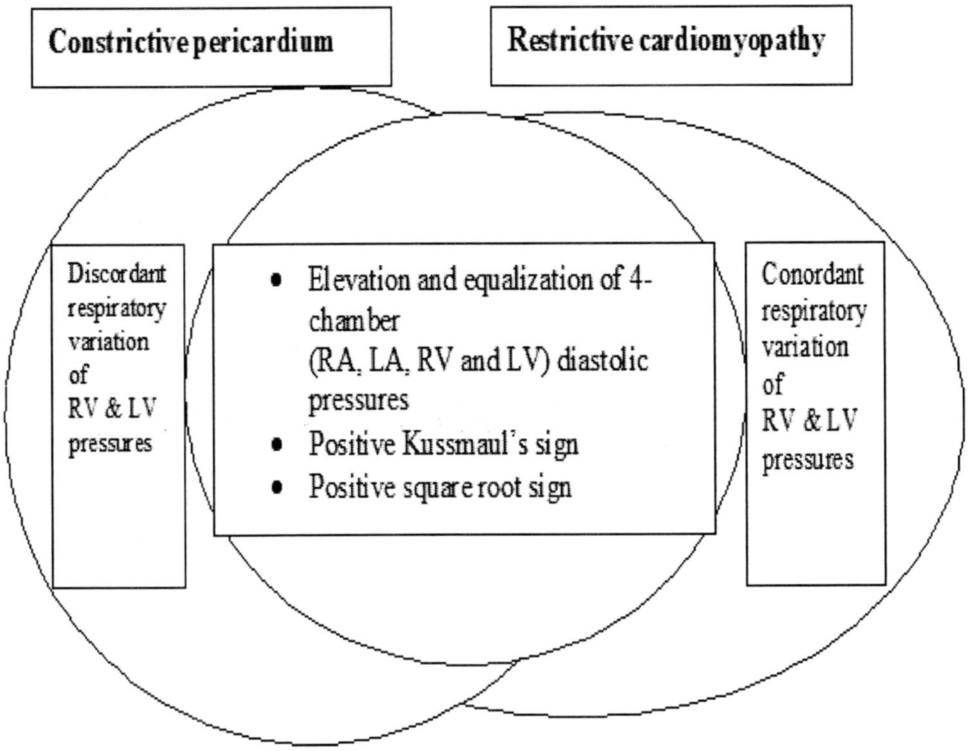

Figure 1. Similarities and dissimilarities between constrictive pericarditis and restrictive cardiomyopathy.

References

[1] Shah PK. Clinical applications of bedside hemodynamics monitoring using the Swan-Ganz catheter. *Physiologist* 1983; 26(1):43-5.

[2] Bonow RO, Carabello B, de Leon AC Jr, Edmunds LH Jr, Fedderly BJ, Freed MD, et al. Guidelines for the management of patients with valvular heart disease: executive summary. A report of the American College of Cardiology/American Heart Association Task Force on Practice Guidelines (Committee on Management of Patients with Valvular Heart Disease). *Circulation*. 1998; 98:1949-84.

[3] Gorlin, R, Gorlin, SG. Hydraulic formula for calculation of the area of the stenotic mitral valve, other cardiac valves, and central circulatory shunts. *Am. Heart J.* 1951; 41:1.

[4] Hakki AH, Iskandrian A, Benis C, Kimbris D, Mintz GS, Segal BL Brice C: A simplified valve formula for the calculation of stenotic cardiac valve areas. *Circulation* 1981; 63:1050-1055.

[5] Cannon, JD Jr, Zile, MR, Crawford, FA Jr, Carabello, BA. Aortic valve resistance as an adjunct to the Gorlin formula in assessing the severity of aortic stenosis in symptomatic patients. *J. Am. Coll Cardiol.* 1992; 20:1517.

[6] Cannon, SR, Richards, KL, Crawford, M. Hydraulic estimation of stenotic orifice area: a correction of the Gorlin formula. *Circulation* 1985; 71:1170.

[7] Carabello, BA. Advances in the hemodynamic assessment of stenotic cardiac valves. *J. Am. Coll Cardiol.* 1987; 10:912.

[8] Kern, MJ. Avoiding pitfalls in hemodynamic diagnosis. *ACC Current Journal Review*, Knoebel, SB (Ed) June 1997.

[9] Task Force on Practice Guidelines (Committee on Management of Patients with Valvular Heart Disease). ACC/AHA guidelines for the management of patients with valvular heart disease: a report of the Am College of Cardiology/Am. Heart Association. *J. Am. Coll Cardiol.* 1998; 32: 1486–1588.

[10] Kern M J, Aguirre F V. Interpretation of cardiac pathophysiology from pressure waveform analysis: Mitral valve gradients Part II. *Catheterization and Cardiovascular Diagnosis* 1992; 27(1): 52-56.

[11] Kern, MJ. 1991. The Cardiac Catheterization *Handbook. Mosby Year Book.* 116p. analysis.

[12] Snyder, RW, Glamann, B, Lange, RA, et al. Predictive value of prominent pulmonary arterial wedge v waves in assessing the presence and severity of mitral regurgitation. *Am. J. Cardiol.* 1994; 73:568.

[13] DeCristofaro, D, Liu, CK. The hemodynamics of cardiac tamponade and blood volume overload in dogs. *Cardiovasc. Res.* 1969; 3:292.

[14] Hansen, AT, Eskildsen, P, Gotzsche, H. Pressure curves from the right auricle and the right ventricle in chronic constrictive pericarditis. *Circulation* 1951; 3:881.

[15] Hancock EW. On the elastic and rigid forms of constrictive pericarditis. *Am. Heart J.* 1980; 100:917.

[16] Siegel R J, Shan P K, Fishbein M C. Idiopathic restrictive cardiomyopathy. *Circulation* 1984; 70(2): 165-169.

In: Drug Toxicity: New Research
Editor: Cam E. Vellotis, pp.89-187
ISBN 978-1-60456-320-7

Chapter 5

Rapid Efficacy and Favorable Toxicity of Artemisinin Derivatives Related to Drug Pharmacokinetic Profiles

Qigui Li and Peter J. Weina
Department of Pharmacology, Division of Experimental Therapeutics,
Walter Reed Army Institute of Research, Silver Spring 20910, USA

1. Abstract

Artemisinin and its developed derivatives, dihydroartemisinin (DHA), artemether (AM), arteether (AE), artesunate (AS), and artelinate (AL), are highly effective antimalarials with a favorable safety profile. Their pharmacodynamic effects against many stages of the malaria life cycle, from young asexual forms (ring) to early sexual forms (gametocytes), account for their rapid activity, which may protect them from resistance, In the past two decades, toxicity studies have shown a dose-dependent neurotoxic effect in animal species administered intramuscularly or intragastrically with artemisinins, especially with oil-soluble AM and AE. In contrast, few neurotoxic effects are induced by water-soluble AS and AL, which have never produced any CNS side-effects in animal species after intravenous injection. Pharmacokinetic profiles demonstrate that drug exposure time plays a more important role in producing neurotoxicity than drug exposure level, production of the more active metabolite (DHA), or drug location in the CNS system. In addition, it has been demonstrated that at a below human therapeutic dose, injectable AS can cause fetal death due to a build up of high peak concentration of AS during the sensitive period of the early gestation days (GD) in animals. To date, however, the neurotoxicity and reprotoxicity have not been convincingly established in humans treated with any of artemisinins. Fatal neurotoxicity can be avoided by reducing the drug exposure time that varies greatly between the different artemisinin compounds. Also reproductive toxicity can be avoided by limiting the exposure of artemisinins during this sensitive period in fetal development (GD 9–14 in rats and GD 15 to week 6 in humans).

Pharmacokinetic/pharmacodynamic evaluations demonstrate that the rapid efficacy of artemisinins is principally due to the drug peak concentration (Cmax) and their antimalarial potency. Other pharmacokinetic parameters, such as drug exposure level (AUC) and drug exposure time (half-life) tend to be of minor significance. The fundamental and reliable measures of efficacy in cure and mortality rates for uncomplicated and severe malaria show that current artemisinins (AS, AM, and DHA) have great role in artemisinin-based combination therapy (ACT) or monotherapy and provide a clear-cut advantage over other antimalarials currently in use. The artemisinin derivatives in combination with standard antimalarials are now being promoted as the best therapeutic option for treating drug-resistant malaria and retarding the development of resistant. There is clear evidence that combinations improve efficacy without increasing toxicity.

Most recently, a decrease in mortality (34.7%) has been demonstrated in a large study using intravenous AS, as opposed to the standard of care quinine injection. Artemisinins as a group are poorly efficacious at curing malaria as monotherapy. However, this shortfall has been overcome by using ACTs and AS injection in combination or in sequential administration with slower acting antimalarial drugs. When considering the demonstrated rapid parasite killing of parasites and variance between individual patients in both pharmacokinetics and pharmacodynamics, initial monotherapy and larger loading dose of AS injection may be needed to ensure that the maximum effect is obtained in all patients with severe and complicated malaria.

2. Introduction

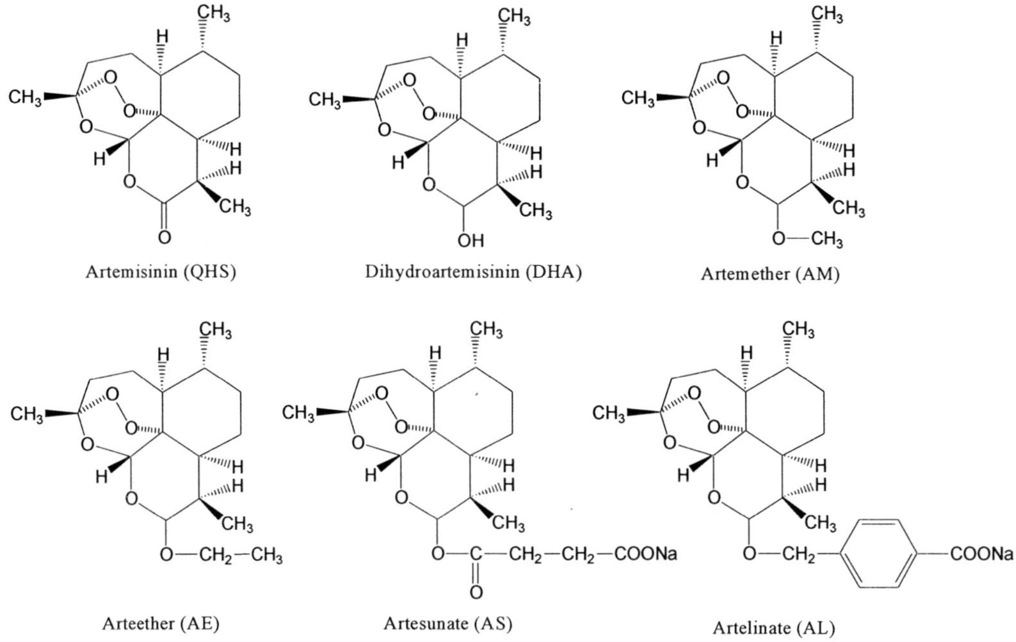

Figure 1. Structures of artemisinin (QHS) and its five derivatives, dihydroartemisinin (DHA), artemether (AM), arteether (AE), artesunate (AS) and artelinate (AL).

Artemisinin (QHS) has been identified as the active antimalarial principle of *qinghao*, a plant used for centuries to treat malaria in China. QHS and its developed derivatives, dihydroartemisinin (DHA), artemether (AM), arteether (AE), and artesunate (AS), are in use for the treatment of uncomplicated, complicated or severe malarias, including multidrug resistant *falciparum* malaria. Another derivative of QHS, artelinate (AL), is in the development of pre-clinical stage. These compounds have several advantages including the more rapid clearance of parasites in the periphery, more rapid resolution of fever, less toxicity and reduction in the transmission potential of *falciparum* malaria. Also, there have been no reports of parasite resistance to date. The chemical structures of the five-artemisinin derivatives and their parent, QHS, are presented in figure 1.

2.1. Efficacy Potency of Five Artemisinin Analogues *In Vitro* and *In Vivo*

Our *in vitro* testing [1] recently reported the relative antimalarial potency of artemisinin and control compounds against W-2 (chloroquine-resistant clone of *P. falciparum*) parasites are 0.004 (chloroquine) < 0.29 (mefloquine) < 0.72 (AL) < 1.0 (QHS) < 1.84 (AM) < 2.41 (AE) < 3.01 (AS) < 3.59 (DHA), and against D-6 (mefloquine-resistant clone of *P. falciparum*) parasites are 0.12 (mefloquine) < 0.16 (chloroquine) < 0.32 (AL) < 1.0 (QHS) < 1.22 (AM) < 1.87 (AE) < 2.48 (AS) < 2.99 (DHA). Artemisinin drugs were also evaluated against Chinese, Philippine and African isolates and clones of *P. falciparum*, and data showed a very similar order of antimalarial potency for the artemisinin derivatives (table 1) [2-4].

Table 1. In *vitro* sensitivity profile with 50% inhibitory concentration (IC_{50}) of artemisinin derivatives and positive control drugs against chloroquine-resistant clone of *P. falciparum* from Indochina (W2), mefloquine-resistant clone of *P. falciparum* from Sierra Leone (D6), Philippine and African isolators of *P. falciparum* by an isotopic microdilution drug sensitivity test using tritium-labeled hypoxanthine [1-3]

Compounds	W2 [1] ng/ml (n = 6)	D6 [1] ng/ml (n = 6)	Philippine [2] nM (n = 23-38)	Africa [3] nM (Range)
Artemisinin	0.83 ± 0.10	1.49 ± 0.04	2.8 ± 1.4	9.31 - 58.2
Dihydroartemisinin	0.28 ± 0.06	0.30 ± 0.09		
Artemether	0.48 ± 0.07	0.73 ± 0.24	1.4 ± 1.3	5.97 - 22.7
Arteether	0.37 ± 0.09	0.48 ± 0.14	0.9 ± 0.5	5.71 – 24.8
rtesunate	0.35 ± 0.12	0.36 ± 0.05	0.9 ± 0.5	
Artelinic acid	1.24 ± 0.15	2.78 ± 0.76		4.66 – 22.5
Chloroquine	202.7 ± 38.1	5.75 ± 1.23	43 ± 17	34.9 – 1670
Mefloquine	3.08 ± 0.90	7.24 ± 2.40	2 ± 0.5	20.8 – 97.1

Values are mean ± SD; W-2: Indochina clone, resistant to chloroquine, sensitive to mefloquine. D-6: Sierra Leone clone, sensitive to chloroquine, resistant to mefloquine.

Results indicated that DHA and AS were shown to be more highly effective than other artemisinin derivatives. Stage-specific activity of the five-artemisinin analogues differed from that of quinine-type antimalarials, and each derivative displayed a unique stage-specific profile. DHA was highly effective against all parasite stages of *P. falciparum* isolates and clones, in most cases achieving 100% growth inhibition within 2-4 h of exposure [5]. QHS, and to a lesser extent AM, were most active against rings and schizonts, demonstrating relatively little activity against trophozoites stage of *Plasmodium falciparum* [5-7]. AE, AS, and AL were most effective against the late-stage ring parasites and trophozoites stages of *P. falciparum, P. cynomolgi, P. vinckei petteri and P. berghei* [8-15]. Compared with DHA, other artemisinin drugs including artemisinin itself only achieve 60-80% growth inhibition that lasted 3-10 hours longer (table 2).

Table 2. Stage-specific sensitivity and growth inhibition of artemisinin derivatives with different isolates and clones of *Plasmodium falciparum* in vitro [5-15]

Drugs effects	Erythrocytic stages			Gametocyto-cidal effects	Parasite growth inhibitory with drug exposure time (hr)*		
	Ring	Tropho-zoites	Schizonts		100%	60-80%	30-50%
QHS	+	+	+	+	6-12	6-10	1-3
DHA	++	++	++	+	2-4		1-2
AM	++		+			8-10	1-6
AE	++	+		+			
AS	++	+		+			
AL	+	+		+		3-6	

*Drug concentration in the culture exposure tests was 10^{-5}-10^{-6} M. QHS = artemisinin, DHA = Dihydroartemisinin, AM = Artemether, AE = Arteether, AS = Artesunate, AL = Artelinate

In general, the stage dependency of drug effects decreased with increasing drug concentrations and exposure times. Stage specificity of drug effect was particularly dependent on exposure time for the artemisinin drugs [9]. The stage-specific sensitivities and growth inhibitions of the artemisinin drugs are summarized in table 2. Only DHA was rapidly effective against all stages of the parasite life cycle and completely inhibited the parasite growth within the shortest exposure time (2-4 hr). Since AS is prodrug of DHA in intro and in vivo [16], these results confirm the greater in vitro potency of DHA compared to the other artemisinin derivatives.

In vivo studies in animal species using the *P. berghei*-infected mouse model, the *P. falciparum*-infected Aotus monkey, and the *P. cynomolgi* infection in rhesus monkey have confirmed that artemisinin and derivatives are highly effective antimalarial compounds. In the mouse model (table 3), the dose of AM and AE curing 50% of infected mice (CD_{50}) had a mean value of 55 mg/kg following single subcutaneous injection [17]. The mean dose for AS and AL was 421 and 211 mg/kg, respectively, after daily for 3 consecutive days subcutaneously [18], suggesting that AL showed two-fold greater antimalarial activity than AS in mice via this route of administration. In the Aotus monkey model, the ED_{50} were 7.1 mg/kg for AM and 11.8 mg/kg for AE during 3 days treatments [17]. In addition, AE is curative at a dose of 5 mg/kg for 3 days after intramuscular administration against blood-induced *P. cynomolgi* infection in rhesus monkey [19]. The curative dose of AS is 3.3 mg/kg initially and then 1.7 mg/kg at 8 and 24 hr after the first intravenous dose in rhesus monkeys infected with *P. coatneyi* [20].

The comparison of the therapeutic potential in monotherapy of artemisinin drugs in humans for 3-5 days treatments is summarized in table 4 [21-43]. The rates of recrudescence, fever, and parasite clearances are traditional parameters for the efficacy of the antimalarial drugs in humans. These three parameters exhibit the therapeutic potential of intramuscular AE with sesame oil (Artemotil), which has much less efficacy [21, 22] compared to that of intramuscular AM [23-32], oral and intravenous AS [33, 34], and the oral DHA [35-38], or even than that of intramuscular α/β-arteether formulated with peanut oil [39-43] in India. It is clear that the efficacy of artemisinins *in vivo* (animal species and humans) is different compared to that of artemisinin drugs *in vitro*.

Table 3. In *vivo* sensitivity profiles with 50% curative total dose (CD_{50}, mg/kg) in mice (mg/kg) of artemisinin and its derivatives against *P. berghei* by an isotopic microdilution drug sensitivity test using tritium-labeled hypoxanthine [17-20]

Compounds	Intragastric (b.i.d x 5D)	Subcutaneous (Single)	Subcutaneous (Daily x 3D)
Artemisinin	469 (365-641)	778 (348-1737)	161 (102-259)
Dihydroartemisinin	85 (66-109)	-	
Artemether		52-71	
Arteether		30-72	
Artesunate	170 (132-217)	-	421 (273-875)
Artelinic acid	170 (132-217)	-	211 (129-376)

Values are given as median (95% confidence limits).

2.2. Basic Pharmacokinetic Parameters of Five Artemisinin Derivatives

The pharmacokinetics of artemisinin and its five derivatives are not yet known in very much detail in humans, but it has been clearly defined in animal species [44-49]. The five-artemisinin analogues have been compared under the same conditions in rats following intravenous, intramuscular, and intragastric administration. The intravenous results showed the basic parameters of PK for the five compounds in table 5, and the intravenous results of DHA, AM and AE were first reported with cremophore formulation [44]. All five artemisinin derivatives exhibited a rapid elimination (0.4-1.4 hr) and biphasic decline in plasma concentration after intravenous administration.

The data shows that AL has the highest plasma level, the slowest elimination half-life, the lowest volume of distribution, and the slowest total clearance when compared with the other four artemisinins. Considering that the dose of AM or DHA is 140 or 147% the dose of artelinic acid in molecular weight, the equal-molecular weight is analyzed in deriving the results. When C_{max} and AUC are recalculated on a μM basis, AL C_{max} and AUC are still higher than other four-artemisinin analogues (table 5). AL was not only stable in vitro in aqueous solution and biological fluid, but also stable in vivo for biotransformation [18, 45, 50, 51]. The data also shows that AE and AS, which was converted almost immediately into DHA and other metabolites, had very low C_{max} and AUC when compared with the other three drugs, suggesting that these two compounds had been rapidly and extensively metabolized in rats. Although AM and AE are oil-soluble agents with very similar chemical strictures (Figure 1), AM showed better pharmacokinetic profiles with higher C_{max} (6231 ng/ml) and AUC (1857 ng·h/ml) than that AE with 3724 ng/ml of C_{max} and 842 ng·h/ml of AUC at a same dose level.

Table 4. Summary of 54 clinical trials of artemisinin derivatives monotherapy in treatment of patients with uncomplicated, complicated, and severe malarias. Values are given mean ± SD. [21-43]

Drug and Regimen	PCT (hr)	FCT (hr)	% of Recru descence	Clinical Trials No.
AE with sesame oil (Artemotil) [21,22]				
(IM 3.2 mg/kg-1.6 mg/kg x 4)	70.2	81.0	40.0	1
(IM 4.8 mg/kg-1.6 mg/kg x 5)	59.2	61.5	22.2	1
AM [23-32]				
(IM 3.2 mg/kg-1.6 mg/kg x 4)	28.3 ± 13.0	38.8 ± 4.4	8.6 ± 6.2	8
(Oral 200 mg-100 mg/kg x 5)	39.7 ± 2.2	34.8 ± 6.9	5.2 ± 2.2	9
AS [33, 34]				
(IV and oral in various regimens)	30.3 ± 10.7	35.9 ± 11.1	7.5 ± 3.1	23
DHA [35-38]				
(Oral in various regimens)	49.1 ± 7.5	33.8 ± 7.7	6.0 ± 1.8	7
AE with peanut oil [39-43]				
(IM 150 mg daily for 3 days)	37.8 ± 12.2	49.9 ± 16.2	9.4 ± 4.1	5

IM = intramuscular, IV = intravenous, PCT = parasite clearance time, FCT = Fever clearance time.

Table 5. Comparison of main pharmacokinetic parameters of artemisinin derivatives (DHA, AM, AE, AS and AL) at 10 mg/kg in rats following single intravenous injection. Values are mean ± SD (n = 4) [44]

Parameters	DHA	AM	AE	AS	AL
MW =	284.9	298.4	312.4	384.4	418.5
Dose (mg/kg)	10	10	10	10	10
Dose (μM/kg)	35.1	33.5	32.0	26.0	23.9
IV Vehicles	CMP	1:3 CMP/saline		0.9% saline (pH 8.5)*	
C_{max}					
(ng/ml)	6683 ± 2405	6231 ± 1837	3724 ± 430	2106 ± 399	12706 ±1010
(μM)	23.5 ± 13.0	20.9 ± 6.2	11.9 ± 1.4	5.5 ± 1.0	30.4 ± 2.2
AUC					
(ng•h/ml)	3184 ± 659	1857 ± 432	842 ± 154	738 ± 114	5481 ± 1754
(μM•h)	11.2 ± 2.3	6.2 ± 1.4	2.7 ± 0.5	1.9 ± 0.3	13.1 ± 3.8
Vss					
(liter)	0.50 ± 0.19	0.67 ± 0.11	0.72 ± 0.09	0.87 ± 0.35	0.39 ± 0.12
CL					
(ml/min/kg)	55.4 ± 9.7	91.8 ± 21.0	200.0 ± 31.0	190.9 ± 30.3	32.1 ± 8.0
t1/2					
(distribution, h)	0.22 ± 0.04	0.10 ± 0.01	0.10 ± 0.02	0.15 ± 0.02	0.19 ± 0.08
t1/2					
(elimination, h)	0.95 ± 0.21	0.53 ± 0.14	0.45 ± 0.03	0.35 ± 0.08	1.35 ± 0.45

CMP = Cremophore EL, DHA = Dihydroartemisinin, AM = Artemether, AE = Arteether, AS = Artesunic acid , AL = Artelinic acid, MW = Molecular weight, IV = intravenous; *pH adjusted to 8.5 with 1N $NaHCO_3$.

2.3. Neurotoxicity of Artemisinins in Animal Species

CNS neurotoxicity has been demonstrated in mice, rats, dogs, and rhesus monkeys that have been repeatedly administered with oil-soluble analogues of AM or AE at multiple doses of 5-24 mg/kg /day [52-55]. Studies show that AM and AE are toxic to the central nervous system and induce neuropathologic changes in these animals. The neurotoxic findings produced by artemisinins in animal species are summarized in table 6. Neuropathology has been detected in dogs given an AE dose of 5.0 – 6.75 mg/kg daily for 28 days [56-58]. The same neuropathology was found in rats at a dose of 12.5 mg/kg of AE given daily for 7 days [59] and in monkeys at 8 mg/kg of AE for 14 days [55]. However, clinical signs (ataxia and shaking) of neurotoxicity appeared at significantly higher doses in dogs (20 mg/kg, 7 days), in rats (50 mg/kg, 7 days), and in monkeys (24 mg/kg, 14 days) [54-56, 60]. This suggests that by the time neurological signs are observed in those animals, the drug concentrations are already three or four times higher than the doses known to cause neuropathologic changes. In other words, the doses to produce clinical and neurotoxic signs are much higher (3- to 4-fold) than that to generate the neuropathological findings confirmed in those animal species.

Table 6. Neurotoxicity findings in pathological and behavioral evaluation in animal species treated with dihydroartemisinin (DHA), artemether (AM), arteether (AE), artesunate (AS) and artelinate (AL) following multiple intramuscular (IM) and intragastric or oral administrations (n = 4-20) [53-65]

Drug	Species	Pathological Neurotoxicity				Behavioral Neurotoxicity			
		Dose mg/kg	Route	Regimen	Refs	Dose mg/kg	Route	Regimen	Refs
AE	Rats	12.5	IM	7 daily	[53, 59]	50	IM	7 daily	[60]
	Dogs	5-7	IM	28 daily	[56-58]	20	IM	7 daily	[56]
	Monkeys	8	IM	14 daily	[55]	24	IM	14 daily	[55]
AM	Dog	20	IM	8 daily	[66]				
	Mice					150	IM	28 daily	[62, 64]
	Mice					300	oral	28 daily	
	Mice	300	oral	28 twice daily	[63]				
AS	Mice					250	IM	28 daily	[62, 64]
	Mice					200	oral	28 daily	[62, 64]
	Mice	300	oral	28 twice daily	[63]				
AL	Rats	160	oral	9 daily	[61]				
DHA	Mice	200	oral	28 daily	[63]	200	oral	28 daily	[63]

DHA = dihydroartemisinin, AM = artemether, AE = arteether, AS = artesunic acid, AL = artelinic acid; IM = intramuscular, Refs = References.

Despite extensive studies with AM and AE neurotoxicity, there is limited evidence of neurotoxicity in animals related to the water soluble artemisinin derivatives, for example AS, the most widely used artemisinin in humans. AL, another water-soluble artemisinin derivative, has also been reported to have some pathological neurotoxicity in rats following intragastric dose at 160 mg/kg daily for 9 days [61]. These studies help us see that the neurotoxicity of oil-soluble artemisinins is more potent than that of water-soluble analogues (table 6). The neurotoxicity of AL has been investigated in beagle dogs following daily oral administration at 25, 100, and 300 mg/kg dose levels for 14 days. No behavioral neurotoxicity has been observed in these beagle dogs at these doses. The considerable lack of toxicity detected in these dogs very well may be caused by very low oral bioavailability at these doses. Actually, in the highest dose level (300 mg/kg), the animals only received one-fifth of total dose due to the very low bioavailability (22%, our unpublished data). A recent study looked at AM, AS, and DHA orally administered daily for 28 days has helped us compare the two groups. There were little clinical or neuropathologic evidence of the neurotoxicity found at high dose levels of over 200 mg/kg/day in mice for the 3 drugs [62-64]. At the highest doses of intramuscular AM and AS, there was neurotoxicity and behavioral deficits of potentially irreversible abnormalities in balance and equilibrium. AM was determined to have much greater neurotoxicity than intramuscular AS though [64, 65].

The water-soluble artemisinin derivatives, AS and AL, were designed for intravenous injection. To date, no neurotoxicity (pathologic or behavioural) has been observed in animal species following intravenous administration at any repeated doses up to maximum tolerated doses (MTD). The MTDs of AS and AL are 240 and 80 mg/kg, respectively, following intravenous injection daily in rats for 3 days, but no neurotoxicity was detected in these animals [66]. In another study, intravenous AS had no effect on the neurotoxic scores at 120 mg/kg in sodium carbonate daily for 7 days (our unpublished data). After one intramuscular injection, a high dose of 420 mg/kg of AS and AL did not produce any neuronal necrosis in the rats. Also, up to 200 mg/kg of AS used orally daily for 5-7 days did not exhibit neuronal changes or any specific clinical signs [56].

Although artemisinin agents, mainly oil-soluble drugs, induced fatal neurotoxicity in animal models, a striking fact in treating patients with the artemisinins is the lack of any serious adverse events, despite careful monitoring in several clinical studies. Severe malarial infection itself, particularly cerebral malaria in multi-drug resistant strains in the developing world, often leaves patients with decreases in neural function. This development has made characterization of potential neurotoxic effects of the artemisinin derivatives very difficult to ascertain, even though these drugs are clinically utilized in ever growing numbers [67-69]. In a study of 3500 patients in Thailand, evidence of serious toxicity was not noticed [70]. From other reports, rare neurological side effects have been noted in humans receiving artemisinin drugs [71-76], and these findings were difficult to dissect from effects due to the concomitant malarial infection.

2.4. Neurotoxicity of Artemisinins in Humans?

A number of studies indicate that no neuralgic side effects are noted in humans from QHS, AM, AS, and DHA treatments. Even AE was safely used from phase I to III clinical trial studies [77-79]. However, a 36-year-old American geologist had neurological symptoms two days after completing AS treatment with worsening ataxia and slurred speech nine days after completing AS treatment [80]. Two months later, the patient still had slurred speech; a wide-based, ataxic gait; and impaired heel-to-shin and rapid alternating movement. He was re-treated with oral quinine and doxycycline after testing positive again for *Plasmodium* species (too scant to speciate) in a smear. Four months later, his ataxia was moderately improved, and his speech was nearly normal. In another case report, a 39-year-old man who returned from Sierra Leone with probable extrapyramidal syndrome that was self-limiting. He had an undetermined febrile illness for which he had received inappropriately long and repeated courses of both AS and chloroquine [81, 82]. Franco-Paredes et al. concluded that the patient's condition "suggests neurotoxicity due to multiple courses of AS therapy, perhaps compounded by chloroquine therapy [83]. However, Newton et al. pointed out that the patient was most likely suffering from the adverse effects of excessive chloroquine [84].

Certainly, these two reports do not constitute proof of any causal association, but the possibility that repeated administration of artemisinin drugs in malaria endemic areas will result in cumulative damage cannot be ruled out [85], especially since these drugs are often freely available for use in tropical countries [86]. However, another four patients experienced neuropsychiatric adverse events. One patient with history of epilepsy, seizure-free for 10 years, had an episode of tonic-clonic seizures; one patient suffered from anxiety, palpitations and sleep disturbance; one developed frank psychosis and another, depression. These patients were also receiving mefloquine though, a known cause of neuropsychiatric disturbances [87].

In the Gambian children with cerebral malaria described by van Hensbrock [23], intramuscular AM was associated with more convulsions (39 vs. 28%, P = 0.01) and more prolonged coma than was intramuscular quinine (26 vs. 20 hr, P = 0.05). Similar results were found in Vietnamese adults [24]. Survival analysis indicated a significant divergence in the times to recovery from coma among patients who remained unconscious for more than two days. In these patients, treatment with AM was associated with slower recovery than that of quinine dosing (66 vs. 48 hr, P = 0.003). Although in the current reports there was no increase in neurological sequelae in patients after multiple treatments with AM, significantly prolonged coma in both studies and increased incidence of convulsions in the AM group of Gamnian children indicates the need for further attentiveness and active investigation of the neurological side effects of artemisinin drugs. A recent report from Mozambique describes a small but significant and irreversible hearing loss in patients exposed to AM-lumefantrine [88, 89]. The results of this trial are controversial though as the treatment group had both malaria and treatment with AM-lumefantrine and the control group had neither. In another case control study, there were no differences in the test results between cases and controls. There was no neurophysiologic evidence of auditory trainstem toxicity that could be attributed to AM-lumefantrine in this study population [90].

Either intravenous followed by oral AS, or oral followed by intravenous AS were given at a dose of 2 mg/kg for 2 days to patients with uncomplicated acute *P. falciparum* malaria [91]. At the time of presentation the patients had been ill for a median of 3 days (range, 1 to 10 days) with fever, headache, anorexia, nausea, and vomiting. No adverse effects of the study drug were observed. In another trial, quinine plus tretracycline versus oral AS given at a total dose of 700 mg over 5 days was studied in patients with acute uncomplicated falciparum malaria [92]. The occurrence of adverse effects, such as tinnitus, was significantly higher in the quinine-tetracycline group. Nausea and dizziness were rather commonly associated with the AS group in this study. Toxicity has also been observed after 5 days of multiple intramuscular doses with AE. One person out of 14 subjects developed shiverers, clammy hands and feet, dizziness, headache, nausea and a 'metallic taste' 1 hr after the injection; the symptoms lasted about one hour and then were resolved spontaneously [93]. In view of their potential for neurological adverse effects, artemisinin analogues after multiple treatments should be borne in mind. Karbwang [92], Kager [93], Hoffeman [94], and Park [95] expressed concern about the potential neurotoxicity of all artemisinin derivatives, which are the drugs of choice for treating severe malaria caused by parasites with suspected resistance to chloroquine and quinine.

2.5. Reproductive Toxicity of Artemisinins in Animals

The artemisinin derivatives (mainly AM and AS) have been extensively studied in animals and in humans, and the experience in human pregnancy are encouraging. However, artemisinins have been shown to be very toxic to animal embryos in repeated preclinical studies. This preclinical data included in vivo embryo–fetal developmental toxicity studies carried out on mice, rats, hamsters, guinea pig, and rabbits, by different laboratories using for the most part ICH-compliant protocols [96-103].

Early study of QHS and AM were conducted in mice, rats and rabbits that were intramuscularly from gestation day (GD) 6 to 15 to observe for reproductive toxicity. The no observed adverse effect level (NOAEL) was 5.4 mg/kg in mice, 2.7 mg/kg in rats and 0.7 mg/kg/day in rabbits; above these doses, there were increased resorptions of fetuses: 100% resorption at 21.4 mg/kg/day in mice, > 90% resorption at 10.7 mg/kg/day in rats and >90% resorption at 2.7 mg/kg/day in rabbits [96, 97]. By subcutaneous administration, the study of AS was dosed in rats from GD 6 to 15, and the developmental retardation of sterna and ribs was noted in surviving fetuses in groups treated with 0.54 mg/kg of AS respectively. The dose that induced 50% fetuses resorbed (ED_{50}) was 0.58 mg/kg [98]. When rats were given a dose of 26 mg/kg/day at GD 1–6, 82.3% of fetuses survived. When the same dose was given in early organogenesis, GD 6–8, only 17.1% of fetuses survived, and treatment occurring after GD 8 resulted in 100% fetal resorption [98]. Recently, our study of AS was also performed in rats following intravenous and intramuscular injection from GD 5 to 15. The ED_{50} of AS after intravenous dosing was 0.61 mg/kg [99].

In experiments carried out in mice, hamsters, guinea pigs and rabbits both DHA and AS intragastrically, intramuscularly, or subcutaneously showed from mild to severe embryolethality effect. In mice and rabbits they caused embryo absorption whereas in hamsters and guinea pigs they induced abortion [100]. In rats, oral AS was administered from GD 6–19. The primary reported effect was embryo–fetal loss manifested as abortion in rabbits and resorption in both rats and rabbits. The no or low adverse effect levels were in the range of 5 to 7 mg/kg/day AS [101]. All preclinical studies of the reproductive toxicity in animal species are summarized in table 7. AS has the greatest toxicity to animal embryos by routes of subcutaneous, intramuscular and intravenous injections with less than 1 mg/kg of the ED_{50}, which is lower than therapeutic dose of 2-4 mg/kg in humans. [103]

Table 7. Embryotoxic effects (NOAEL and ED_{50}) of artemisinin (QHS), dihydroartemisinin (DHA), artemether (AM), artesunate (AS) given intragastrically, intramuscularly, subcutaneously, and intravenously on pregnant animal species (female mice, rats, hamster, guinea pig, and rabbits) [97-102]

Animals (Drugs)	Dose Duration (daily)	Dose Regimens	Dosing Routes	No-observed-adverse-effect-level (NOAEL) Oral	IM	SC	IV	ED_{50} (95% CL) (mg/kg)
Mice (AM) [97]	GD6-15	Multiple x 10	IM		5.4			11.3 (10.6-12.0)
(DHA) [100]	GD7	Single	SC			10		32.8 (27.7-38.9)
Rats (QHS) [96]	GD1-6	Multiple x 6	Oral	5.6				11.5 (10.5-12.2)
(DHA) [102]	GD9.5, 10.5	Single	Oral	7.5				NA
(AM) [97]	GD6-15	Multiple x 10	IM		2.7			6.13 (4.52-8.26)
(AM) [97]	GD6-15	Multiple x 10	Oral	2.5				14.4 (10.4-17.8)
(AS) [98]	GD6-15	Multiple x 10	SC			0.2		0.58 (0.55-0.61)*
(AS) [99]	GD6-18	Multiple x 11	IM		0.5		0.4	0.61 (0.59-0.62)*
(AS) [101]	GD6-17	Multiple x 12	Oral	5-7				7.74 (6.92-8.57)
Hamster (DHA) [100]	GD7	Singl	SC			4.2		6.06 (5.90-6.21)
(DHA) [100]	GD7	Singl	Oral	20				51.0 (37.9-68.7)
(AS) [100]	GD5	Singl	SC			0.35		1.0 (0.9-1.2)*
Guinea Pig (DHA) [100]	GD18	Single	IM		2.5			18.3 (13.9-24.2)
Rabbits (AM) [97]	GD7-18	Multiple x 12	IM		0.7			NA
(AS) [101]	GD7-19	Multiple x 13	Oral	5-7				NA
(DHA) [100]	GD9	Single	IM		5			7.57 (7.48-7.67)

DHA = Dihydroartemisinin; AM = Artemether; AS = Artesunate; IM = intramuscular; SC = subcutaneous; IV = intravenous; ED_{50} = drug concentration induces 50% fetus resorbed; GD = gestation day (The day of mating was defined as day 0 of gestation.); * The severe toxic effects were detected in the animals treated with AS after single or multiple intramuscular, intravenous or subcutaneous injections. Values of ED_{50} are given as median (95% confidence limits). NA = not available.

Some recent studies found that tissue damage in embryos exposed to DHA affect primarily red blood cells during yolk sac hematopoiesis and higher concentrations and/or longer exposure inhibited angiogenesis [102, 104, 105]. Another study in rats showed that AS subcutaneous injection at a dose of 40 mg/kg/d during days 6-10 of gestation significantly decreased the concentration of serum progesterone in early pregnant rats and discontinued the degeneration of decidual cells and fetuses [106]. In cell culture, AS significantly decreased rat embryonic and placental glutathione peroxidase (GSH-Px) and increased malondialdehyde (MDA) level in these tissues [107].

The WHO expert panel judged from their review of these and 28 other experimental laboratory reports that in animals "all the artemisinin analogues have been associated with embryolethality over a narrow dose range and that there are instances of effects on development of the cardiovascular system, the axial skeleton and the limbs", but that "these do not suggest the nature of the toxic action." They considered that "because the safety data are limited, artemisinin compounds should only be used in the second and third trimester when other treatments are considered unsuited" [108].

Thus, an important population at high risk for malaria will continue to be excluded from treatment with artemisinin based combination therapy unless these treatments are shown to be effective and safe in pregnancy. Two early reports in China on pregnant women described that the effects of QHS, AM or AS were not found evident of drug toxicity [109, 110]. There were 94 cases of first trimester exposure to AS identified in the published literature [111, 112] and no unexpected adverse effects were reported. In areas of multi-drug resistance, only treatments based on artemisinin compounds were effective, and pregnant women have been treated for malaria with these drugs throughout pregnancy. Data from limited series of pregnant women (2,045 cases) exposed to artemisinin compounds, including a small number (108 cases) in the first trimester, did not show an increase in the rates of abortion or stillbirth or evidence of abnormalities. There were no clinically significant adverse effect of the drugs, on the outcomes of the pregnancies, or the development (neurological and physical) of the infants, including 44 infants exposed during the first trimester [112-120]. Treatment with AS during pregnancy is associated with higher birthweight, which may have resulted from clearance of malaria parasites, as placental malaria is associated with reduced birthweight [121]. However, the influence of confounding factors should not be excluded.

2.6. Current Use of Artemisinins Alone and Combination Regimens

In view of the fact that certain artemisinin drugs have produced fatal neurotoxicity and reproductive toxicities (in animals only), high recrudescent rate, poor oral bioavailability, and short half-lives, especially, intramuscular AE and AM were not successful in the clinical trials by monotherapy [21-24]. Artemisinin-based combination therapies (ACTs) are most preferred for their enhancement of efficacy [122-124], lower malaria incidence and their potential to lower the rate at which resistance emerges and spreads [125, 126]. Four ACTs recommended by a WHO Expert Consultative Group in 2001 are AM-lumefantrine (Coartem), AS-mefloquine (Artequin), AS-amodiaquine, and AS-sulfadoxine/pyrimethamine

[127]. Recently, WHO has endorsed ACTs as the "policy standard" for all malaria infections in areas where *P. falciparum* is the predominant infecting species [128].

The rapid parasite clearance of artemisinin drugs in the treatment of early cases of uncomplicated malaria with ACTs may prevent its progression to severe disease with consequent reduction in severe cases and mortality rate. AM-Lumefantrine was the first registered, fixed, ACT treatment, and constitutes about 70% of all current clinically-used ACTs [129]. It is highly effective when given twice a day for three days (6-dose) and with a small amount of fat [130, 131]. This is because lumefantrine has to be given with food (preferably containing fat) to ensure adequate absorption and thus efficacy. In an initial study with a 4-dose AM-lumefantrine regimen, there was a relatively high rate of late treatment failure (E1) [132]. In the study in an area with high-grade mefloquine resistance, the 6-dose AM-lumefantrine regimen was associated with a 28% treatment failure at 14 days (E3) [133]. Another ACT treatment, AS-mefloquine, has been used in South-East Asian countries such as Thailand and Cambodia, widely since 1994 and remains highly effective for uncomplicated falciparum malaria. Under the WHO system of efficacy assessment, more than 95% of patients will remain free of malaria 28 days after such treatment (E2) [134, 135]. However, the failure rate of AS-mefloquine combination has been reported to be up to 13% in Thailand and Cambodia [136], and the neuropsychiatric effects of mefloquine as well as its relative expense are problematic [137].

Monotherapy with the artemisinins was significantly decreased after 2001 to prevent the experiencing resistance. For complicated and severe malaria, however, intravenous AS, as monotherapy, is still in first line treatment for both adults and children in Asian countries [138], and some areas in Africa [139]. Trying to replace quinine (which has been the principal drug used to treat severe malaria for nearly 400 years) with a more effective, less expensive, and better tolerated drug [140], an initial trial using intramuscular AM demonstrated less toxicity but no clear mortality benefit over quinine [141, 142]. More recent trials have used intravenous AS with a more favorable pharmacokinetic profile [143, 144]. The SEAQUAMAT trial, a multicentre randomized trial conducted in Bangladesh, Thailand, Myanmar, Indonesia, India and Vietnam, recently reported a 34.7% reduction in all cause mortality associated with intravenous AS compared with intravenous quinine [138, 145, 146]. This is the largest trial ever performed in severe malaria and the first to demonstrate conclusively a mortality benefit over standard quinine therapy. There is convincing evidence that for those who do develop severe malaria, intravenous AS will reduce the risk of death by one-third when compared to quinine therapy. For the 202 children included in the trial, artesunate injection was equally safe and effective [145].

Almost immediately intravenous AS was recommended for patients with severe malaria by The European Network on Imported Infections Disease Surveillance (TropNetEurop) [147]. The most recent advance in antimalarial chemotherapy has been the use of artemisinin derivatives, especially intravenous AS, which may well revolutionize the management of complicated and severe malaria [148]. Therefore, we still need AS monotherapy [149]. However, there is currently no product available that is produced under good manufacturing practice (GMP) conditions. Walter Reed Army Institute of Research (WRAIR) has being developed a novel cGMP injection of AS since 2003, which is in the process of US FDA approval [66, 150].

2.7. The Objectives of the Chapter

Several perplexities continue to vex us with the artemisinins [151]. Why does this neurotoxicity mostly occur in animals treated with oil-soluble artemisinins (with sesame oil vehicle), but not or less with water-soluble agents? Why does the neurotoxicity induced by artemisinins depending on drug exposure time but not on drug exposure level? Why does the neurotoxicity and reproductive toxicity so easily observed in animal models not occur in humans getting equal or even higher doses of the drug? Why does the efficacy of artemisinins depend upon drug peak concentration (C_{max}) but not drug exposure level or time? In this review based on Walter Reed Army Institute of Research and other research data from recent two decades, the pharmacokinetic characteristics will be evaluated and discussed that may shed light on some of these questions. Principally, the discussion will be: 1) neurotoxicity concerning drug pharmacokinetics; 2) pharmacokinetic role in reproductive toxicity; 3) relationship between drug efficacy and pharmacokinetics; and 4) how to maintain rapid efficacy and avoid lethal toxicities. This review will also summarise current artemisinin (and its derivatives) developments and outline clinical research on efficacy and toxicity that aims to bring artemisinin-based combinations to those that need them most.

3. Neurotoxicity Concerning Drug Pharmacokinetics

3.1. The Role of DHA in Neurotoxicity

DHA is obtained by sodium borohydride reduction of artemisinin, an endoperoxide containing sesquiterpene lactone; this was isolated by Chinese researchers and characterized as the antimalarial principle of the plant *Artemisia annua.* Through *in-vitro* bioassay tests, DHA has been shown to be 1.4-5.2 folds more active than other artemisinins [1-3, 18-20] but has also been shown to be 2-4 folds more toxic than other artemisinins in vitro and in vivo [152-156]. Due to its poor solubility in water or oils, DHA has only been formulated as an oral preparation and has been used primarily as a semisynthetic compound for derivatization to other oil soluble and water-soluble artemisinins [33]. The effectiveness of AS has been attributed to its rapid and extensive hydrolysis to DHA [16, 44, 143, 157, 158). The efficacy of AM and AE has also been credited to the conversion to DHA, but their conversion rates were significantly lower and less complete than in AS [16, 44]. AL is a very stable artemisinin agent *in vitro* and *in vivo*, and has almost no biotransformation to DHA in animal species [18, 45].

Thus, evaluating the conversion rates of various artemisinin drugs is very important for assessing the risk of neurotoxicity for the four compounds that are the focus of this article. A conversion evaluation of AM, AE, AS, or AL to DHA is summarized in table 8 [27, 29, 65, 159-176]. The summary shown illustrates that the conversion of artemisinin drugs to DHA in humans, which seem to be much more efficient than that in other animal species. Compared to the data from animal species and humans treated with AM or AS, the ratios of AUC_{DHA} to

$AUC_{AM\ or\ AS}$ are significantly higher in humans (0.4-9.7) than in animal species (0.04-2.7), suggesting that the human hydrolysis system is more active and complete.

Table 8. Mean ratios of AUC_{DHA} (an active metabolite) /$AUC_{AM\ or\ AE,\ AS,\ and\ AL}$, and the concentration values of $AUC_{DHA}/AUC_{AM\ or\ AE,\ AS,\ and\ AL}$ in ng·h/ml as the conversion evaluation of artemisinin derivatives (AM, AE, AS, and AL) to DHA in animal species and humans. [27, 157-163]

Drugs	Animal Species		Humans	
	Rats [44]	Dogs	Volunteers	Patients
Artemether (AM)				
Intravenous	0.04 (65/1857)			
Intramuscular	0.07 (71/1007)		0.41–1.62 [a]	1.06 [b]
Oral	0.10 (38/366)		1.12-7.69 [c]	1.42–8.55 [d]
Arteether (AE)				
Intravenous	0.04 (29/842)			
Intramuscular	0.15 (43/286)	0.23 (181/804) [159]		
Oral	0.17 (50/298			
Artesunate (AS)				
Intravenous	0.64 (474/738)	0.50 (778/1533)[160]		2.81–8.12 [e]
Intramuscular	0.31 (236/773)	0.73 (1109/1521)[160]		
Oral	2.74 (595/217)	0.45 (299/660) [160]	4.29–5.36 [f]	6.35–9.71 [g]
Rectal			2.31[170]	
Artelinic acid (AL)				
Intravenous	0.01 (63/12706)	0.001 (7/11262) [45]		
Intramuscular	0.01 (44/5023)	0.003 (23/10195) [45]		
Oral	0.03 (62/1650)	0.002 (14/8849) [45]		

References: [a] = [27, 161], [b] = [162], [c] = [161-171], [d] = [161-172], [e] = [158, 173], [f] = [174-176], [g] = [91, 157, 158, 161, 176]; DHA = dihydroartemisinin.

In the animal species, the conversion rates are different with the four artemisinin agents. The highest hydrolysis found for AS are in rats and dogs with the DHA/AS ratio in the range of 0.31-2.74, whereas less than 0.23 of the ratio of DHA to their parent drugs have been measured for AM and AE. Moreover, the ratio in the range of 0.001-0.03 for AL conversion to DHA calculated in rats and dogs, suggests that DHA should not contribute as much toxicity for the 3 drugs (AM, AE, and AL) as that for AS (table 6). The concentration with AUC data has demonstrated that DHA hydrolyzed from AS is in the range of 236–596 ng·h/ml compared to that from AM and AE in the range of 29-71 ng·h/ml at same dose level in rats [44]. However, while AM and AE induce neurotoxicity in the animals, AS does not [177]. Similar results are observed in dogs, 1109 ng·h/ml of DHA is produced from AS at a dose of 10 mg/kg without neurotoxicity symptoms [160], whereas 312 and 181 ng·h/ml of DHA from AM and AE, respectively, at a dose of 20 (AM) and 15 (AE) mg/kg has resulted in fatal neurotoxicity following intramuscular injection for the drugs [65, 159].

Data from our recent work found the maximum tolerant dose (MTD) for AS to be 240 mg/kg daily for 3 days after intravenous injection [66]. The animals were sacrificed at 24 hrs (1 day) and 192 hrs (8 days) after last dose. Histopathological evaluation demonstrated mild and moderate tubular necrosis in uninfected rats treated with AS 240 mg/kg; interestingly, fewer pathological lesions (minimal tubular necrosis) were observed in malaria infected rats.

Renal injury was reversible in all cases by day 8 after cessation of dosing and no neurotoxicity was found in any case with all intravenous regimens [66]. In this case, the AUC of 6984–15768 ng·h/ml of DHA, which is converted from AS, can be simulated daily in this regimen of rats according to our previous study [44]. Although DHA is 2-4 folds more active and more toxic than other artemisinin derivatives [152-156], the high level of DHA generated from AS does not seem to have a role in neurotoxic induction in animal species.

In other comparative studies of toxicokinetics and hydrolysis, AL and AS were administered to malaria-infected rats using 3 daily equimolar doses (96 μmoles/kg) via intravenous administration. Plasma concentration of AS with a daily dose of 36.7 mg/kg was one-third less on day 3 than on day 1, resembling that of its active metabolite, DHA. The results were similar for other artemisinin drugs, but not for AL. Toxicokinetic parameters of AL were very comparable from day 1 to day 3 at the same molecular doses of AS at 40.6 mg/kg. AS was the pro-drug of DHA with a DHA/AS ratio of 5.26 compared to the ratio of 0.01 for DHA/AL. Other toxicokinetic parameters revealed that the total $AUC_{1\text{-}3\ days}$ (84.4 $\mu g\cdot h\ ml^{-1}$) of AL was 5-fold higher than that of AS (15.7 μg·h/ml of AS plus DHA). In this study, the two drugs did not produce any CNS toxicity [178], but the general toxicity of AL was 3-fold greater than that of AS in malaria-infected rats [179]. The minimum doses of AS and AL producing parasitemia suppression were 2.3 and 2.5 mg/kg, respectively. The suppressive doses for decreasing the parasitemia by half (SD_{50}) were 7.4 and 8.6 mg/kg, respectively. The MTD for artesunate was 240 mg/kg with a therapeutic index of 32.6, whereas the MTD for AL was 80 mg/kg with a therapeutic index of 9.3 [179]. It is barely comprehensible that AS with 4893 ng·h/ml of DHA was not only significantly safer than AL with only 160 ng·h/ml of DHA, but it also did not produce neurotoxicity [178].

Therefore, we believe that DHA is not an important factor in neurotoxicity induction in animal species even though DHA is 2-4 times more toxic than other artemisinin derivatives in direct in vitro and in vivo studies [152-156].

3.2. The Role of Drug Distribution in the CNS

Data on the distribution of artemisinin analogues in the brain have few available studies, and of the published data, their methods all differ significantly. So to date, there are no comparative published results for quantitative analysis of the artemisinin drugs in brain tissue.

Using the thin-layer chromatography densitometry method, artemisinin (QHS), AM, and AS are found to cross the blood-brain and blood-placenta barriers with intravenous injection in rats [180]. QHS seems easier to detect in the brain after oral administration than after intravenous injection [181]. By radioimmunoassay, the highest level of AS was found in the rat intestine 10 minutes after intravenous administration, followed by the brain, liver, kidney, and other organs, in decreasing order. After one hour, the drug levels dropped significantly but not uniformly in all tissues, with high levels still remaining in the brain, fat, intestine and serum [182]. The highest levels were found in rat brains 5 minutes after intravenous injection. Moderate levels of AM were also found in the heart, lung and skeletal muscles, while liver and kidney levels were low [183].

At 24 h after intramuscular injection of ^{14}C-arteether, the tissue homogenate method was used to identify that the highest levels of radioactivity were present in the intestinal tracts, liver, kidneys, and spleen. Lower amounts of radioactivity were found in brown fat and brain. The lowest levels of radioactivity were present in the heart, testes, muscle and residual carcass. High-performance liquid chromatographic data from this work indicated that three metabolites of arteether, but not arteether itself, could cross the blood-brain barrier (BBB). The calculated apparent concentration in the whole brain was 0.89% of the total radioactivity after intramuscular injection of 25mg/kg arteether [our unpublished data].

Autoradiographs of rats sacrificed 1 h following administration of ^{14}C-AL showed widespread distribution of the radiolabel. The relative activity of tissues (as density per unit area) were intestinal tract > liver > kidney > bone marrow > spleen > brown fat and salivary glands > heart and testes > brain. At 48 h, the relative activities were as follows: intestinal content > spleen > kidney > liver > salivary glands > brown fat and bone marrow > testes > brain. The low residual activity found in the brain appeared uniformly distributed. Autoradiographic evidence confirmed the presence of ^{14}C-AL in the brain from 1 to 192 h. However, the presence of ^{14}C-AL in the brain was at a lower level than the presence of ^{14}C-AL in most other tissues. There was no evidence of a label concentration in any area of the brain that was visible in the whole body sections. It was found that ^{14}C-labelled AL could not easily penetrate through the blood-brain barrier. An apparent concentration of 0.1% of total radioactivity/brain was calculated from an intravenous and oral administration of 10 mg/kg AL [178].

More recently, a neurotoxic dose range study showed that neuronal damage occurred in all beagle dogs at 40 and 80 mg/kg of AM following multiple intramuscular daily treatments. At 20 mg/kg, minimal neuronal effects occurred in 5 out of 8 dogs. Two hours after the 8th administration (on day 8), only low levels of AM were found in cerebrospinal fluid (CSF) with 25, 60, and 71 ng/ml for 20, 40, and 80 mg/kg dosing, respectively [65]. AM levels in the CSF were < 10% of plasma concentration.

These limited and incomparable data indicates that the oil-soluble derivatives, AE (0.89% of total dose in brain) and AM (10% of plasma level in CSF) seem to have the ability to cross the BBB more readily than water-soluble artemisinin compounds, like AL (0.1% of total dose). If this is true, then the differential neurotoxicity of AE and AM with the water soluble forms is easily understood. However, this deduction is not supported by the observation that AS, a water-soluble drug, has the ability to easily cross the BBB. The largest fraction of AS has been found in rat brain after intravenous administration by radioimmunoassay [182]. Recently it was found that the levels of ^{14}C-AS in rat brain were higher (>2-fold) than that in plasma; the AUCs of radioactivity in brain and plasma were 70.7 and 29.4 μg·h/g, respectively. During a 192 hour period, 1.27% of total radioactivity dose was detected in the rat brain. The half-life of ^{14}C-AS in brain tissue was 94.2 hours, significantly longer than that in plasma with only a 63.7 hour half-life [184]. These results indicated that the resident time of ^{14}C-AS was longer in the brain than in plasma. This may reflect a "sink effect" of DHA uptake transfer by lipid-rich brain structures [185].

If the absence of AS in CSF is consistent with its low lipid solubility and a decrease of concentration in plasma after intravenous injection [143], then the types of metabolites present in the brain tissue are unknown [184]. Whether these metabolites in the brain are associated with neurotoxicity is also unknown. Artesunate is converted stoichiometrically to DHA, concentrations of which peak at 5-10 min [143, 173] in plasma. DHA is highly lipid soluble and has a low molecular mass (284 Da) - both factors favoring penetration of CSF [185]. Since DHA has relatively low solubility in water, it should be able to cross cell membranes and the BBB. After treatment with AS in patients, the parent drug (AS) can not be detected in the CSF. However, DHA levels in the CSF increase with time while DHA levels in plasma decrease. These finding suggest a continuing influx but a slower efflux of DHA in which DHA might accumulate in CSF during frequent AS dosing [185].

Although (i) radiolabeled AS has been shown to easily cross the BBB and have more accumulation in brain tissue when compared to other artemisinins, as described above [180-185], and (ii) other investigators has found increasing DHA levels in CSF (1100-1450 ng/ml) than in plasma (104-120 ng/ml) after intravenous injection of 120 mg AS in malaria patients [186], but no neurotoxicity has been observed. Therefore, while the artemisinin agents distribute in brain tissue and CSF, they do not appear to be a major factor in neurotoxicity.

3.3. The Role of Drug Exposure Levels in Neurotoxicity

Pharmacokinetic (PK) data demonstrate that AE and AM accumulation is observed in the plasma of rats [187], beagle dogs [65], rhesus monkeys (our unpublished data), and humans [188] following multiple intramuscular injections. Data collected from rat studies have demonstrated that the accumulation of AE in plasma is due to a slow and prolonged absorption from the injection sites [187]. The drug formulation, administration route, and plasma accumulation all appear to be associated with both general toxicity and neurotoxicity [62, 64, 177, 187, 189]

3.3.1. Drug Exposure Level in Rats

An accumulation and prolonged exposure of AE in plasma was first reported in rats with severe neurotoxicity due to slow and prolonged absorption in the muscle injection site following daily intramuscular injections of 25 mg/kg for 7 days [187]. The absorption of AE from muscle (at the injection site) was incomplete in the first 48 hours after a single injection. At 24 and 48 hours after dosing, 38% and 22% of the total dose of AE still remained in the injection site, respectively. The amount of AE in muscle rapidly decreased for 1-2 hours and then exhibited a much slower rate of decrease. Half-lives for the fast and slow absorption phases in the muscle were 1.0 hour and 26.3 hours, respectively. It is expected that the remaining dose amount would be absorbed later because an intramuscular total dose of AE with sesame oil should be 100% absorbed in the absence of decomposition or metabolism at the injection site.

The analysis of TK parameters on day 1 was similar to that of the single intramuscular dose. However, after day 1, the kinetic data estimates from days 2-7 showed a notable change in the PK parameter estimated for day 1 (figure 2, top). The elimination $t_{1/2}$ of AE after 7 daily doses was prolonged from 13.7 hours on day 1 to 31.2 hours on day 7, suggesting that the exposure time of AE had been greatly extended. C_{max} of AE (410 ng/ml) on day 7 was found to be three times higher than that on day 1 (130 ng/ml). AUC intramuscular dose was found to be 4.5-fold higher on day 7 at steady state (4367 ng·h/ml) than on day 1 (905 ng·h/ml). This indicates that the exposure concentration of AE has been greatly increased and the system of excretion and biotransformation in the rats may not have been normal [190]. Only a pathophysiological factor could change the slopes of the distribution and elimination due to biotransformation, excretion, and protein or tissue binding [191, 192].

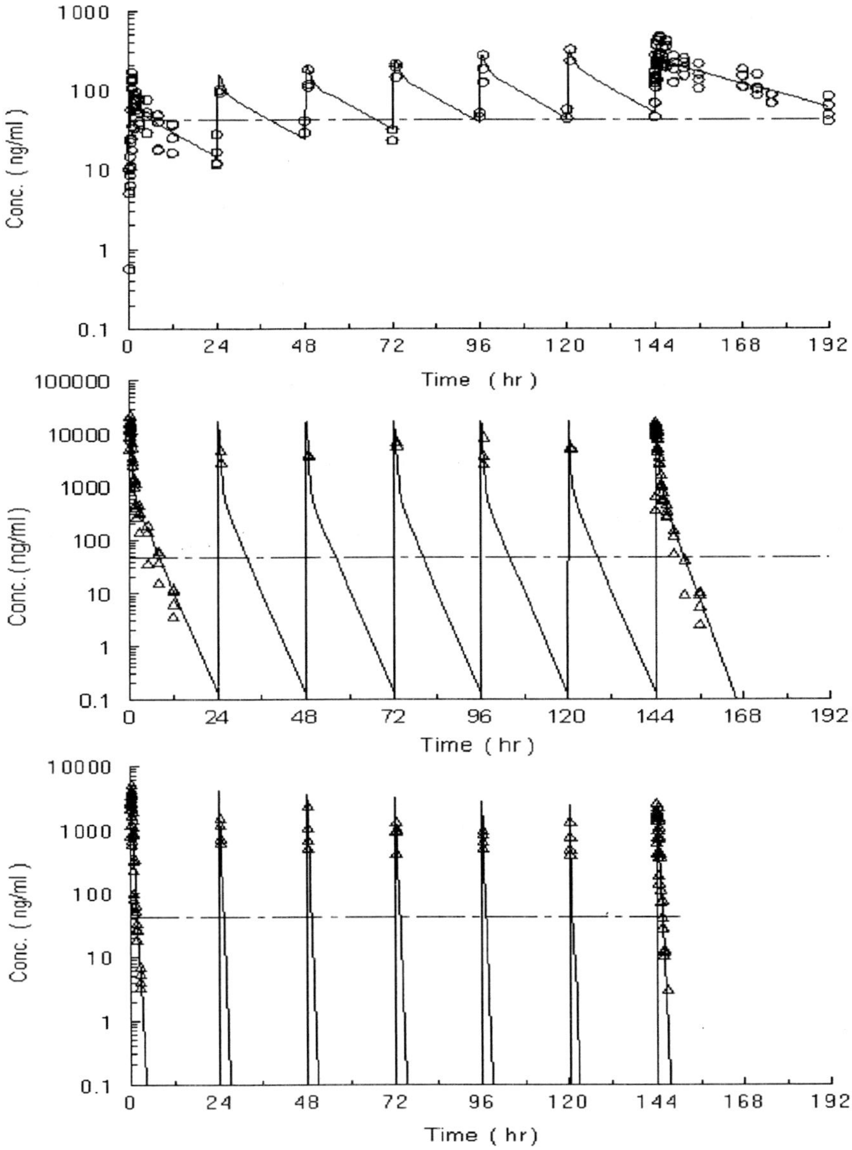

Figure 2. Pharmacokinetic profiles measured by HPLC-ECD (markers) and computer fitted curves (solid line) of 25 mg/kg of arteether with sesame oil (top, n = 4, Reference 187). Artelinate (middle) and artesunate (bottom) with 5% $NaHCO_3$/0.9% saline following daily intramuscular injection 25 mg/kg daily for 7 days in male rats. (n = 3, Reference 202). The minimal detected pathological effect level (MDPEL) from arteether measurement was estimated with 41.32 ng/ml (dashed line) in rats as described in Section 3.4.1.

Table 9. Neurotoxicity effects with exposure concentration (total AUC) and neurotoxic exposure time of artemisinin derivatives at an over 41.32 and 40.92 ng/ml of the minimal detected pathological effect level (MDPEL) of arteether, respectively, after intramuscular or oral administrations in rats (7 days dosing) and dogs (14 days dosing). [65, 152, 159, 187, 193, 194]

Rats	Arteether [187] Intramuscular (Sesame oil)	Arteether [152] Intramuscular (1:2 CRM/saline)	Artelinic acid [193] Intramuscular (5%$NaHCO_3$)	Artesunate [193] Intramuscular (5%$NaHCO_3$)
Dose	25 mg/kg x 7	25 mg/kg x 7	25 mg/kg x 7	25 mg/kg x 7
Neurotoxicity	Severe and death	Moderate	No	No
AUC total 7D, μg·h/ml	16.92 ± 4.04	46.29 ± 2.06	86.84 ± 5.59	8.57 ± 3.34
AUC total 7D (DHA)	3.43 ± 0.76	5.35 ± 0.83	0.56 ± 0.18	5.06 ± 1.21
AUC Day 1 (μg·h/ml)	1.31 ± 0.34	4.17 ± 0.68	12.46 ± 1.85	1.89 ± 0.80
AUC Day 7 (μg·h/ml)	11.37 ± 2.05	7.31 ± 0.59	10.56 ± 0.76	0.99 ± 0.34
C_{max} Day 1 (ng/ml)	130.4 ± 39.0	1227 ± 171	20044 ± 3459	3981 ± 992
C_{max} Day 7 (ng/ml)	410.0 ± 90.9	1826 ± 118	15585 ± 1476	2078 ± 416
Exposure time (hr)	164.28 ± 7.91	102.96 ± 5.26	42.48 ± 6.80	22.26 ± 4.87
Dogs	Artemether [65] Intramuscular (Peanut oil)	Arteether [159] Intramuscular (Sesame oil)	Artelinic acid a Oral (Suspension)	Artelinic acid [194] Oral (Capsules)
Dose	20 mg/kg x 7	15 mg/kg x 14*	20 mg/kg x 14	25 mg/kg x 14
Neurotoxicity	Moderate	Severe and death	No	No
AUC 7 or 14D (μg·h/ml)	32.13	24.39 ± 18.04	231.58 ± 115.81	191.14 ± 90.80
AUC Day 1 (μg·h/ml)	2.39	0.81 ± 0.32	13.97 ± 3.11	10.46 ± 4.89
AUC Day 7 or 14 (μg·h.ml)	5.11	7.09 ± 3.74	12.78 ± 3.37	11.35 ± 5.78
C_{max} Day 1 (ng/ml)	190	90.11 ± 14.74	12360 ± 2706	6279 ± 2995
C_{max} Day 7 (ng/ml)	346	352.7 ± 202.6	9780 ± 2885	7177 ± 6248
Exposure time (hr)	174	277.59 ± 10.67	57.98 ± 14.55	47.41 ± 11.78

[a] = Report from our contract company (Southern Research Institute); DHA = Dihydroartemisinin, CRM = cremophore, AUC = area under the curve.

Drug exposure levels of 25 mg/kg AE after a 7 day treatment was 16.92 ± 4.04 μg·h/ml for the AUC (a total of 7 days of AUC data), which induced severe neurotoxicity and animal death [187]. However, this exposure concentration level of AE was just one-fifth of the total AUC of AL (86.84 ± 5.59) with the same regimen of AE following intramuscular injection [202] (table 9). The clinical observation did not show any neurotoxicity effect in those animals treated with AL (figure 2, middle), even at high AL doses of 100 mg/kg after multiple intramuscular doses in rats [our unpublished data]. Computer simulation indicated that the total AUC for the high dose treatments (100 mg/kg) throughout the 7 days was 341.88 μg·h/ml and was 21 times higher than that of AE treated rats. This result suggests that the 5-21 times higher exposure concentrations of AL did not seem to be a principal independent factor in causing neurotoxicity (Table 9).

In order to demonstrate that the neurotoxicity of AE is related to drug accumulation in blood and is due to the slow and prolonged absorption from the intramuscular injection sites, a study was designed to decrease the accumulation and toxicity of AE through the replacement of traditional sesame oil with a cremophore vehicle [152]. When administered at a daily dose of 25 mg/kg for 7 days, AE blood accumulation with sesame oil (AESO) had a 7.5-fold higher AUC (on last versus first day dosing), while AE with cremophore (AECM) had only a 1.8-fold higher AUC. Although the accumulation of AECM was greatly reduced, its total exposure level (46.29 μg·h/ml) was still 2.7-fold higher than AESO (16.92 μg·h/ml) due to a higher bioavailability of AECM (74.5%) compared with AESO (20.3%) (Table 9, figure 3). While histopathological examinations of the brain demonstrated neurotoxic changes in both groups, the AESO group was significantly more severe than the AECM group. Brain injury scores with AECM were mild to moderate (2.3 to 3.0), but with AESO they were moderate to severe (3.0 to 4.7) on day 7 and day 10, respectively (Table 10). This study further demonstrated that the toxicity of AE was not dependent on its exposure level in rats.

Table 10. Average effects in rat brain areas of repeated arteether (AE) injection with vehicle sesame oil (AESO) and cremophore (AECM) by daily intramuscular dosing of 25 mg/kg for 7 days (n = 3) [152]

	Finding	Vehicle Control	AESO	AECM	Student Test
Day 7	Neuronal chromatolysis	0	3.00 ± 1.00	2.33 ± 1.15	P = 0.092
Day 10	Neuronal chromatolysis	0	4.67 ± 0.58	3.00 ± 1.00	P = 0.019

*Finding were grading as 0 = no significant lesions, 1 = minimal, 2 = mild, 3 = moderate, 4 = marked, and 5 = severe.

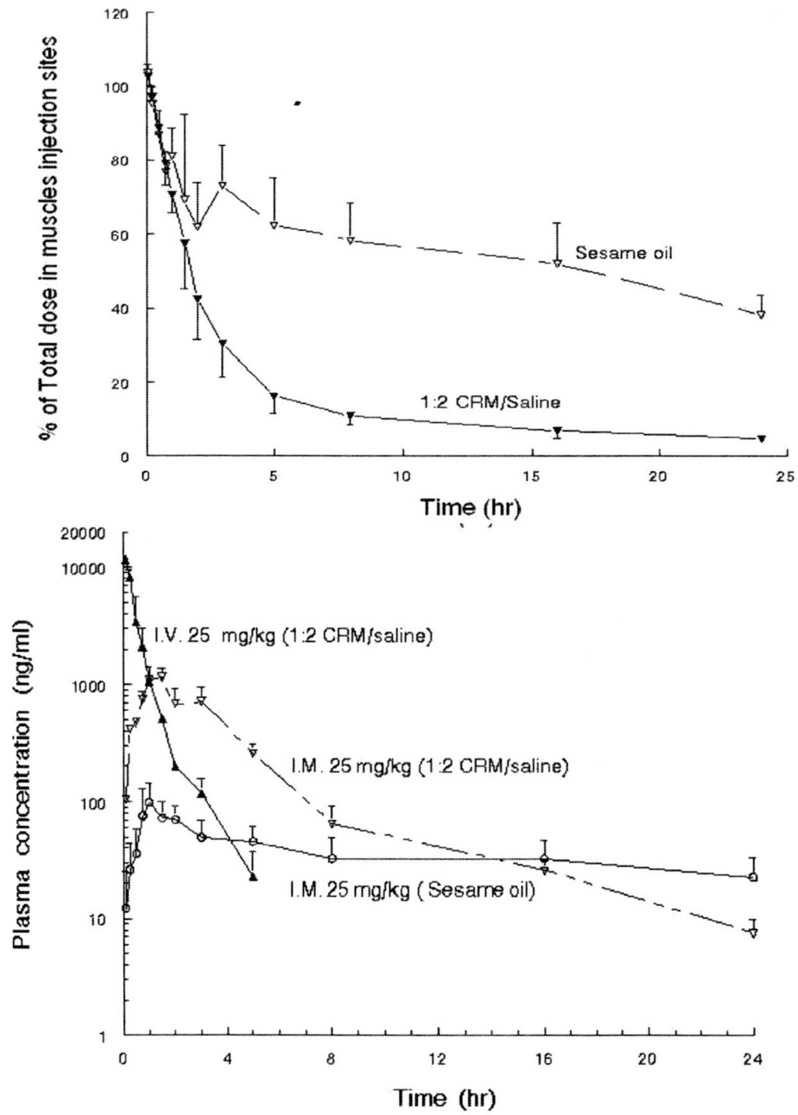

Figure 3. Mean amounts of arteether (AE) in muscle (injection site) measured by HPLC-ECD (top chart, n = 3) and mean plasma concentration-time profiles (bottom chart, n = 3) and by using 25 mg/kg of AE with sesame oil (dashed-line) and with 1:2 cremophore/0.9% saline (sold-line) after 7 days intramuscular injection in male rats [152, 187].

3.3.2. Drug Exposure Level in Dogs

Arteether accumulation was also observed in plasma of beagle dogs with severe neurotoxicity and death after daily intramuscular administration at 15 mg/kg for 14 days [159]. C_{max} of AE (352 ng/ml) was found to be four times higher on the last day (day 14) compared to the C_{max} on day 1 (90 ng/ml). AUC (7.09 μg·h/ml) on the last day was 8.7-fold higher than AUC of the intramuscular dose on the first day (0.81 μg·h/ml) indicating that the exposure concentration of AE had been greatly increased (figure 4, top). The total AUC during the 14 days at 15 mg/kg AE daily intramuscular repeated injection was 24.39 μg·h/ml (Table 9),

Similar accumulation results for AM were reported in dog plasma after daily intramuscular administration of 20, 40, and 80 mg/kg for 7 days [65]. The concentration-time profile of 20 mg/kg AM in the beagle dog is shown in table 9. The analysis of the toxicokinetic (TK) parameters on day 2-7 was changed, with the parameter estimated on day 1. The elimination t½ of AM after 7 daily dosing was prolonged from 9 hours on day 1 to 37 hours on day 7, suggesting that the exposure time of AM had been significantly increased (Figure 5, top). C_{max} of AM (340 ng/ml) doubled on day 7 from that on day 1 (190 ng/ml). AUC (6.79 μg·h/ml) on day 7 was 2.8-fold higher than AUC of the IM dose on day 1 (2.39 μg·h/ml), also indicating that the exposure concentration of AM had been increased.

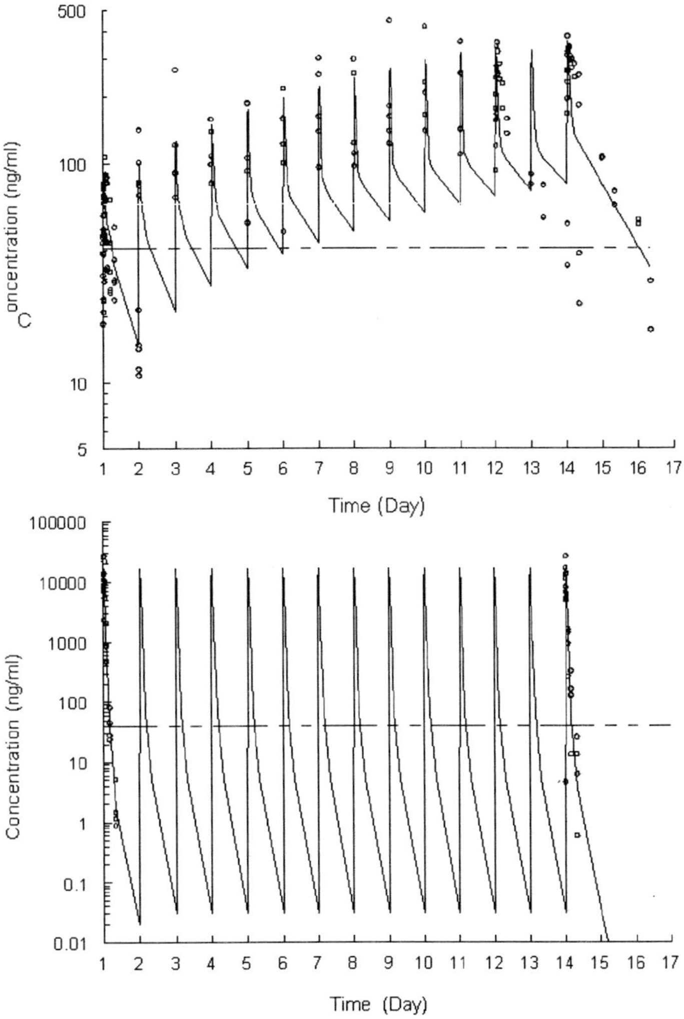

Figure 4. Pharmacokinetic profiles measured by HPLC-ECD (open circle) and computer fitted curves (solid line) of 15 mg/kg of arteether [159] with sesame oil after intramuscular injection (top, n = 5); 20 mg/kg suspension of artelinic acid with carboxymethyl cellulose (CMC) and water (bottom, n = 4) following intragastric administration daily for 14 days in beagle dogs [194]. The minimal detected pathological effect level (MDPEL) of AE was estimated as 40.92 ng/ml (dashed line) in male dogs as described in Section 3.4.2.

Compared to drug exposure levels, much higher plasma concentrations were found in dogs treated with AL following oral administration. An AUC value produced by AL at 20 mg/kg in a suspension formulation was 231.6 ± 115.8 μg·h/ml following daily oral doses for 14 days (figure 4, bottom). However, the value dropped to 191.14 ± 90.80 μg·h/ml for oral AL in a daily 25 mg/kg capsule formulation for 14 days (Table 9). The animals in both groups did not show any clinical toxicity [193]. The two dose regimens in dogs treated with AL showed at least 7 times higher exposure concentrations than those in dogs treated with AE. Neurotoxicity was neither detected in those animals with 20 or 25 mg/kg oral dose levels for 14 days [193, 194], nor in animals treated at even very high AL doses of 320 and 300 mg/kg after multiple oral doses [194, 195]. The drug exposure levels of these treatments suggest that a much higher exposure concentration of AL in the dogs does not produce neurotoxicity compared to AE and AM, which induce neurotoxicity with much lower exposure concentrations (Table 9) in dogs.'

3.3.3. Drug Exposure Level in Monkeys

Similarly, great plasma accumulation of AE was shown in rhesus monkeys' plasma after daily intramuscular administration of 16 mg/kg for 14 days (figure 6, top). The concentration-time profile of 16 mg/kg AE in the monkeys showed that the C_{max} of AE (1230 ± 577 ng/ml) on day 14 was 19-fold higher than that on day 1 (63.36 ± 9.08 ng/ml). AUC (53101 ng·h/ml) on the last dosing day was 60-fold higher than the AUC of the intramuscular dose on the first dosing day (877 ng·h/ml), indicating that the exposure concentration of AE was greatly increased [our unpublished data].

3.3.4. Drug Exposure Level in Humans

Except for AE and AM intramuscular injections with oils, no plasma accumulation is found for all artemisinin drugs by other administration routes in human. On the contrary, four artemisinin drugs (QHS, AS, AM, even DHA) have reported a declining concentration in plasma during multiple oral treatments in malaria patients and health subjects. The C_{max} and AUC values are markedly reduced from one-third to one-seventh on last dose day compared with first day. The decrease in drug exposure during treatment is not disease-related, since the artemisinin drug PK on day 1 is similar to that reported in healthy subjects [95, 196-199]. Similar time-dependent declining of oral AM was also found in animals (figure 5, bottom) [65]. One possible explanation for the decrease in plasma concentration-time during treatment is an increase in metabolic capacity due to auto-induction of hepatic drug-metabolizing enzymes. However, the drug decrease did not occur for AE in sesame oil after intramuscular administration in humans.

Kager reported on the first use of AE in humans on the studies of safety, tolerance and preliminary pharmacokinetics [93]. An initial AE intramuscular dose of 3.2 mg/kg was used in 27 healthy subjects on day 1. The dosage was then decreased to 1.6 mg/kg for four additional days. The PK data showed a long elimination half-life of 25-72 hr, explaining the marked accumulation in plasma observed in the multiple dose injection (figure 6, bottom). Recently, another study reported administering AE by intramuscular injection to human subjects in multiple doses in a clinical treatment trial. Two dose regimens of AE (AE with 3.2 mg/kg intramuscular start and then 1.6 mg/kg for 4 days as low dose regimen, and high dose of AE regimen with 4.8 mg/kg at 0 hr and 1.6 mg/kg at 6, 24, 48, 72, and 96 hr) were administered for the patients with uncomplicated falciparum malaria [21, 200]. Although these dose regimens have been designed as loading (high) and maintaining (low) doses, AE accumulation was still observed in the human plasma for both of those two dose regimens (Table 11).

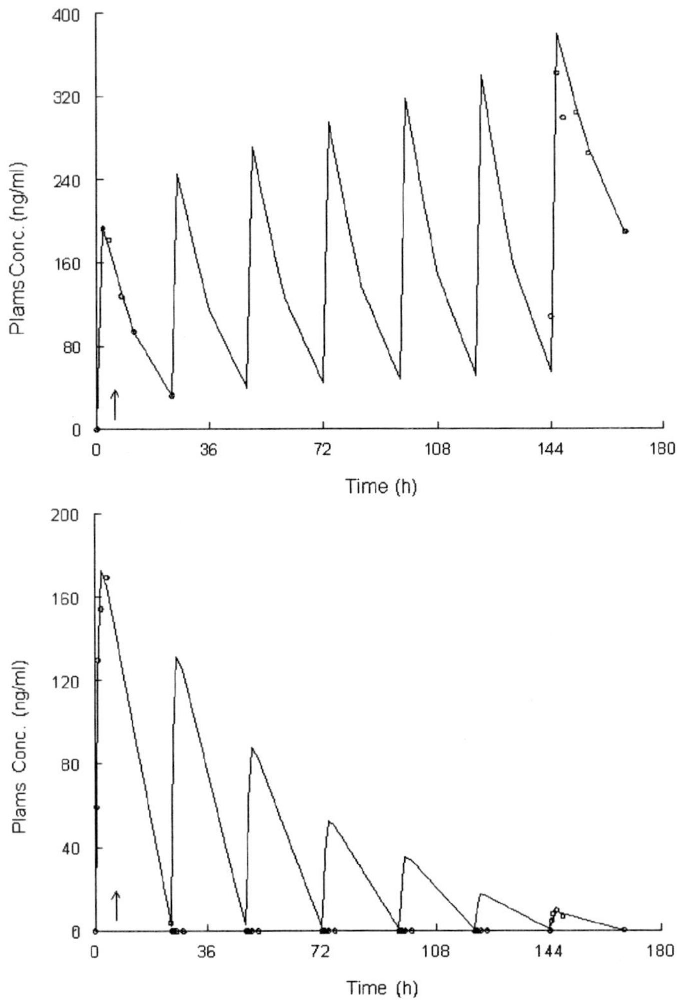

Figure 5. Pharmacokinetic profiles measured by HPLC-ECD (open circle) and computer fitted curves (solid line) of 20 mg/kg of artemether with sesame oil (top, showing drug accumulation) after intramuscular injection and 600 mg/kg of artemether in capsule (bottom, showing drug decline) following oral administration daily for 7 days in beagle dogs. [65].

In the low dose regimen, the elimination t½ of the low dose of AE regimen in human after 5 daily dosing was prolonged from 12.5 hr (day 1) to 40.7 hr (day 5), suggesting that the exposure time of AE had been greatly extended. The C_{max} of AE was two times higher on day 5 (140.8 ng/ml) than that on day 1 (63.6mg/ml). $AUC_{96\text{-}120h}$ (8409 ng·h/ml) on day 5 was 3.5-fold higher than $AUC_{0\text{-}24h}$ of the intramuscular dose on day 1 (2521 ng·h/ml), indicating that the exposure concentration of AE had been greatly accumulated. Similar profiles of the prolonged half-lives and increased C_{max} and AUC were also confirmed in the high dose regimen of AE in humans (table 11). These dose regimens proved to be safe and had potent antimalarial efficacy in reducing parasitemias from the peripheral blood.

3.3.5. Prolonged Absorption Effect on the Accumulation of AE and AM

Many scientists believed that the intramuscular administration of AM and AE was associated with the slowest elimination because the drugs were dissolved in oil (sesame or peanut oil) and, when injected, formed a depot from which drug was slowly released [44, 62, 74, 93]. The inference of slow elimination was recently demonstrated in a rat study, which also found a great deal of accumulation in plasma at injection sites [187]. Following 25 mg/kg of AE in sesame oil daily intramuscular injections for 7 days, the study confirmed and extended the results of earlier studies [44] by demonstrating that the absorption of AE from muscle (injection site) was incomplete. This study also indicated that up to 38% of the total single dose of AE remained in the injection site 24 hr after dosing and 22% of the total single dose still remained in the muscle after 48 hr. The dose amounts of AE remaining in the injection site vs. time are shown in figure 3 (top). The amount of AE rapidly decreased for 2-3 hours and then exhibited a slower decrease. The half-lives for the fast and slow absorption phases were 0.97 ± 0.48 hr and 26.3 ± 1.2 hr, respectively. Following 7 days of multiple dosing of AE (25 mg/kg), 91.4% of a single dose (25 mg/kg) was still left in the muscles from the 7 injection sites 24 hrs after last dose [187].

After intramuscular multiple dosing, accumulation of AE levels in plasma and muscle were evaluated. Plasma concentration after 7 days of dosing increased 3-4 fold, from an increase in C_{max} of 130.4 ng/ml to 410.0 ng/ml to an increase in AUC from 905 ng·h/ml to 4367 ng·h/ml. When compared with single dosing, AE accumulations in the muscle at injection sites increased 2.4-fold after multiple injections from 38% (day 1) to 91.4%, (day 7) of the total single doses following the 7 daily doses. When muscle absorption data from the single dose study was used to simulate the amount of dose remaining in the muscle after 7 days of dosing, 89% of a single dose was calculated to be present, which is similar to the actual measured amount [187]. This suggested that the change in TK observed during day 1 was not due to a change in absorption, but rather a change in body distribution or/and elimination. Therefore, the volume of distribution at a steady state on day 7 (41.8 L) was 40% of the volume on day 1 (104.3 L). Clearance value was increased by 89% from day 1 to day 7, 0.98 L/h to 1.85 L, respectively. The elimination t½ of AE after 7 daily dosing was also prolonged from 13.7 hr (day 1) to 31.2 hr (day 7).

Furthermore, the histopathological study demonstrates that the slow and prolonged absorption of AE in rat muscle is due to a slow release of AE from the sesame oil phase and therefore associates the cytotoxicity of the drug on the muscle cell at the injection site [our unpublished data].

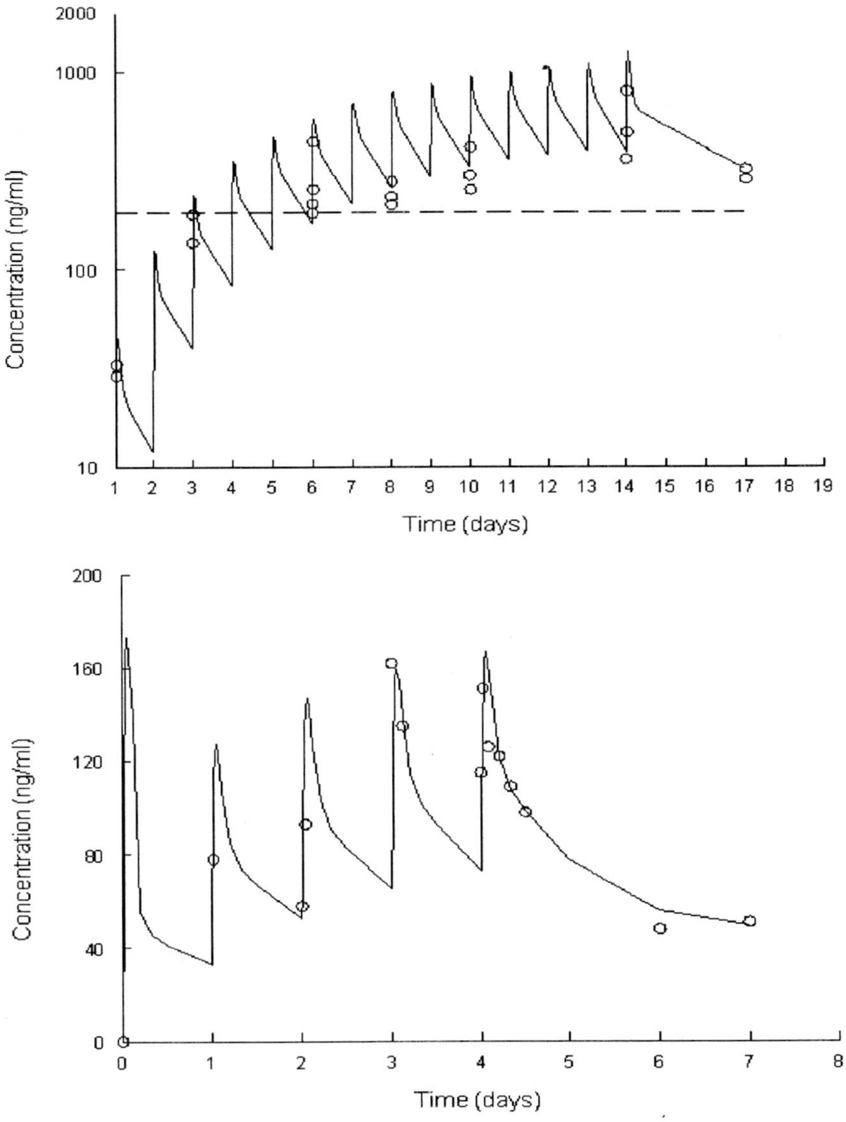

Figure 6. Pharmacokinetic profiles measured by HPLC-ECD (empty diamonds) and computer fitted curves (solid-line) of 16 mg/kg daily for 14 days in rhesus monkeys (top, n = 2) [our unpublished data], and the minimal detected pathological effect level (MDPEL) of AE was estimated as 193.8 ng/ml (dashed line) in male dogs as described in Section 3.4.3. In humans, 3.2 mg/kg in first day and then 1.6 mg/kg for another 4 days of arteether with sesame oil from health subjects (bottom, n = 27) [93]. Both data showed the drug accumulation in monkeys and humans after the 5 days treatments.

Table 11. Main pharmacokinetic parameters of ß-arteether with sesame oil (Artemotil) following multiple intramuscular administration of low dosage regimen (3.2 mg/kg on day 0 and 1.6 mg/kg on day 1-4, n = 11) and high dosage regimen (4.8 mg/kg on day 0 and 1.6 mg/kg on time 6, 24, 48, 72, and 96 hr, n = 44) in Thai patients with severe *P. falciparum* malaria* [200]

Parameters	Day 1	Day 5	Day 1-5	Ratio of Day 5/Day 1
Low dosage regimen (n =11)				
Dose (mg/kg)	3.2	1.6		
Cmax (ng/ml)	63.6 ± 39.9	140.8 ± 74.2		2.9 ± 2.4
$AUC_{inf\text{-} Artemotil}$ (ng·h/ml)	2521 ± 1950	8409 ± 4730	16242 ± 9113	4.5 ± 2.9
$AUC_{inf.\ DHA}$ (ng·h/ml)			2842 ± 1119	
$t_{1/2}$ absorption (h)	3.20 ± 0.64	2.13 ± 1.44		
$t_{1/2}$ elimination (h)	12.53 ± 3.91	40.66 ± 14.82		3.4 ± 1.1
High dosage regimen (n = 44)				
Dose (mg/kg)	6.4	1.6		
Cmax (ng/ml)	110.1 ± 56.9	241.1 ± 121.4		2.7 ± 1.5
$AUC_{inf.\ Artemotil}$ (ng·h/ml)	4702 ± 2964	9484 ± 4365	19782 ± 7725	2.9 ± 1.9
$AUC_{inf.\ DHA}$ (ng·h/ml)			3209 ± 1058	
$t_{1/2}$ absorption (h)	3.18 ± 2.90	3.46 ± 1.96		
$t_{1/2}$ elimination (h)	22.36 ± 9.24	31.62 ± 12.73		2.0 ± 1.3
Patient 151 (who likely got first dosing intravenously, n =1)				
Dose (mg/kg)	6.4	1.6		
Cmax (ng/ml)	2407.5	317.3		0.1
$AUC_{inf.\ Artemotil}$ (ng·h/ml)	12259	7403	24529	0.6
$AUC_{inf.\ DHA}$ (ng·h/ml)			2432	
$t_{1/2}$ elimination (h)	9.4	28.9		3.1

*Values were indicated are the mean ± SD. Min = minutes; AUC = area under the curve; Vss = volume of distribution at steady state; F = fraction of drug absorbed into blood; CL = clearance rate; MRT = mean residence time; DHA = dihydroartemisinin.

3.4. The Role of Drug Exposure Time in Neurotoxicity

3.4.1. Drug Exposure Time in Rats

Genovese et al. [59] found that a minimal daily dose of AE at 6.25 mg/kg for 7 days is the no detectable pathological effect dose (NDPED), which does not produce clinical neurotoxicity in rats. Statistically significant neuropathology in brain stem nuclei was observed in the group of rats (6/6 affected) treated with 12.5 mg/kg. These results demonstrate that AE-induced brainstem neuropathology in rats could occur at the relatively high dose of 12.5 mg/kg (double the NDPED dose) for 7 days (Table 6). The pharmacokinetic parameters and the minimal plasma AE concentration of 41.32 ng/ml at 12.5 mg/kg dose has been determined by our previous studies [152], as the minimal detected pathological effect level (MDPEL) in plasma that should result in clinical neurotoxicity and neuropathology [56, 201].

When calculating the exposure time of AE with sesame oil spent over the MDPEL (41.32 ng/ml) period in rats, neurotoxic exposure time was 164.28 ± 7.91 hours in the 7 day treatment after daily 25 mg/kg intramuscular injections (figure 7, top; table 9). This exposure time affected neurotoxicity is seen at 85.6% of the total dose treatment period (192 hours) with AE [152]. The total exposure time of AE with cremophore was 102.96 hours during the treatment period (192 hours, figure 7, bottom), which was about a third (37%) less than the exposure time of AE with sesame oil (164.28 hours). Neurotoxicity effects in those rats were reduced from severe to moderate, and the drug exposure time seems to be related to the effects of neurotoxicity (table 10) [152].

Compared with AL treatment, drug accumulation and neurotoxicity were not found in animals treated at the same dose (25 mg/kg), same period (7 days) and same conditions as the AE study [187, 202]. The drug exposure period of AL spent over the MDPEL was 42.48 ± 6.80 hours (figure 2, middle, table 9) in rats, which was significantly shorter (4-fold) than the AE study (164.28 hours). Therefore, the animals treated with AL would have avoided the risk and the neurotoxic outcome. An even wider safety margin is seen in animals treated with AS. With the same conditions, 25 mg/kg of AS daily for 7 days generated 22.26 ± 4.87 hours of exposure time in rats (figure 2, bottom; table 9), is 7-fold shorter than that in animals treated with AE (figure 2, top; table 9). This result suggests that the 4-7 time shorter exposure times of AL and AS over the MDPEL compared to the exposure times of AE seem to play a major role in avoiding clinical neurotoxicity.

Changing administration route from intramuscular to intragastric, AL showed moderate neurotoxicity in rats treated with 160 mg/kg daily in 9 multiple doses for 9 days but not in animals with 288 mg/kg every other day in 5 multiple doses for 9 days [61]. When calculating the neurotoxic exposure time we can not have the MDPEL data from animals treated with oral AL. However, there was available with a minimum detectable neurotoxic effect level (MDNEL), defined as the minimal inhibition of gastric emptying on day 5 [61], as this seems to relate to a neurotoxic effect induced by various artemisinins, including: AM, AE, and DHA [152]. In this study, the stomach contents were examined in the rats belonging to the daily 160 mg/kg dosing regimen for AL at 8 and 24 hours post dosing at various time points in the study. The quantity of AL detected in the stomach was expressed as both the amount of drug per gram of stomach contents and as a percentage of a single dose. On days 3, 5, 7, and 9 we detected 0, 46.52, 178.59, and 486.21 μg, respectively, of AL per gram of stomach contents 8 hours after the last dose. The increasing drug remaining in stomach over the course of dosing suggests that gastric emptying is inhibited. This inhibition of gastric emptying progresses from mild inhibition on day 5 to severe inhibition on day 9. This inhibition persisted even at 24 hours post dosing. Twenty-four hours post dosing on days 5, 7, and 9 we found 5.74, 25.50, and 29.11 μg of AL/g, respectively, contents remained in the stomach. It is postulated that this decrease in GI motility could result from a decrease in vagal tone from a decrease in sympathetic outflow [155].

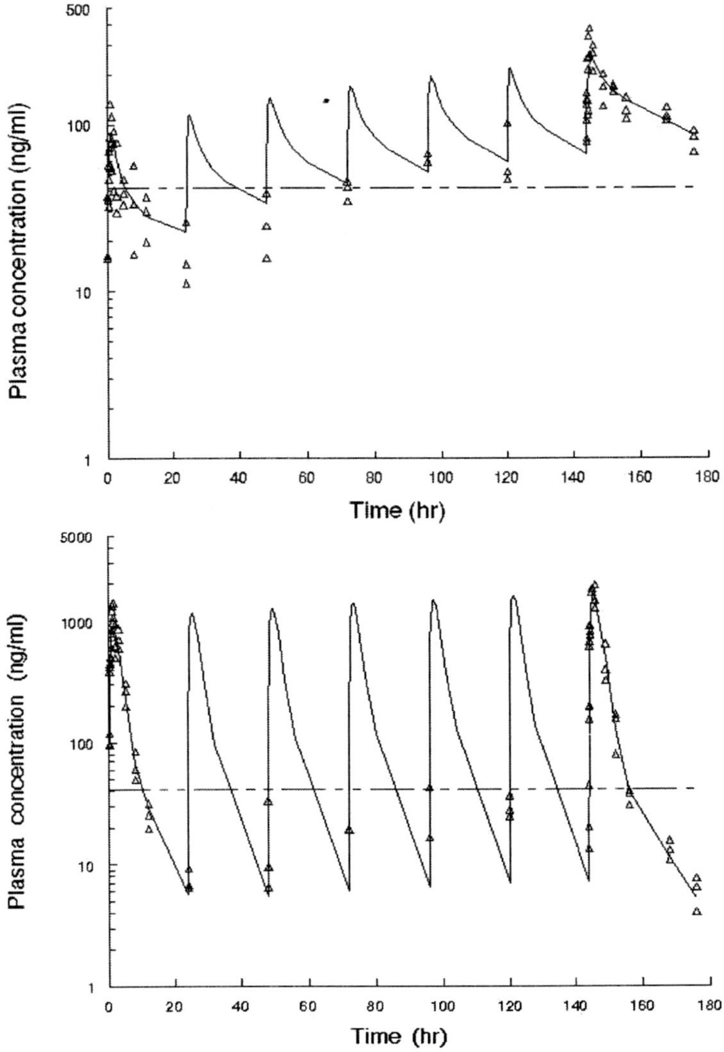

Figure 7. Toxicokinetic profiles in plasma measured by HPLC-ECD (open circle) and computer fitted curves (solid-line) of 25 mg/kg of arteether with sesame oil (AESO, top, n = 3) and arteether with cremophore (AECM, bottom, n = 3) following daily intramuscular injection for 7 days in male rats [152]. The minimal detected pathological effect level (MDPEL) was estimated as 41.32 ng/ml (dashed line) [section 3.4.1].

Therefore, on the day 5 post dosing the beginning inhibition of gastric emptying was defined as an initial neurotoxic effect in the rats with 160 mg/kg regimen. The corresponding plasma concentration of AL on day 5 in minimum was 346.26 ng/ml, which was the minimal anorectic toxicity in the rats. The neurotoxic exposure time with AL's MDNEL (346.26 ng/ml), 186 hours was measured as the exposure period threshold to affect neurotoxicity (Figure 8, top). These results indicate a correlation between neuropathology of rats and a prolonged AL exposure. The AL exposure was related to drug accumulation in the blood resulting from a delayed gastric emptying-induced prolonged absorption of the drugs from the stomach [61]. When rats were treated intermittently with AL at 288 mg/kg every other day in 5 multiple doses for 9 days, the neuronal degeneration was not identified (not significantly different from that of vehicle control group) until day 7 after the last treatment. The neurotoxic exposure time was calculated as 75 hours in the animals (Figure 8, bottom). The data further indicated that by shortening the drug exposure time at MDNEL level, it was possible to reduce the neurotoxic risk in the animal treated with the artemisinins [67].

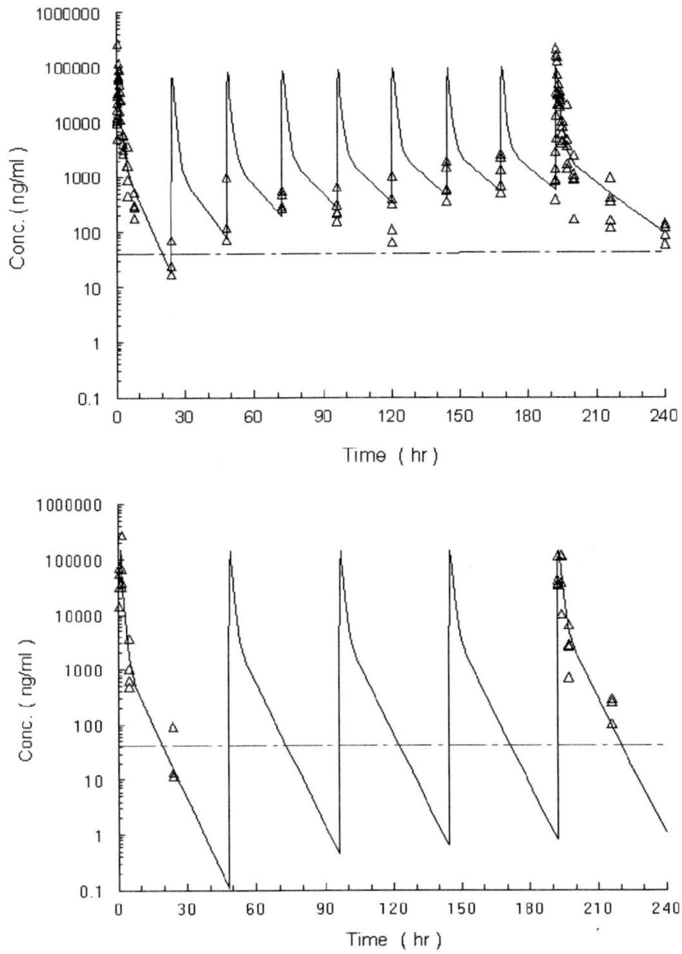

Figure 8. Pharmacokinetic profiles measured by HPLC-ECD (markers) and computer fitted curves (solid line) of artelinic acid (AL) in suspension at 160 mg/kg daily for 9 dosages (top, n = 5), and artelinic acid in suspension at 288 mg/kg every other daily for 5 dosages in rats (bottom, n = 4). The two regimens have same total dose with 1440 mg/kg and same treatment period for 9 days [61]. The minimal detected pathological effect level (MDPEL) from arteether (AE) measurement was estimated as 41.32 ng/ml (dashed line) for rats.

The drug retained in the stomach appears to be a reservoir which delays and prolongs the absorption of AL and results in drug accumulation (high AUC) and prolongs elimination (great Vss and long $t_{1/2}$). This reservoir is very similar to the depot effect seen with the oil-soluble artemisinins (AM and AE) intramuscularly in the injection sites. This accumulation increases the time that the drug levels are above a toxicity threshold and can thereby induce neurotoxicity. In this study, we attempt to correlate the neurotoxic exposure time to the observed histopathological findings to the two dosing groups. We found that the neurotoxic exposure time to be significantly extended for animals in the daily AL treatment cohort (186 hrs) compared to those in the every other day dosing cohort (75 hrs). To determine the neurotoxic exposure time for the two regimens, we calculated the time that the AL plasma level was above the minimum detectable neurotoxic effect level (MDNEL), which defined in this study as the plasma level at the time of onset of the anorectic effect. Although the MDNEL is not a minimum detectable pathological effect level (MDPEL), which defined as the first observation of neuronal injury, as was used in a previous study where AE was shown to produce neurotoxicity when given intramuscularly at 12.5 mg/kg daily for 7 days [152]; its estimation can give us an initial estimation of neurotoxic exposure time and allow us to correlate this exposure time with observed histopathology from different AL dosing regimens. It is clear that in the present study the delayed gastric emptying resulted in AL accumulation in blood and prolonged a neurotoxic exposure time (186 hr) in the 160 mg/kg x 9 rats when compared to 75 hr in 288 mg/kg x 5 animals. It is obvious that the neurotoxic exposure time is a key factor in the neurotoxicity induced by oral AL in rats.

3.4.2. Drug Exposure Time in Dogs

Davidson [58] showed that a minimal daily dose of AE at 3 mg/kg for 28 days is a no detectable pathological effect dose (NDPED) that does not cause neurotoxicity in beagle dogs; this was confirmed by histopathological examinations. AE-induced brainstem neuropathology has been detected though in some dogs with a dose as low as 5 mg/kg/day from Brewer [52, 57], 6.25 mg/kg from Dayan [56], and 6.75 mg/kg from Davidson [58], based on a daily dose for 28 days. Thus, the average of the minimal dose to produce neurotoxicity in dogs should be 6 mg/kg (calculated from the three findings.) The minimal plasma concentration of AE with this low dose (6.0 mg/kg) has been simulated by previous publications in figure 4 (top) [159]. The concentration level of 40.92 ng/ml could be calculated as the MDPEL in plasma that should be the first risk for causing neurotoxicity in dogs.

AE accumulation was also observed in plasma of the beagle dogs after daily intramuscular administration of 15 mg/kg for 14 days [159]. The mean concentration-time profile of AE in the beagle dog is shown in figure 4 (top). The kinetic data from toxicokinetic parameters indicated notable changes on the last dosing day from the pharmacokinetic parameters estimated on day 1. The important change was the elimination $t_{1/2}$ of AE during the two weeks of daily dosing. The elimination was prolonged from 11.9 hours on the first dosing day to 22.5 hours on the last dosing day, suggesting that the exposure time of AE had been doubly extended. Also, a MDPEL (40.92 ng/ml) of AE in beagle dogs first appeared in that study on day 6-7. Therefore, day 6-7 would be the earliest time that neurotoxicity occurred in the beagle dogs, based on the toxicities and the toxicokinetic data analysis.

When estimating the exposure time of AE over the concentration level of 40.92 ng/ml (MDPEL) in dogs with severe neurotoxicity and death, the exposure period was 277.59 ± 10.67 hours in a 14-day study after daily intramuscular injections of 15 mg/kg (table 9). The neurotoxic exposure time of AE was 82.6% of the total dosing treatment period (336 hours).

Compared with AL dosing by suspension or capsules orally, the neurotoxic exposure times were calculated to be 57.98 ± 14.55 hours for AL suspension (figure 4, bottom), and 47.41 ± 11.78 hours for AL capsules (table 9). All animals treated with AL were not observed to have any neurotoxicity [194].

The evaluations from above strongly support the findings that neurotoxicity is exposure time dependent in the animal species regardless of formulation and administration route. As a result, the artemisinins exposure time in animal species has an imperative role in the induction of neurotoxicity. Other factors of the pharmacokinetic parameters, such as drug distribution in the brain, toxicity of active metabolite (DHA), or drug exposure level, tend to be of minor importance.

3.4.3. Drug Exposure Time in Monkeys

AE was present in rhesus monkeys plasma after daily intramuscular administrations of 16 mg/kg for 14 days [our unpublished data]. The concentration-time profile of 16 mg/kg AE in the monkeys showed that the C_{max} of AE (1230 ± 577 ng/ml) on day 14 was 19 fold higher than that on day 1 (63.36 ± 9.08 ng/ml). AUC (53101 ng·h/ml) on the last dosing day was 60-fold higher than the AUC of the intramuscular dose on the first dosing day (877 ng·h/ml), indicating that the exposure concentration of AE had been increased (figure 6, top). Since AE-induced brainstem neuropathology in monkeys occurred at a minimal dose of 8 mg/kg daily doses for 14 days [55], the minimal plasma concentration of AE 193.8 ng/ml with this low dose (8.0 mg/kg) had been simulated by our unpublished data, as the minimal detectable pathological effect level (MDPEL) in plasma that should be at first to risk causing neurotoxicity in monkeys. The MDPEL value (193.8 ng/ml) of monkeys is 4-fold greater than that of rats (41.32 ng/ml) and dogs (40.92 ng/ml), indicating that the rat and dog seems to be more sensitive than monkey species to suffer neurotoxicity.

3.5. Drug Exposure Time Resulting in Neurotoxicity

To date, there have been no neurological side effects noted in humans due to DHA, QHS, AM, AE and AS treatments. After intramuscular administration, AE and AM provide a longer exposure time in humans the same way they did in animal species (rats, dogs and monkeys) [21, 188, 200]. The conversion of AM and AS to DHA in human is much higher than that in animal species [156-171], but why humans are able to avert the fatal neurotoxicity described in animal species is unknown. This review finds that the drug exposure time is the principle factor in the induction of neurotoxicity in rats, dogs and monkeys. The minimal detected pathological effect level (MDPEL) has been used to measure the exposure period at neurotoxic effect levels in the animals in the present discussion. When using the rats (41.32 ng/ml) or monkeys (193.8 ng/ml) MDPEL to calculate human samples treated with AE with regimen of 4.8 mg/kg at 0 hr and 1.6 mg/kg at 6 hr and then daily in 2-5 day following intramuscular injection, the 162.4 or 33.2 hours (figure 9, top), respectively, of drug exposure time is estimated during the 5 days treatment in the subjects [200]. However, in the 42 patients treated with this regimen there was a failure to detect any neurotoxicity even under the very carefully monitored design in those clinical trials. With regard to acute toxicity, monkeys have fewer responsive than rats, whereas humans appear to be less sensitive than animals [203, 204] and humans have much better repair capabilities than do animals [205].

Other possible explanations for the neurotoxicity discrepancy observed between animal and human can be:

i) The therapeutic dose (2-4 mg/kg) in humans is never higher than the minimal dose that exhibited neuropathologic findings in rats (12.5 mg/kg for 7 days), dogs (6 mg/kg for 28 days), or monkeys (8 mg/kg for 14 days). Also, it is never higher than the minimal doses that showed clinical signs in rats (50 mg/kg for 7 days), in dogs (20 mg/kg for 7 days), or in monkeys (24 mg/kg for 14 days), all of which are 3-4 times higher than the doses resulting in neuropathologic findings;
ii) The treatment period (3-7 days) in humans is never longer than the minimal time for the development of neurotoxicity in rats (7 days), dogs (28 days), or monkeys (14 days);
iii) Many of the patients followed had been seriously ill with cerebral malaria due to severe *falciparum* infection. The resulting evidence may lead to future studies on whether the pattern of neurotoxicity occurred from the illness or from the drug(s);
iv) A number of early reports did not pay sufficient attention to the feasibility of associating brain damage and neurological disorders in patients with such treatments of malaria; and
v) Post-marketing surveillance is limited in developing countries and the potential neurological side-effects of the drug are not recorded.

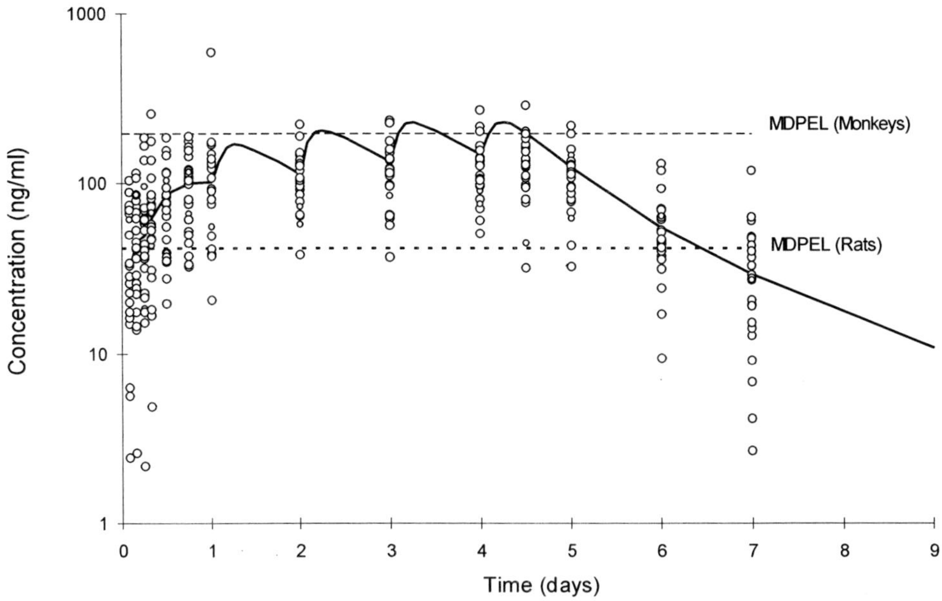

Figure 9 (Continued)

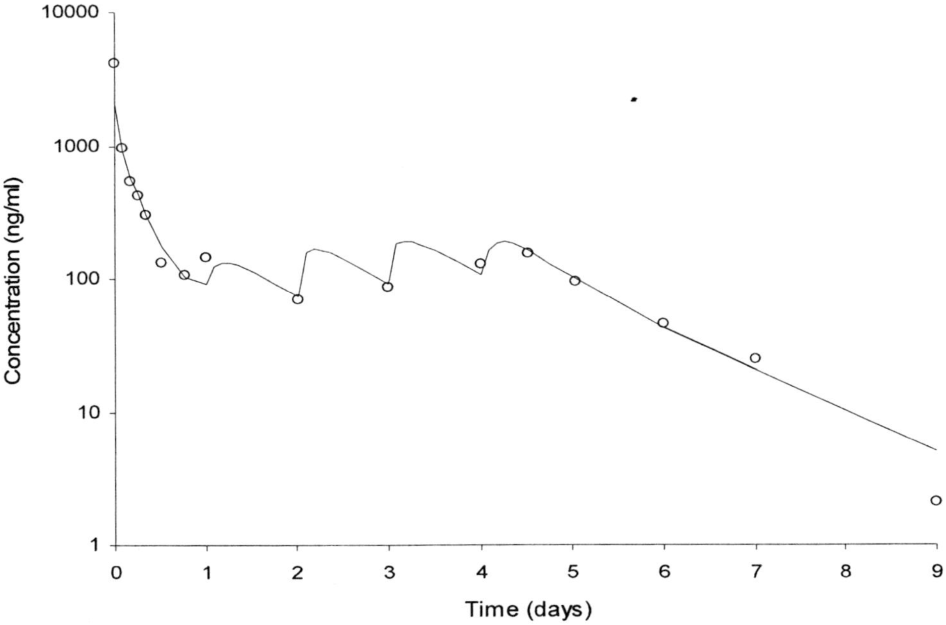

Figure 9. Pharmacokinetic profiles in plasma measured by HPLC-ECD (open circle) and computer fitted curves (solid-line) of 4.8 mg/kg at 0 hour and 1.6 mg/kg at 6, 24, 48, 72, and 96 hours of arteether (AE) with sesame oil in 42 patients summary as intramuscular administration (top chart), and in a single patient (bottom chart), who seemed to be injected into vessel as intravenous injection at first dosing and appeared a great efficacy [200].

In conclusion, the drug exposure time of artemisinins is the principle factor responsible for the induction of neurotoxicity in animal species. Therefore, the active metabolites (DHA), the drug distributed in CNS, and/or the drug exposure levels do not play important roles in inducing neurotoxicity. The oil-soluble artemisinins, AM and AE, possess the ability to induce fatal neurotoxicity because their sesame oil vehicle delays and prolongs the absorption from the intramuscular injection sites leading to an enormous drug accumulation, notably extending the exposure time to the toxic effect level. This would indicate that relinquishment of sesame oil as a vehicle should be considered. The water-soluble artemisinins, AS and AL, have very short half-lives and produce limited exposure time in animal species and humans, indicating that once-daily oral or intravenous administrations of AS are relatively safe.

4. Drug Pharmacokinetic Role in Reproductive Toxicity

4.1. Pharmacokinetics of Artemisinins and other Antimalarials in Pregnancy

Physiological changes in pregnancy – beginning during the first trimester, and most marked during the third trimester – alter the absorption, distribution and clearance of drugs. In addition, most drugs gain access to the feto-placental unit. These changes are detailed below before considering specific effects for individual classes of drugs. The pharmacokinetics of antimalarials is altered in pregnancy. This is the consequence of multiple factors: expansion of the distribution volume, increase in clearance, change in the protein binding, lipid distribution and absorption of drugs, as well as influence of hormonal changes on the drug metabolism [206].

4.1.1. Drug Absorption

Gastric emptying and small intestine motility are reduced in pregnancy due to elevation of progesterone. The elevation may increase T_{max} and reduce C_{max}, although effects on total bioavailability may be relatively minor. An increase in gastric pH, due to a reduction in H^+ secretion and an increase in mucus production may increase the ionization of weak acids, reducing absorption of acid material more than that of weak bases. Such effects are unlikely to be important during repeated dosing. They may, however, reduce the efficacy of a single dose of an oral drug such as an analgesic or anti-emetic for which T_{max} and C_{max} are important. A more practical problem for drug absorption is the nausea and vomiting associated with pregnancy. If nausea is reduced in the evening its effects on absorption can be minimized by deferring dosing until the evening (in the case of once-daily dosing). For example, dose optimizations for antimalarial drugs, such as AS, are needed in pregnancy [207].

4.1.2. Drug Distribution

During pregnancy there is an expansion of intravascular (plasma volume) and extra-vascular (breasts, uterus, peripheral edema) water content. Thus, total body water increases, creating a larger space within which hydrophilic drugs may distribute, i.e. increasing V_d. As a result of this apparent dilution, C_{max} of many antimalarial drugs is reduced, although the clinical effect of the reduction is compensated by changes in protein-binding. Total plasma concentration of albumin-bound drugs decreases as a result of haemodilution and the subsequent fall in plasma albumin concentration. In addition, steroid and placental hormones displace drugs from their protein-binding sites. There is the possibility of a rise in free (active) drug concentration of agents that are normally albumin-bound. This would be expected to produce an increased drug effect. However, the unbound drug is distributed, metabolized and excreted; therefore, the free concentration of drug is little influenced. These changes in protein binding are of clinical importance when monitoring plasma concentrations of drugs. Although body fat increases, creating a larger volume of distribution for lipophilic drugs - this has little practical importance.

4.1.3. Drug Metabolism snd Elimination

Some enzymes of the hepatic cytochrome P-450 and G6PD systems are induced by estrogen/progesterone, resulting in a higher rate of metabolism (and hence elimination) of drugs. For example, primaquine (8 aminoquinoline) is not prescribed in pregnancy because of the intravascular hemolysis risk in the mother and the fetus. This risk is linked to the dose administered and the degree of G6PD deficiency [208]. Clearance of drugs (such as artemisinins) that are secreted via the biliary system may be attenuated due to the cholestatic property of estrogen [209]. Some extra-hepatic enzymes, such as cholinesterase, have diminished activity during pregnancy. Renal blood flow is increased by 60 ± 80% during pregnancy, and glomerular filtration rate rises by 50%, leading to enhanced elimination of drugs that are normally excreted unchanged - for example, mefloquine and halofantrine [209]. This leads to slightly lower steady-state drug concentrations; however this rarely necessitates increasing the dosage [210].

4.1.4. Feto-Placental Unit

Drug transfer occurs mainly via diffusion across the placenta, thus favouring the movement of lipophilic agents; the rate-limiting step is placental blood flow.

Protein-bound drugs do not cross the placenta. Both the immature fetal liver and the placenta can metabolize drugs. Immature phase I (hydrolysis, oxidation and reduction) and phase II (conjugation) metabolism can only occur in the fetus early gestation post-conception. Some antibiotics (tetracycline and doxycycline) are used in combination with quinine or artesunate in areas of multi-drug resistance [211]. Use of these antibiotics in human pregnancy is associated with disturbances of bone growth of the fetus [212] and with irreversible teeth coloration when given in the late gestation [213]. Congenital cataract has also been reported [214]. Furthermore, the hepatotoxicity of tetracycline is increased in pregnancy [215] and fatal fatty liver degeneration occurs when large doses are used [216]. Most antimalarial drugs are weak bases and are mainly non-ionized (lipophilic), diffuse across the placental barrier and become ionized in the more acidic fetal blood, leading to a net movement from the maternal to fetal system.

4.1.5. Pharmacokinetic Role of Artemisinins in Pregnancy

These physiological changes in pregnancy can cause a decrease in plasma concentrations and AUCs, resulting in reduced efficacy. Few studies in women have been published for artemisinins and other antimalarials. For example, chloroquine in oral treatment [217] by using prophylaxis [218], oral mefoloquine [219], oral progunil [220, 221], oral atovaquone [118], as well as oral DHA [207] all have altered kinetics in pregnancy, and plsama levels are significantly lower than in non-pregnant patients with malaria [118, 207, 217-221]. This is likely due to increased clearance, larger volume of distribution and perhaps altered absorption following the oral administration. A similar observation is also found in animal studies for oral administration of AS [101]. It is clear that oral dosages of these antimalarials need to be adapted to keep efficacy when given to pregnant patients and animals with malaria [210].

However, the pharmacokinetic parameters for the antimalarial agents show no significant difference between pregnant and non-pregnant women and animal species after intravenous or intramuscular injections [91, 222, 223]. The pharmacokinetics of chloroquine is determined in pregnant and non-pregnant rabbits following intravenous administration. Chloroquine rapidly crossed the placenta, resulting in equivalent fetal and maternal blood concentrations 15-30 min after dosing the mother. The subsequent 1 and 2 hr fetal blood concentrations are about two-fold higher than the corresponding maternal blood concentrations. The desethylchloroquine metabolite blood concentrations are low relative to the drug, although the metabolite is detected in all blood samples including the initial 5 min maternal blood samples and 15 min fetal blood samples. Comparing the pharmacokinetics of chloroquine in the pregnant and non-pregnant animals reveals no difference in total body clearance. However, there is an approximately two-fold decrease in the apparent volumes of distribution and terminal half life in the pregnant rabbits. Because of the relatively large inter-animal variability of these parameters, the differences are not statistically significant ($p > 0.05$), but do indicate a trend toward changes in chloroquine pharmacokinetics during pregnancy [223].

4.1.5.1. Pharmacokinetics of AS in Pregnant and Non-Pregnant Rats

Preclinical studies of the reproductive toxicity in animal species (table 7) suggested that AS contains the greatest toxicity to animal embryos by routes of subcutaneous and intramuscular injections (single or multiple doses) with less than 1 mg/kg of the ED_{50}, which is much lower than the therapeutic dose (2-4 mg/kg) in humans. The comparative pharmacokinetics of AS was determined in pregnant and non-pregnant rats following 3 daily multiple intramuscular administrations [224]. Since the bioequivalence of AS by intravenous regimen was fulfilled for AS by intramuscular injection in rats [224], the results after intramuscular regimen could refer to a study by intravenous administration. Comparing the pharmacokinetics of AS in the pregnant and non-pregnant animals revealed no difference in plasma concentrations, body volume distributions, and total body clearance only one day after injection.

However, the pharmacokinetic parameters changed significantly on day 3 and on the conversion of AS to DHA during the 3 days of treatments. On day 3, the plasma concentration of AS decreased from C_{max} 8668 ng/ml on day 1 to 5037 ng/ml on day 3 and from AUC 3984 ng·h/ml on day 1 to 2239 ng·h/ml on day 3 in the non-pregnant rats, but no significant changes showed in pregnant animals (table 12). The body volume distribution (Vss) and total body clearance (CL) remarkably increased two-fold from Vss/F 2325 ml/kg on day 1 to 4624 ml/kg on day 3 and from CL/F 139.7 ml/min/kg on day 1 to 231.7 ml/min/kg on day 3 in non-pregnant rats, but there was no significant difference showed in pregnant animals [99, 224].

Similar no-change results of pharmacokinetics were exhibited for DHA, an active metabolite of AS, from day 1 to day 3 in the pregnant rats. The AUC value of DHA was even higher on day 3 (4820 ng·h/ml) than that on day 1 (3681 ng·h/ml). However, the significant decrease of plasma concentration in non-pregnant animals was on day 3 when compared to day 1 in values of C_{max} and AUC (table 12). In addition, the conversion rates of AS to DHA were much greater in pregnant rats than that in non-pregnant rats. The ratios of AUC_{DHA}/AUC_{AS} were 0.99-1.02 for pregnant rats and 0.42-0.48 for non-pregnant animals, indicating that the total AUC from day 1 to 3 (15049 ng·h/ml) in pregnant rats was more 3-fold higher than that (4015 ng·h/ml) in non-pregnant rats [224].

Table 12. Main pharmacokinetic parameters of artesunate (AS) and dihydroartemisinin (DHA), an active metabolite of AS, following multiple intramuscular administration of 30 mg/kg daily for 3 days (on GD11-13) in pregnant (n = 3) and non-pregnant rats (n = 4)* [99]

Parameters	Pregnant Rats		Non-pregnant Rats	
	GD 11	GD 13	Day 1	Day 3
Artesunate (AS)				
Cmax (ng/ml)	16545 ± 2873	14927 ± 7292	8668 ± 1068	5037 ± 805
Tmax (hr)	0.08	0.08	0.15 ± 0.04	0.23 ± 0.08
$AUC_{inf.}$ (ng·h/ml)	3749 ± 311	4758 ± 849	3984 ± 620	2239 ± 470
$t_{1/2}$ absorption (h)	0.08 ± 0.02	0.10 ± 0.02	0.13 ± 0.02	0.13 ± 0.04
$t_{1/2}$ elimination (h)	0.35 ± 0.02	0.49 ± 0.09	0.43 ± 0.02	0.41 ± 0.05
Vss/F (ml/kg)	2133 ± 589	2378 ± 769	2325 ± 511	4624 ± 827
CL/F (ml/min/kg)	133.3 ± 13.2	107.7 ± 25.1	139.7 ± 24.0	231.7 ± 58.8
$AUC_{D1\text{-}3\ total}$ (ng·h/ml)		13630 ±1952		8893 ± 1690
AUC_{Day3}/AUC_{Day1}		1.27 ± 0.23		0.61 ± 0.12
Dihydroartemisinin (DHA)				
Cmax (ng/ml)	10335 ± 1475	9087 ± 1437	3049 ± 1499	2409 ± 344
Tmax (hr)	0.08	0.14 ± 0.06	0.23 ± 0.08	0.25 ± 0.07
$AUC_{inf.}$ (ng·h/ml)	3681 ± 238	4820 ± 625	1636 ± 273	1049 ± 95
$t_{1/2}$ absorption (h)	0.08 ± 0.01	0.10 ± 0.01	0.13 ± 0.01	0.11 ± 0.02
$t_{1/2}$ elimination (h)	0.37 ± 0.04	0.53 ± 0.13	0.51 ± 0.09	0.53 ± 0.14
Vss/F (ml/kg)	3164 ± 305	3342 ± 395	10314 ± 4081	8450 ± 3734
CL/F (ml/min/kg)	135.8 ± 12.9	106.3 ±13.5	321.5 ± 63.1	393.6 ± 183.6
$AUC_{D1\text{-}3\ total}$ (ng·h/ml)		15049 ± 3092		4015 ± 326
AUC_{Day3}/AUC_{Day1}		1.48 ± 0.29		0.66 ± 0.16
Ratio AUC_{DHA}/AUC_{AS}	0.99 ± 0.09	1.02 ± 0.11	0.42 ± 0.10	0.48 ± 0.07

* Values were indicated are the mean ± SD. min = minutes; AUC = area under the curve; Vss = volume of distribution at steady state; F = fraction of drug absorbed into blood; CL = clearance rate; MRT = mean residence time; GD = gestation day.

As described previously, four artemisinin drugs (QHS, AS, AM, even DQHS) have reported a declining concentration in plasma during multiple oral treatments in malaria patients and health subjects. The C_{max} and AUC values are markedly reduced from one-third to one-seventh on last dose day compared to the first day. The decrease in drug exposure during treatment is not disease-related, since the artemisinin drug PK on day 1 is similar to that reported in healthy subjects [95, 196-199]. One possible explanation for the decrease in plasma concentration-time during treatment is an increase in metabolic capacity due to auto-induction of hepatic drug-metabolizing enzymes. The declining results are also demonstrated in rats following intramuscular and intravenous injections of AS [178, 202]. Why didn't the concentrations decrease after multiple doses of AS were given to pregnant rats?

4.1.5.2. Tissue Distribution of Radiolabeled as in Pregnant Rats

Tissue distribution and pharmacokinetics of $[^{14}C]$ artesunate (^{14}C-AS) related material following single intravenous administration were reported recently in pregnant Sprague-Dawley rats using quantitative whole-body autoradiography [225]. After dosing, rats were deeply anesthetized with isofluorane, euthanized, and frozen by submersion in a bath of hexane cooled to approximately -70°C with solid carbon dioxide at 0.5, 3, 8, 24, 48, 72, 96, and 192. Carcasses were stored at approximately -20°C prior to preparation for whole-body autoradiography. Sagittal, whole body sections, which were approximately 40 μm thick, were obtained from each rat, and were supported using adhesive tape (Scotch Tape No. 8210, 3M Ltd., St. Paul, MN, USA). Sections were taken of various levels from each carcass until samples of the following tissues or biological matrices along with QC blood standards were obtained (where possible): Adipose (brown and white), adrenal gland, bile (in bile duct), blood (cardiac), brain (cerebrum, cerebellum), bone, bone marrow, epididymis, esophagus, uveal tract of the eye and lens, Harderian gland, heart, kidney cortex and medulla, large intestine (and contents), liver, lung, lymph node, nasal turbinates, pancreas, pituitary gland, prostate gland, salivary gland, seminal vesicles, skeletal muscle, skin, amnion, amniotic fluid, fetal body, mammary, ovary, placenta, uterus, vagina, stomach (and contents), small intestine (and contents), spleen, spinal cord, testis, thymus, thyroid, and urinary bladder (and contents).

Sections were allowed to dry by sublimation in the cryomicrotome at -20°C for approximately 2 days. Sections were then mounted on cardboard backing and exposed along with [^{14}C] spiked blood calibration standards to [^{14}C] sensitive imaging plates (Molecular Dynamics, Sunnyvale, CA, USA). The imaging plates and sections were enclosed in exposure cassettes and were allowed to be exposed in a lead safe at room temperature for four days. At the end of the exposure time, the sections were removed from the imaging plate. The plates were then scanned and the images stored onto a dedicated QPS computer server using the Typhoon 9410, phosphor image acquisition system (Molecular Dynamics, Sunnyvale, CA, USA).

Quantification, relative to the calibration standards, was performed by image densitometry using MCID image analysis software (Imaging Research, St. Catherine's, Ontario, Canada). Image optical density data was acquired as MDC/mm2. The autoradiographic standard image data (calibration and internal standards) were sampled using the MCID software to create a calibrated standard curve and to verify section thickness uniformity. The actual whole body sections were used as a reference to identify tissues. Specified tissues, organs, and fluids regions of each image were analyzed, and the tissue concentrations were interpolated from each standard curve as microcuries per gram. Tissue concentration data were determined for the tissues and/or contents listed previously. Tissue concentrations were converted to microgram equivalents per gram of tissue based on the specific activity of the test material [226-228].

Upper and lower limits of quantitation were determined and employed for these data. The results and conclusions described in this report are based on digital images that were selected from a complete set of autoradiographs. The clarity observed in the digital images may not be apparent in reproductions obtained by photocopying.

Similar to our previous publication in male rats [209], the mean terminal half-lives of radioactivity in blood (97.73 h) and other tissues (131.69 hr on average) in the present study were greatly prolonged compared with that of unchanged AS (0.43 h) and unchanged DHA (0.75 h), an active metabolite of AS. The drug was widely distributed after 0.5 hr in select tissues and the total amount of radioactivity in all measured tissues per gram was 217.19 μg equivalents (table 13). The highest concentration of radiolabel was found in small intestine contents (81.21 μg equivalents), followed by the bile (13.22 μg equivalents), small intestine (8.85 μg equivalents), liver (8.12 μg equivalents) and the rest. At the same time point, the total radioactivity was 17.41 μg equivalents detected in feto-placental unit (amnion, amniotic fluid, fetal body, mammary, ovary, placenta, uterus and vagina), indicating that ^{14}C-AS could rapidly cross the placenta and are deposited in fetal pigmented tissues [225].

Three hours after the injection, the radioactivity level in all tissues had increased up to 271.0 μg equivalents; the remarkable increase of radioactivity level in other tissues at 3 hours may relate to the re-distribution from tissues or enterohepatic circulation [209]. However, the drug distribution slightly decreased in productive tissues from 17.41 μg equivalents (0.5 hr) to 14.20 μg equivalents (3 hr). From 8 to 192 hours, measured radioactivity level rapidly declined in all tissues except for the spleen and bone marrow (table 13). At 192 hours after dosing, residual activity (close to 3.58% of total amount collected) was still detected in some tissues and the highest levels of radioactivity were measured in the spleen, bone marrow, kidney, bile (in duct), and adrenal gland; trace amounts were also found in other tissues. The total $AUC_{0\text{-}192h}$ of the radioactivity in all measured tissues of pregnant rats was 22879 μg equivalents·h/g, and only 6.54% (1480 μg equivalents·h/g) of the total radioactivity was present in the feto-placental tissues. During the treatment period, measured levels of radioactivity were more than 2-4 fold higher in the ovary, placenta, and uterus, respectively, than in blood; the AUC of radioactivity from 0 to 192 hours was 555, 367 and 216 μg equivalents·h/g in the ovary, placenta, and uterus, respectively, but 134 μg equivalents·h/ml in the plasma. The half-life of radioactivity was measured in the blood at 97.73 hr, whereas that in the ovary, placenta, and uterus were 159.90, 200.55, and 152.60 hr, respectively, suggesting that ^{14}C-AS remained in those reproductive tissues longer than in blood [225].

4.2. Damage to the Angiogenesis of Embryos Induced by Artemisinins

Artemisinin derivatives are not currently recommended for use during the first trimester of pregnancy in women because the derivatives cause embryo death and some abnormalities in early pregnancy in animals [96-103]. In order to better understand the mechanism of the developmental toxicity in animals, the main animal experiments have been listed here for the discussion.

With big doses (40 mg/kg subcutaneously on day 6-10 of gestation), Lou and Zhou observed that AS significantly decreased the concentration of serum progesterone in early pregnant rats; decidual cells and fetuses of treated groups were found to be degenerated at day 11. Drug was shown to directly damage the decidual cells. Similar results were found in human decidual cell cultures with AS for 48 h. The damage of AS on the decidua and placenta may be the mechanism of its contragestational action [106]. These results also suggested that in order to examine the effect and mechanism of AS on embryo development, rat embryo and placental glutathione peroxidase (GSH-Px) and malondialdehyde (MDA) must be identified by using dithionitrobenzene (DTNB) direct method and thiobarbituric acid (TBA). They found that AS induced developmental toxicity in rat embryos and placenta by neutralizing the antioxidant defense mechanism [107].

Table 13. Mean concentrations and main pharmacokinetic parameters of ^{14}C-AS following single intravenous injections at 5 mg/160 μCi/kg in the tissue or organs of the pregnant rats by quantitative whole body autoradiograph (QWBA) [225]

Tissue Type	Tissue	Cmax μg/g	$t_{1/2}$ hr	AUC μg·h/g	% total AUC
Adipose	Adipose (brown & white)	6.49	118.72	807.67	3.53
Alimentary Canal	Large Intestine	1.82	99.08	173.41	0.76
	Large Intestine (contents)	7.34	49.00	617.83	2.70
	Stomach & Contents	3.44	141.53	361.46	1.58
	Small Intestine	9.47	68.61	204.78	0.90
	Small Intestine (contents)	120.35	27.55	3172.53	13.87
Central Nervous System	Brain	2.11	155.21	88.84	0.39
	Spinal Cord	2.72	168.31	127.65	0.56
Dermal	Skin	1.71	100.77	111.97	0.49
Endocrine	Adrenal Gland	7.59	207.79	1145.58	5.01
	Pituitary Gland	2.93	172.50	213.82	0.93
	Thyroid Gland	2.58	139.81	323.57	1.41
Excretory/ Metabolic	Bile (in duct)	16.84	153.87	1387.64	6.07
	Renal Cortex	6.71	179.10	1490.90	6.52
	Renal Medulla	6.19	117.97	326.73	1.43
	Liver	9.06	160.42	903.65	3.95
	Urinary Bladder	23.66	74.39	674.17	2.95
	Urinary Bladder (contents)	44.27	41.79	592.24	2.59
Ocular	Eye Uveal Tract	1.08	71.83	45.09	0.20
	Eye Lens	0.29	70.75	17.22	0.08
Reproductive	Amnion & Amniotic Fluid	1.56	76.91	64.32	0.28
	Fetal Body	2.26	83.63	80.91	0.35
	Mammary	2.99	120.76	100.03	0.44
	Ovary	5.84	159.90	555.13	2.43
	Placenta	3.21	200.55	366.77	1.60
	Uterus	2.19	152.60	215.58	0.94
	Vagina	1.46	88.96	96.98	0.42
Respiratory Tract	Lung	2.13	93.92	135.31	0.59
	Nasal Turbinates	4.27	155.33	311.18	1.36
Secretary	Harderian Gland	4.34	78.01	157.18	0.69
	Pancreas	2.96	142.56	235.57	1.03
	Salivary Gland	2.34	206.18	313.67	1.37
Skeletal/ Muscular	Bone	0.32	171.66	25.79	0.11
	Heart	2.96	166.21	405.69	1.77
	Skeletal Muscle	1.91	158.88	135.96	0.59
Vascular/ Lymphatic	Blood (cardiac)	1.57	97.73	133.50	0.58
	Bone Marrow	9.76	359.31	2822.62	12.34
	Lymph Nodes	2.27	200.63	357.48	1.56
	Spleen	8.68	246.06	3359.66	14.68
	Thymus	1.75	175.93	219.16	0.96
			Mean 131.69	Total AUC 22879.22	Total % 100

*The procedures described in this paper were performed in accordance with Quest Pharmaceutical Services, L.L.C. (QPS, Newark, DE). This study was not conducted in compliance with the Food and Drug Administration Good Laboratory Practice Regulations and was not inspected by the quality Assurance department of QPS.

Chen et al. reported that AS [105] and DHA [229] were found to inhibit angiogenesis in vivo and in vitro. The anti-angiogenic effect in vivo was evaluated in nude mice by means of human ovarian cancer HO-8910 implantation and immunohistochemical staining, vascular endothelial growth factor (VEGF) and VEGF receptor KDR/flk-1. The in vitro effect of AS was tested on models of angiogenesis, namely, proliferation, migration and tube formation of human umbilical vein endothelial cells (HUVEC). The results showed that AS and DHA significantly inhibit angiogenesis in a dose-dependent form. Additionally, the inhibitory effect of AS and DHA on HVUEC proliferation was stronger than that on Hela, JAR, HO-8910 cancer cells, NIH-3T3 fibroblast cells and human endometrial cells, indicating that AS and DHA were selectively against HUVEC. These findings and the known low toxicity of AS and DHA are clues that artemisinins may be a promising angiogenesis inhibitor [105, 229].

The effects of DHA in rat's whole embryo cultures (WEC) were recently conducted by Longo et al. [104]. DHA was added to the culture medium for the entire 48-hour culture, 1.5 hours after the beginning or 1.5 hours before the end of the culture dose of 0.01–2 μg/ml. DHA affected primarily red blood cells during yolk sac hematopoiesis. Higher concentrations and longer exposure inhibited angiogenesis. More studies the inhibition of angiogenesis by artemisinins were conducted by various investigators [230-235]. AS strongly reduced angiogenesis in vivo in terms of vascularization of Matrigel plugs injected subcutaneously into syngenic mice. Based on these studies, AS represents a promising candidate drug for the treatment of the highly angiogenic Kaposi's sarcoma. As a low-cost drug, it might be of particular interest to areas of Kaposi's sarcoma endemics. These results and the known low toxicity are clues that AS and DHA may be promising novel candidates for cancer chemotherapy [232, 235].

It is clear that the embryotoxicity and contragestational effect of artemisinins (AS and DHA) in pregnant animal species is mainly due to the angiogenesis and the expressions of vascular endothelial growth factor on embryos and fetuses. Further research has demonstrated that the embryotoxicity of artemisinins is drug exposure level dependent [104, 229].

4.3. Artemisinins Exposure Level and Time on Inhibition of Angiogenesis

To study the effects of DHA on embryonic development, a rat whole embryo culture (WEC) study was conducted by Longo et al. [104]. This model allowed the investigation of early embryonic developmental stages, which reportedly were highly susceptible to artemisinin compounds in vivo, in the absence of maternal interaction. Ultimately, the WEC study was conducted in order to understand better the mechanism of the developmental toxicity and to identify the initial target of action of DHA.

On gestation day 9, pregnant female rats were euthanized to extract embryos (9.5 days of age, 1–3 somites). The extracted embryos were randomly distributed to experimental groups and cultured in a 25-ml glass bottle (5 embryos/bottle) containing 5 ml of heat-inactivated sterile rat serum. DHA was dissolved in DMSO and added to the culture medium (5 μl/bottle) in order to obtain a range of final concentrations of 10 – 2000 ng/ml. Group 1: control, DMSO 0.1% from GD 9.5 to 11.5; Group 2: DHA 10, 50, 100, 500, 1000 and 2000 ng/ml from GD 9.5 to 11.5; Group 3: DHA 50, 100, 500, 1000 and 2000 ng/ml at GD 9.5 for 1.5 h, thereafter the medium was changed and embryos were cultured in normal serum until GD 11.5; Group 4: DHA 1000 and 2000 ng/ml at GD 11, 1.5 hr before the end of the culture. At the end of the culture period, the embryos (11.5 days old) were transferred into Tyrode's salt solution (Sigma) and examined under the stereomicroscope.

All embryos exposed to DHA for 48 hr at all concentrations were alive at the end of the culture period. At DHA concentrations ≥ 50 ng/ml, the visceral yolk sac was well vascularized but pale; yolk sac vessel formation and circulation appeared normal but blood was visibly paler than in controls. This effect increased in proportion to increasing DHA concentrations. At concentrations ≥ 500 ng/ml, the vasculature was also affected. Vessel diameter was reduced, small anastomotic vessels were not visible, and the number of circulating cells was further reduced. At 1 µg/ml, yolk sac vasculature and circulating cells were markedly reduced and at 2000 ng/ml only a few poorly organized yolk sac vessels were present.

The allantois, although well developed up to the DHA concentration of 500 ng/ml, showed pale umbilical vessels starting from 50 ng/ml. At 1 µg/ml, the allantois was present but attached ectopically to the yolk sac (fusion with the chorion did not occur near the ectoplacental cone but in other regions of the yolk sac). At 2000 ng/ml, the allantois was lying free in the exocelom. At DHA ≥ 1000 ng/ml, the heart-rate was reduced and irregular. Analysis of cytospin blood preparations showed a reduction in the number of RBCs starting at concentrations ≥ 100 ng/ml, and deformed or damaged RBCs at concentrations ≥ 500 ng/ml. At 2000 ng/ml, DHA induced complete embryonic disruption with multiple non-specific abnormalities. Histological examination showed areas of cell death in the branchial arches, in the mesenchyme of the caudal region and near the dorsal aorta at 100, 500 and 1000 ng/ml. Complete tissue disorganization was detected at 2000 ng/ml. Histological examination confirmed the reduced presence of RBCs in the heart and aorta of embryos exposed to DHA at 100 ng/ml concentrations. For embryos exposed to DHA for 48 hr, the no observed adverse effect level (NOAEL) was 10 ng/ml.

Similar observation of the embryotoxicity was also found at 1.5 hr after culture with DHA. The embryos exposed to DHA at all concentrations tested were alive at the end of the culture period and had normal heart rate. At DHA concentrations ≥ 100 ng/ml, the visceral yolk sac, although well vascularized, was pale; yolk sac vessel formation and circulation appeared normal, but blood was visibly paler than in control embryos. This effect was more obvious with increasing concentrations. Starting from 1µg/ml, the circulation was also affected, and small anastomotic vessels were not visible. The allantois, although well developed at all concentrations tested, showed pale umbilical vessels starting from 100 ng/ml and cases of ectopy from 1000 ng/ml. At DHA concentrations ≥ 2000 ng/ml, the heart rate was reduced and irregular in the majority of embryos. The analysis of cytospin blood preparations showed a clear reduction in the number of RBCs starting from 500 ng/ml and deformed or damaged RBCs from 1000 ng/ml. For embryos exposed to DHA for 1.5 h at the start of the culture, the NOAEL was 50 ng/ml.

The results evidently indicated that the drug exposure level is more important to induce the embryotoxicity than drug exposure time; this was evident because the AS and DHA have very short half lives [44] in clinical therapy. When concentrations of DHA were increased to100 ng/ml for 1.5 hr, the initial damage could be seen on the embryos. At 500 ng/ml, the analysis of cytospin blood preparations showed a clear reduction in the number of RBCs. At 1000 ng/ml level, the significant ectopy, irregular heart rate, and deformed or damaged RBCs were observed and detected. Those indicators would be great references for the clinical monitoring on the embryotoxicity induced by artemisinins. The literature on human trials and animal experiments concluded that a range of 1000-2000 ng/ml was an acceptable estimation of median AS or DHA maximum concentration [162-176].

4.4. Drug Sensitivity Period in Pregnant Animals and in Pregnant Women

Although the drug exposure level is a major factor in the development of embryotoxicity in animals, the sensitive duration period of the embryos during the gestation is another important factor for the toxic investigation. In most studies in the rat, treatment usually started around implantation on day 6 and continued thereafter. A common effect seen was a dose-related increase in post-implantation loss with total resorptions at higher dose levels. Some studies show instances of morphological abnormalities at doses that cause fetal resorption, without maternal toxicity. All studies using AS, AM or AE show a steep dose–response curve and some have demonstrated marked sensitivity to the day of dosing between Days 9–14 of gestation in the rat. In particular, in Chinese studies on rats, with AS, a dose of 0.4 mg/kg produced no increase in resorptions (5.8%), but 0.8 mg/kg caused 98% resorption [98]. Total resorption was also induced by AS at 25 mg/kg SC, when administered during GD 9–11 or 12–14, while no effect was seen when treatment was given prior to GD 8 or after GD 14. Further comparative in vivo experiments with AS, DHA, AM and AE indicate that the critical period for induction of resorption is GD 9–14; GD 10 is identified as the most sensitive day [104].

From day 9.5 of gestation in rats (day 7.5 in mice) and day 15 in humans, simple diffusion is no longer sufficient to meet the increasing demand for oxygen supply of the growing embryo. At that point, undifferentiated mesenchyme on the yolk sac condenses to form angiogenetic cell clusters, the blood islands that give rise to hematopoietic stem cells (the precursors of the blood cells) and angioblasts (the precursors of blood vessels). As soon as a capillary network is created, mature erythroid cells formed within the yolk sac enter the embryos and reach the vitelline vessels. Hematopoiesis within the yolk sac occurs in rats during GD 9–14 (GD 7–12 in mice) and in humans between GD 15 and 6 weeks of gestation, when it is replaced by late embryonic, fetal and subsequently definitive adult sites of hematopoiesis (the liver, spleen and bone marrow) [236]. The effects of exposure to artemisinins during this special period of organogenesis can be noticed especially on the embryotoxicity.

During the development period embraced by this experiment, it becomes more apparent that a transition occurs from predominantly anaerobic to aerobic glycolysis, with active Krebs cycle and oxidative phosphorylation; this requires significantly higher oxygen concentrations as well as an adequate circulation. Accordingly, culture conditions are changed from 5 to 20% O_2. Under the latter conditions, the probability of reactive oxygen species (ROS) formation is increased. The visceral yolk sac has a protective role for the embryo proper by removing ROS and antioxidant defenses increase several times in the yolk sac from GD 9 to 13 [237].

Longo's results are compatible with the hypothesis that DHA also affects RBC precursors (hemoangioblasts) and the Wolffian blood islands, thus explaining why hematopoiesis as well as vasculogenesis and angiogenesis are affected, although with different sensitivities. Some of the features observed in embryos seem to point to similar mechanisms as those described above for the malaria parasite. Embryonic RBCs derived from the yolk sac have transferrin receptors as they react with anti-rat CD71 monoclonal antibody. Moreover, some of the in vivo studies reported fetal growth retardation, delayed skeletal development and cardiovascular malformations in the animals [97-107]. The damage to the hematopoietic system and angiogenetic process may all be induced by exposure to those artemisinins. Finally, the days of marked sensitivity correspond to the period of yolk sac hematopoiesis, which occurs during GD 9–14 in rats and, correspondingly, GD 15 to week 6 in humans.

4.5. Drug Exposure Duration and Peak Level Concerning the Reprotoxicity

The adverse impact of malaria in pregnant women is largely caused by *P. falciparum*; approximately 90% of clinical cases globally occur in sub-Saharan Africa. Every year there are approximately 50 million pregnancies in women living in malarious areas [222]. Artemisinins have been used to treat pregnant women since 1987 [110]. Data from limited clinical trials in pregnant women (2101 cases) exposed to artemisinin compounds, including a small number (108 cases) in the first trimester, do not show an increase in the rates of abortion or stillbirth or evidence of abnormalities. There were no clinically significant adverse effects of the drug, neither in the outcomes of the pregnancies, nor in the development (neurological and physical) of the infants, including 44 infants exposed during the first trimester [109-120, 238, 239]. Are artemisinins really not toxic to either the women, the fetuses during pregnancy, or to the infants during lactation? Without other relevant human pharmacokinetic data, it is difficult to quantify the risk of possible embryonic death or teratogenicity with exposure to artemisinin compounds in the first trimester in women. However, the two factors of the pharmacokinetic characteristics (including tissue distribution) and the drug sensitive period of the embryos during the gestation (summarized above) may assist us in avoiding the low birth weight, abortion, and even potentially fetal death for pregnant women requiring malaria therapy.

In the summary of embryotoxicity in animals (table 7), the severe toxic effects were detected in the animals treated with AS after single or multiple intravenous, intramuscular or subcutaneous injections. The three ED_{50} doses (0.58-1.0 mg/kg) are all below human therapeutic dose (2-4 mg/kg). Other dosage regimens of AS, AM and DHA produced the high ED_{50} doses with values of 6.1-32.8 mg/kg in those animal species, which seems to be safe in clinical usage because those dosages are higher than the human therapeutic doses with wide safety margin. Why is the situation so severe such that there is AS only following the single or multiple injections intravenously, intramuscularly and subcutaneously? The possible explanations could be:

1 The administration is during the days of marked sensitivity corresponding to the period of yolk sac hematopoiesis, which occurs during GD 9–14 in rats;

2 The bioequivalences of AS by intramuscular and subcutaneous administration are fulfilled for AS by intravenous injection in rats [224], and the 3 administrations of AS can produce a significantly higher peak concentration than AS, AM, and DHA after oral administration or AM with oil vehicle after intramuscular injection in rats [44]. Again, the data revealed that the peak concentration is a major issue that causes the toxicity;

3 As with multiple administrations, a single subcutaneous injection of AS also induced severe embryotoxicity in hamsters, demonstrating that the drug exposure level (even with just one exposure) is the principal role for persuading the toxicity when compared to longer drug exposure time with multiple doses;

4 When the peak concentrations are high in the blood, the concentration could be even higher in the location of the feto-placental unit because the drug distribution of AS in feto-placental tissues was always higher (2-4 folds) than that in the blood of the pregnant rats [225].

To treat women with artemisinins, a recent WHO consultation has recommended that: i) because of the limited experience with artemisinins in pregnancy they should only be used when other treatments are considered unsuitable; ii) presently, they cannot be recommended for treatment of malaria in the first trimester. They should not, however, be withheld if they are considered lifesaving for the mother; iii) to further document the safety of artemisinin compounds in pregnancy, careful follow-up is required, with documentation of pregnancy outcome and the subsequent development of the child whenever possible; and iv) to guide further development of policies on the use of artemisinin derivatives during pregnancy, alone or in combination, there is an urgent need for further research/documentation of their efficacy and safety for use as therapy for malaria [108].

In accordance with WHO recommendations and the new research described above, the two major issues for considering artemisinin drug use in a program for prevention or management of malaria in pregnant women are safety and effectiveness. First, the exposure to artemisinins should be avoided during the early sensitive days (GD 15 to week 6 in humans), which is the critical period for induction of embryo damage and resorption, to protect pregnant women from malaria with treatment of artemisinin derivatives. This is essentially the same recommendation as WHO consult above that the artemisinin drugs should not be used in the first trimester of pregnancy in women. Secondly, WHO recommends that artemisinin compounds should only be used in the second and third trimester when other treatments are considered unsuited. However, we feel that oral doses or oral doses in combination regimens could be used to treat pregnant women at in the first trimester when other treatments are considered unsuited, because the oral regiments provides a lower peak concentrations, and that can make the agents safer than intravenous or intramuscular injection of AS. In fact, reprotoxicity was not found in humans treated with artemisinins during the past twenty years; this conclusion resulted from the more than 90% of pregnant women treated orally or intramuscularly with AM in sesame oil over that period whose tests resulted in a much low plasma concentration and prolonged absorption from muscle [65, 109-120].

In addition, further studies to define the precise mechanism of damage in animal models are warranted. Reliable pharmacovigilance on the use of these drugs in pregnancy and the careful monitoring of safety after exposure in the first trimester of pregnancy, when treatment may occur inadvertently or be necessary to save life even with injection AS, are needed.

To date, there have been no convincingly documented cases of embryotoxicity or other reprotoxicity side effects noted in humans due to QHS, DHA, AM and AS treatments [109-120, 238, 239]. After the four oral drugs and one intramuscular drug (AM) administration, the conversion of AM and AS to DHA in humans was been much higher than that in animal species although they produced lower peak concentrations in plasma [156-171]. It remains unknown how humans have been able to avert the death embryotoxicity described in animal species. Data from limited clinical trials in pregnant women (2,101 cases) exposed to artemisinin compounds, including a small number (108 cases) in the first trimester, have not shown an increase in the rates of abortion or stillbirth; they have also not shown evidence of abnormalities. With regard to acute toxicity, humans appear to be less sensitive than animals [203, 204] and humans have much better repair capabilities than do animals [205]. Other possible considerations for the reprotoxicity discrepancy observed between animal and human:

I. The animal data revealed that only intramuscular or subcutaneous (including intravenous) AS causes reprotoxicity at lower dose than the therapeutic dose (2-4 mg/kg) in humans. Other doses in different regimens (oral or intramuscular AM) are safe at higher levels than the therapeutic doses. Since more than 90% of pregnant patients have been treated with oral or intramuscular AM in our counted trials (2101 cases), it may be the reason for the lack of toxicity observed;
II. Many of the pregnant patients followed have been seriously ill with malaria, which is responsible for 5-12% low birth weight (LBW), 35% of LBW that is preventable during pregnancy [240], and contributes to 70,000-200,000 infant deaths each year [241]. The resulting evidence may lead to future studies on whether the pattern of reprotoxicity has occurred from the illness or from the drug(s) [238, 242];
III. A number of early reports have not paid much attention to the feasibility of associating low birth weight, abortion, and/or infant disorders in patients with such treatment of malaria with artemisinins; and
IV. Post-marketing surveillance has been limited in developing countries, and the potential reproductive side-effects of the drug have not been well recorded.

5. Relationship between Drug Efficacy and Pharmacokinetics

Artemisinin derivatives have been found to kill not only asexual blood stages, but also early stages of gametocytes of *P. falciparum* [243-246]. DHA is highly effective against all parasitical blood stages [5] and gametocytes of *P. falciparum* [247]. Other artemisinin drugs (AM, AE, AS and AL) are most active against rings and schizonts stages but are not as active against trophozoites stage of *P. falciparum, P. cynomolgi, P. vinckei petteri and P. berghei*

[5-15]. The results of clinical trials to date indicate that artemisinins are relatively non-toxic and rapidly effective against multi-drug resistant strains of *P. falciparum* [248, 249]. However, patients treated with artemisinin drugs alone have been found to exhibit high recrudescence rates [250]. The pharmacodynamic properties of these drugs have been relatively addressed with pharmacokinetic findings [161, 164, 166, 250].

5.1. Drug Exposure Level and Time Affect on Efficacy *In Vitro*

At dose range 10^{-7}-10^{-5} M (30 –3000 ng/ml), synchronous culture study showed that artemisinin was extremely effective against both of ring and schizonts stages, demonstrating 100% growth inhibition of these stages within 4-6 h. The inhibitory effects of AM were more gradual, requiring 8-10 hr of exposure time to achieve 70% growth inhibition of the ring stage and 40-50% inhibition of schizonts stage. DHA is found to be highly effective against all stages of the parasite, in most cases achieving 100% growth inhibition by 2-4 hr [5].

Classically, *in vitro* studies have addressed the effect of drug exposure against *P. Falciparum* for 48 hr (one life cycle). Recently, more life cycles of *P. falciparum* study on drug exposure time and concentration had been investigated [9, 251]. The parasite viability after exposure to artemisinin was assessed to explore any killing or suppressive effect of the compound in relation to its concentrations and exposure time. Concentration of 10^{-6}-10^{-5} M (280-2800 ng/ml) artemisinin showed a parasitical effect after only 3 hr of drug exposure, whereas 10^{-7} M (28 ng/ml) artemisinin required 24 hr of exposure for a cidal effect. At concentration of 10^{-8} M (2.8 ng/ml), artemisinin had no appreciable effect on the parasites. If the concentration was increased to 3 x 10^{-8} M (8.4 ng/ml), (with drug exposure time extending to 72-96 hr and the parasitemia reducing below the starting level of 0.5%), then the long exposure time to the lower concentration could be as effective as the high concentration [251].

It is clear that the low dose will increase the exposure time, and the high dose will shorten the treatment period. At a 10^{-8} or 10^{-7} dose level (3-30 ng/ml), artemisinin drugs require 24-96 hr of constant exposure to kill all parasites (IC_{99}). Therefore, the low dose range cannot be selected for artemisinin drugs in human treatments in malaria because 1) the artemisinins have very short half-life and 2) longer exposure time of artemisinins is a principle factor leading to fatal neurotoxicity because the exposure time is more likely responsible than other PK parameters resulting in fatal neurotoxicity.

Survival of the patient is obviously key in treating patients with severe and complicated malaria. Using a low effective dose would delay the treatment time period and should not be allowed. A high loading dose would best achieve switching off all the parasite's vital functions as soon as possible [252]. There is currently no evidence that rapid parasite killing with high doses is harmful. Similarly, there is no evidence of a Jarisch-Herxheimer reaction in malaria and therapeutic blood drug concentrations can be readily achieved without risking toxicity [247].

Because of these factors, the plasma concentration of the artemisinin derivatives in human against *P. falciparum* should be at least 10^{-6}-10^{-5} (300-3000 ng/ml) or higher for AS or DHA, the more potent of the artemisinin compounds. The concentration should be even higher for AE or AM, and ideally should be higher for AL due to its the lowest antimalarial potency among the five agents [1]. The relative antimalarial potency of artemisinin compounds against W-2 parasites is 0.72 (AL) < 1.0 (QHS) < 1.84 (AM) < 2.41 (AE) < 3.01 (AS) < 3.59 (DHA), and the potency against D-6 parasites is 0.32 (AL) < 1.0 (QHS) < 1.22 (AM) < 1.87 (AE) < 2.48 (AS) < 2.99 (DHA). In fact, higher plasma concentration of AS at 21098 ng/ml in humans [our unpublished data] and AL at 20044 ng/ml in animals did not result in the any toxicity, as discussed in section 3.3 (table 9).

5.2. Drug Exposure Level and Time Affect on Efficacy *In Vivo*

Human and animal species studies have shown unambiguously that artemisinin derivatives are very potent drugs against *falciparum* and *vivax* malaria. These drugs initiate immediate decreases in parasitemia and, in most studies; clinical recovery of the patient is faster than with other antimalarials. However, a high recrudescence (about 30-50% for 3 days, 6-15% fro 5 days, and 2-6% for 7 days regimens) is still a major disadvantage for all of these compounds after monotherapy [12, 33]. Although the clinical significance of the rapid killing advantage, in terms of mortality, has yet to be determined by using other artemisinins drugs [23, 24, 74], at least one published study has shown the potential in decreasing mortality. The SEAQUAMAT trial, a multicentre randomized trial conducted in Bangladesh, Thailand, Myanmar, Indonesia, India and Vietnam, recently reported a 34.7% reduction in mortality associated with intravenous AS compared with intravenous quinine [138, 145, 146].

Efficacy in Malaria (Animal Models)

Injectable AS is being developed as a potential agent for the treatment of severe and complicated malaria. A risk assessment of the therapeutic index and related hematological changes of AS and AL following daily intravenous injection for 3 days has been conducted in *P. berghei* infected and uninfected rats. The minimum doses of AS and AL for parasitemia suppression were 2.3 and 2.5 mg/kg, respectively, and the suppressive doses for decreasing parasitemia by half (SD_{50}) were 7.4 and 8.6 mg/kg, respectively. There seemed to be no significant difference between these two water-soluble compounds at suppressive dose levels [179].

However, with regards to parasite clearance time (PCT), equimolar doses of 96 μmoles/kg, AS (36.7 mg/kg) cleared parasitemia in 7 out of 18 rats with a 39% clearance rate. At this dose, the PCT of AS was 52.8 hrs and clearance time lasted only 2.7 days with recrudescence back in the 7 animals. Accordingly, AS did not clear 0.339% (Emax) of parasitemia in rats treated at this dose level. The EC_{50} was 8.86 hrs, and the area under the effect curve (AUEC) was 536 % of parasitemia·hr for this dosage of AS/$NaHCO_3$ in the 7 rats. Using the same equimolar dose of 96 μmoles/kg, AL (40.6 mg/kg) cleared the parasitemia in all of 19 rats with 100% clearance rate. At this dose level, the PCT of AL was 57.2 hrs with clearance lasting for 3.2 days before recrudescence. Computer fitting revealed that E_0 was 6.2 ± 2.3%, whereas Emax was measured at 0.008 ± 0.01% of parasitemia. The EC_{50} was 10.9 hrs, and the area under the effect curve (AUEC) was 313 % of parasitemia·hr for this dosage of AL [179].

It is comprehensible from this data that at the equimolar dose of AL (with 100% clearance) has much great efficacy than that of AS (with 39% clearance) in the malaria infected rat. However, the *in vitro* data indicate that, AS has a 5-8 fold greater antimalarial activity than AL (Section 5.1.). Why do the results contrast between *in vitro* and *in vivo* data? A pharmacokinetic analysis may provide the answer to the question. The comparative pharmacokinetics and hydrolysis studies of intravenously administered AL and AS were performed in malaria-infected rats using 3 daily equimolar doses (96 μmoles/kg). The drug concentration of AS with daily doses of 36.7 mg/kg was one-third less on day 3 than on day 1, and the mean Cmax of AS on day 1 was 16,492 ng/ml and 1,377 ng/ml on day 3. Similar to its active metabolite, DHA, it had peak plasma drug concentrations of 10,842 and 6,485 ng/ml on days 1 and 3, respectively, suggesting an auto-induction of hepatic drug-metabolizing enzymes for AS [95, 196-199].

The auto-induction of the enzymes were similar for other artemisinin drugs (QHS, DHA, AE and AM) [95, 196-199], but not for AL. Pharmacokinetic parameters of AL were very comparable from day 1 to day 3 with same AS molecular dose at 40.6 mg/kg. The mean Cmax of AL on day 1 was 48,453 ng/ml and 44,101ng/ml on day 3. AS is the pro-drug of DHA with a DHA/AS ratio of 5.26 compared to a ratio of 0.01 for DHA/AL. Although total $AUC_{1\text{-}3D}$ of 13,051 ng·h/ml DHA was produced by AS compared to 524 ng·h/ml DHA by AL, the peak level of AL was still 2-fold and 6-fold higher than that of AS plus DHA concentrations on day 1 and day 3, respectively. The increase in AL's peak concentration can explain why AL has a much great efficacy than AS *in vivo* (figure 10). Other pharmacokinetic parameters revealed that the total $AUC_{1\text{-}3}$ days (84.4 μg·h/ml) of AL was 5-fold higher than that of AS (15.7 μg·h/ml of AS plus DHA). The elimination half-life of AL (7.1 h) was much longer than that of AS (0.36 h) or DHA (0.72 h) (table 14). The remarkable alteration of the pharmacokinetic shape of AL may be caused by poor conversion rates to DHA and an enterohepatic circulation, which has been confirmed by pharmacokinetics and tissue distribution studies [178, 209]. Compared to AS, higher drug peak and AUC values of AL in the rat blood may be the cause of its increased efficacy in vivo.

To evaluate the efficacy of AE and AM with two different intramuscular vehicles, sesame oil and cremophore, efficacy and pharmacokinetic investigation have been performed in rats [152]. AE and AM showed comparable efficacy against *P. berghei* when used cremophore vehicle to replace sesame oil following intramuscular treatment. The results of 50% cure dose (CD_{50}) were significantly different between the sesame oil and cremophore. AE and AM with sesame oil had the similar CD_{50} values of 34.1 (1.3-66.9) and 35.6 (7.6-63.6) mg/kg, respectively. However, the drugs with cremophore had 14.2 (6.8-21.5) and 21.0 (18.5-23.4) mg/kg for AE and AM, respectively, in malaria mice (table 15). The results showed that AE and AM formulated in cremophore had a significantly higher efficacy than the sesame oil formulation following the three daily multiple intramuscular injections in mice.

Table 14. Toxicokinetic parameters of artesunate (AS) and artelinate (AL) at 96 μmoles/kg following multiple intravenous injections daily for three days in *P. berghei* infected rats by using Culex automated blood sampler. [178]

TK Parameters	AS (36.7 mg/kg , n = 4)		AL (40.6 mg/kg, n = 6)	
	Parent drug (AS)	Metabolite (DHA)	Parent drug (AL)	Metabolite (DHA)
Day 1				
Cmax (ng/ml)	16492 ± 4205	10842 ± 1950	48453 ± 7177	124.2 ± 36.2
Tmax (h)	0	0.19 ± 0.03	0	0.33 ± 0.18
$AUC_{inf.}$ (ng·h/ml)	1324 ± 242	4893 ± 779	25857 ± 2114	160.4 ± 86.2
$t_{1/2}$ distribution (h)	0.04 ± 0.01	0.20 ± 0.02	0.29 ± 0.06	
$t_{1/2}$ elimination (h)	0.36 ± 0.03	0.72 ± 0.05	7.05 ± 2.01	
Vss (liter/kg)	8.10 ± 1.70	-	4.57 ± 2.01	
CL (ml/min/kg)	474.2 ± 89.8	-	25.93 ± 2.10	
MRT (h)	0.62 ± 0.33	0.43 ± 0.04	2.89 ± 1.11	
Day 3				
Cmax (ng/ml)	1377 ± 898	6485 ± 1053	44101 ± 21452	116.6 ± 74.3
Tmax (h)	0	0.18 ± 0.06	0	0.26 ± 0.12
$AUC_{inf.}$ (ng·h/ml)	490.6 ± 314.0	3327 ± 743	24650 ± 8663	204.2 ± 134
$t_{1/2}$ distribution (h)	0.12 ± 0.07	0.21 ± 0.02	0.30 ± 0.08	
$t_{1/2}$ elimination (h)	0.46 ± 0.06	0.65 ± 0.06	6.06 ± 0.64	
Vss (liter)	76.87 ± 8.54	-	5.24 ± 3.50	
CL (ml/min/kg)	2172 ± 1274	-	29.40 ± 8.24	
MRT (h)	0.53 ± 0.01	0.60 ± 0.11	2.78 ± 1.34	
Total $AUC_{1\text{-}3D}$ (ng·h/ml)	2717 ± 809	13051 ± 1926	84406 ± 19703	524 ± 277
Ratio of DHA/AS or DHA/AL (1-3D)		5.26 ± 2.22		0.01 ± 0.00

TK = toxicokinetics, DHA = dihydroartemisinin, MRT = Mean residence time; D = days.

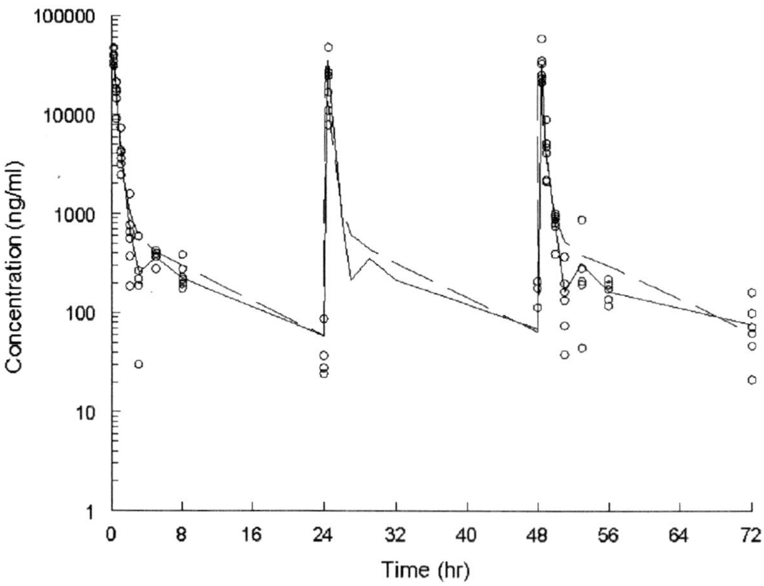

Figure 10 (Continued)

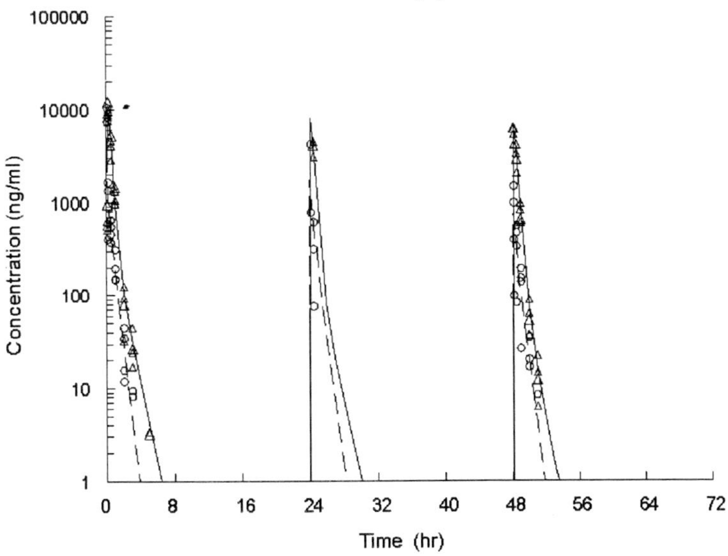

Figure 10. Individual plasma concentration-time profiles of artelinate (AL) measured by LC/MS/MS (markers) and mean concentration (solid line) as well as computer fitted curves (dashed line) by pharmacokinetic parameters at daily dosage of 40.6 mg/kg intravenously for three days in malaria-infected rats (top, n = 6). Individual plasma concentration-time profiles of artesunate (AS) measured by HPLC-ECD (markers) and computer fitted curves for parent drug, AS (dashed line), and its active metabolite, DHA (solid line), by pharmacokinetic parameters at dosage of 36.7 mg/kg once daily intravenously for 3 days in *P. berghei* infected male rats.(bottom, n = 4) [178].

Table 15. Antimalarial activity (50% cure dose, CD_{50})* and corresponding 95% confidence interval (95% CI) of arteether and artemether given intramuscularly in daily dose for 3 days against P. berghei in female mice (n = 8 for each dose level) [152]

Drug	Arteether (CD_{50})		Artemether (CD_{50})	
	mg/kg	95%CI	mg/kg	95%CI
Sesame oil formulation	34.1	1.3-66.9	35.6	7.6-63.6
Cremophore formulation	14.2	6.8-21.5	21.0	18.5-23.4

* When the mice have survived and showed negative smears at 60 days, they were considered cured.

The mean plasma concentration-time profile (n = 3) of AE formulated with sesame oil (AESO) and 1:2 cremophore/0.9% saline (AECM) after single intravenous and intramuscular doses is shown in figure 3 (bottom). AE with sesame oil and cremophore data showed a biphasic pattern of disposition and was fitted by a two-compartment open model after either intravenous or intramuscular injection. The concentration-time profiles of AE with the two vehicles are shown in figure 7 after daily intramuscular for 7 days with the multiple administrations. The trough plasma concentrations increased significantly up to the last dosing in AESO treated rats, but not in AECM rats. Obviously, the drug accumulated (7.5-fold) in the plasma of animals administered with AESO (comparing the 7th dosing day to the first dosing day). In the AECM rats, the AE level increased slightly (1.8-fold) on day 7 over that on day 1 following the multiple dosing.

Significant differences in pharmacokinetic parameters between AECM and AESO are summarized in table 16 after multiple intramuscular doses of 25 mg/kg. Plasma peak concentration on day 1 indicated that the Cmax of AECM (1227 ± 171 ng/ml) was more than 13-fold higher than that of AESO (92.2 ± 19.9 ng/ml). The area under the curve (AUC) of AECM (4165 ± 676 ng·h/ml) was about 4-fold greater than that of AESO (1135 ± 277 ng·h/ml) on day 1. Total AUC of AECM (46286 ± 2061 ng·h/ml) during the 7-day dosing period was about 2.7-fold higher than that of AESO (16922 ± 4038 ng·h/ml). The elimination half-life was 7.0 ± 0.9 hr for AECM and 17.7 ± 2.7 hr for AESO on day 1. Based on the AUC data, the bioavailability of AECM was 74.5 ± 12.1% and 20.3 ± 5.0% for AESO after a single intramuscular injection. The data suggested that AECM, a less oily formulation, was more easily absorbed by the muscle with a higher Cmax and AUC, which may be the explanation of its increased efficacy.

Table 16. Pharmacokinetic parameters of arteether (AE) and dihydroartemisinin, a metabolite of AE, following single intravenous (25 mg/kg), and multiple intramuscular (25 mg/kg) administration with sesame oil and 1:2 cremophore (CRM)/0.9% saline daily for 7 days in male rats (n = 3-7) [152]

Dosing Parameters	IV single	Intramuscular Multiple			
	Vehicle:	Sesame oil (AESO)		1:2 Cremophore/saline (AECM)	
	CRM/Saline	Day 1	Day 7	Day 1	Day 7
Arteether					
Cmax (ng/ml)	14482 ±1023	92.2 ± 19.9	311.9 ± 54.6	1227 ± 171	1826 ± 118
Tmax (min)	0	1.42 ± 0.63	1.67 ± 0.58	1.33 ± 0.29	1.33 ± 0.58
AUC (ng·h/ml)	5593 ± 591	1135 ± 277	8527 ± 1006	4165 ± 676	7312 ± 588
AUC_{D1-8} (ng·h/ml)			16922 ± 4038		46286 ± 2061
Vss (liter)	0.98 ± 0.25	150.2 ± 33.7	54.1 ± 7.8	8.70 ± 1.21	5.06 ± 0.27
Cl (ml/min/kg)	71.3 ± 9.11	73.7 ± 2.8	147.9 ± 6.19	76.3 ± 2.9	76.0 ± 1.9
$t_{1/2}$ distribution (h)	0.22 ± 0.04	0.71 ± 0.47	1.08 ± 0.49	1.00 ± 0.04	1.18 ± 0.14
$t_{1/2}$ elimination (h)	0.82 ± 0.05	17.66 ± 2.68	29.57 ± 2.07	6.96 ± 0.93	9.06 ± 1.69
MAT (h)	-	0.76 ± 0.40	0.87 ± 0.39	1.04 ± 0.03	1.07 ± 0.10
MRT (h)	0.74 ± 0.18	23.56 ± 3.42	41.51 ± 2.84	6.21 ± 0.66	5.83 ± 0.09
Bioavailability (%)	100	20.3 ± 5.0	152.4 ± 17.9	74.5 ± 12.1	130.7 ± 10.5
% of single daily dose in muscle		37.6 ± 8.2	91.4 ± 11.6	4.7 ± 1.8	17.3 ± 3.3
Dihydroartemisinin (DHA, a metabolite of AE)					
Cmax (ng/ml)	815.8 ±164.2	16.02 ± 4.05	123.8 ± 28.9	171.1 ± 79.4	188.4 ± 91.0
Tmax (min)	0	0.92 ± 0.14	0.86 ± 0.35	0.92 ± 0.14	1.33 ± 0.29
AUC (ng·h/ml)	350.0 ± 97.1	117.1 ± 33.0	790.3 ± 220.6	607.7 ± 101.5	708.2 ± 29.2
AUC_{D1-8} (ng·h/ml)			3427 ± 759		5346 ± 831
$t_{1/2}$ elimination (h)	1.08 ± 0.16	9.17 ± 2.54	14.47 ± 2.17	4.71 ± 0.71	6.64 ± 1.25
Ratio of DQHS/AE	0.06 ± 0.02	0.09 ± 0.03	0.08 ± 0.03	0.14 ± 0.03	0.11 ± 0.01

* On day 1 the amount of dose in the muscle was measured at 24 h after first dosing, and on day 7 the amount of dose was measured at 24h after last dosing. IV = intravenous, CRM/saline = 1:2 cremophore/0.9% saline.

The *in vivo* efficacy model shows that AE and AM formulated with cremophore had a significantly higher efficacy than that with sesame oil. It is apparent that the higher plasma concentration of AE produced by cremophore formulation has prinçiple role in the increased efficacy. Plasma concentration showed that the C_{max} and AUC of AECM were about 13-fold and 5-fold, respectively, higher than that of AESO on day 1. Even the total AUC of AECM (46286 ng·h/ml) during the 7-day period was 2.7-fold higher than with AESO (16922 ng·h/ml). The much higher level of AE exposure in the rats using a cremophore vehicle truly contributed to the antimalarial efficacy, and without a doubt, the antimalarial efficacy is drug concentration dependent [5, 9, 251, 252], especially with the 13-fold higher peak concentration.

Efficacy in Malaria (Human Studies)

Karbwang reported on four patients, not cured of their malaria by the oral AM regimen used in his study, that had significantly lower plasma concentrations of DHA, an active metabolite of AM [25] than others in the study. Using the same AM dose amount, a much lower C_{max} (196 ng/ml at 6 h and 54 ng/ml at 12 h) of DHA was measured in the four patients than the Cmax (354 ng/ml at 6 h and 158 ng/ml at 12h) of DHA in 46 other subjects. Also, a lower AUC (834 ng·h/ml) of DHA was detected in these 4 patients but not in the remaining 46 patients (3684 ng·h/ml). Concentrations of the parent drug, AM, was not much different in these four patients (1044 ng·h/ml) when compared to the other subjects (1272 ng·h/ml). It is unknown how those patients resulted in such low DHA concentrations, but these low levels of DHA may be the cause for the treatment failure. The four patients, in whom most parasites may have been more mature, may have required higher concentrations of AM/DHA than patients with similar numbers of parasites.

More recently, Sharma reported on two patients who died with a very high degree of parasitemia (16% and 50%) and cerebral malaria. The dose regimen of AM at 80 mg was intramuscularly injected twice on first day and then once daily for another four days [253]. Intramuscular formulation of AM resulted in very low plasma concentration and low bioavailability [85] due to the prolonged absorption from the injection site [187]. This study showed that using a low dose regimen (total 480 mg) may not have enough drug concentration to cure the heavy parasitemia in these patients.

During a phase III clinical trial of intramuscular Artemotil (AE), a patient had inadvertently obtained a full or fractional intravenous injection with the intramuscular formulation on the first day of treatment. The difference in concentration profiles vs. time of AE and DHA for patient number 151 from the high dose group is shown in figure 9 (bottom). As first dosing, AE seemed to be accidentally injected in patient 151 through a vessel instead of the muscle. This resulted in an intravenous injection profile with very high C_{max} concentration right after injection and a rapid distribution phase. AE and DHA plasma concentrations decreased significantly after first dosing with an elimination $t_{1/2}$ of 1.1 hr in the first 6 hrs. After the second intramuscular injection at the 6th hour, the elimination $t_{1/2}$ of AE was immediately extended to 9.35 hr as a daily half-life. The Cmax (2407 ng/ml) was shown to be about 22-fold higher in patient 151 than the mean value (110 ng/ml) reported in other patients in high dose group. AUC value (12259 ng·h/ml) was 2 times higher than the mean value (7403 ng·h/ml) shown in other subjects. The same results were also reported for increasing DHA levels in patient 151. To be expected, this patient was successfully cure at 36 hr (PCT) and 4 hr (FCT) compared with other patients with 64.4 hr (PCT) and 70.1 hr (FCT) [200]. The clinical cure indicated that the intravenous formulation, like AS injection, is very important in the rapid treatment of malaria with high peak concentration (C_{max}), especially in the severe and complicated malaria. In the meantime, the C_{max} (22-fold) could have also been an important factor in the observed increase of drug efficacy.

Other cases of oral or intramuscular administration of AS and AM were compared in malaria patients [144, 254]. The first-dose pharmacokinetic properties of intramuscular AS at 2.4 mg/kg immediately followed by 1.2 mg/kg daily and AM at 3.2 mg/kg intramuscular start, followed by 1.6 mg/kg daily were compared in Vietnamese adults with severe falciparum malaria. A total of 19 patients were studied; 9 received AS, and 10 received AM. Intramuscular AS was rapidly absorbed. Concentrations of AS in plasma peaked between 523 and 3221 ng/ml (median, 2193 ng/ml) within 20 min of injection and then declined with a median (range) half-life of 30 (3 to 67) min. AS was hydrolyzed rapidly and completely to the biologically active metabolite DHA. Peak DHA concentrations in plasma ranged between 488 and 2011 ng/ml (median, 869 ng/ml) and declined with a t1/2 of 52 (26 to 69) min. The median times for fever and parasite clearance were 65 h and 38.2 h, respectively, in the AS group. All patients survived.

In contrast, AM was slowly and erratically absorbed. The absorption profile appeared biphasic. Maximum AM concentrations in plasma ranged between 20 ng/ml and 487 ng/ml (median, 171 ng/ml) and occurred at a median (range) of 10 (1.5 to 24) h. There was relatively little conversion to DHA. After intramuscular injection in cases of severe malaria, absorption of the water-soluble AS is rapid and extensive, whereas the absorption of the oil-based AM is slow and erratic with relatively little conversion to the more active DHA. The median times to fever and parasite clearance were 56 h and 48 h, respectively, in the AM group. Two out of ten patients died in the process (20% mortality). Based on this pharmacological study, parenteral AS seems preferable to AM as an initial antimalarial therapy, particularly in seriously ill patients. Also, with the peak concentration (2193 ng/ml) of AS being 13-fold higher than that (171 ng/ml) of AM, it indicates that a high peak concentration contributes greatly in improving efficacy and reducing mortality.

After oral dose, despite a 29% lower molar dose, oral AS administration result in a significantly larger drug concentration. It also resulted in higher antimalarial activity than after oral AM ($P \leq 0.02$). The mean (95% CI) oral antimalarial bioavailability of AM, relative to oral AS, corrected for molar dose was 58% (40–76). The mean (95% CI) relative antimalarial bioavailability of AM was lower on the first day of treatment, 31% (17–100), compared to the second day, 72% (44–118) ($P = 0.018$). In *vivo* parasite clearance and time above the *in vitro* IC_{90} were similar for the two drugs, despite considerable differences in C_{max} and AUC. The oral antimalarial potency following AM was significantly lower than that after AS. AM oral antimalarial bioavailability was reduced in acute malaria. Oral AS provided greater antimalarial activity than AM at the same molar dose [254].

All of the evidence shows that higher plasma concentration (C_{max} and AUC), especially the peak concentration (C_{max}), will greatly increase the efficacy and clinical therapeutic potentials of artemisinin drugs. As discussed above, from the severity of these complications, *P. falciparum* malaria constitutes a medical emergency, and appropriate treatment should be initiated as soon as infection is suspected. The appropriate treatment means that enough high dose regimens should be given as to provide a successful therapeutic efficacy for the malaria patients. It is known that 84% of all malaria related deaths occurs within 24 hr of hospital admission in African children [255]. Therefore, first exposure concentrations of artemisinin drugs are very clinically important.

5.3. Therapeutic Efficacy of Artemisinins in Monotherapy

The therapeutic potentials of all artemisinin drugs in monotherapy with 54 clinical trials have been summarized in the treatment for malaria with various dose regiments (table 4). Successful (or 100% cure) treatment is found neither in the 3-5 day treatments nor the high dose (4.8 mg/kg) regimens with monotherapy [21-45, 256]. The rates of recrudescence, fever, and parasite clearances are traditional evaluations for the efficacy of the antimalarial drugs in humans. These three parameters exhibit the therapeutic potential of intravenous, intramuscular and oral agents in various regimens. Results have shown that AE in sesame oil vehicle is not superior to that of the oral DHA, oral and intravenous AS, intramuscular AM, or even intramuscular α/β-arteether formulated with peanut oil.

With these data, and their known mode of rapid action, the artemisinin group of antimalarials is considered to be highly and independently effective compared with other traditional malaria drugs. Although there is no evidence that drug resistance has occurred *in vivo*, short treatment courses (3-5 days) are associated with high recrudescence rates. The data that emerges from all available artemisinin drugs is that given a dose sufficient to induce initial parasite clearance and clinical recovery, the duration of therapy is the ultimate determinant for recrudescence. The rates of recrudescence (30-50% for 3 day regimen, 6-15% for 5 day regimen, and 2-6% for 7 day regimen) continues to be a big problem for all these compounds described previously [12, 33]. It has been suggested that preventing recrudescence does not have the highest priority, but that a recrudescence should rather be treated with the same regimen again. Eventually, all patients would be radically cured with this strategy. The potential risk of development of resistance and recrudescence urges us to look for combination regimens that offer radical cure instead.

Reduction of parasitemia measured as the parasite clearance time (PCT), along with the fever clearance time (FCT) are primary measures of initial drug effect in *vivo*. Reviews of this therapeutic efficacy from multiple clinical studies demonstrate that when given alone (monotherapy) AM (oral and intramuscular administration), AS (oral and intravenous dosing), and DHA (oral) appear to have same effects for reducing PCT and FCT with various dose regimens (table 4). The finding that therapeutic potentials of AM and AS in oral formulation could be equal to DHA may be contributed to the great conversion rate of AM and AS to DHA in human and high peak concentrations as described above. AE after intramuscular injection appears to have fewer efficacies than the other 4 drugs, even with high dosage regimen or compared with AM intramuscular formulation (table 4), which may have much lower blood concentration due to slow and prolong absorption [144, 254, 257].

Parasitemia count and clearance time (PCT) do not always accurately reflect the total burden of parasitised red blood cells, but better parameters are not available. All artemisinin compounds induce a remarkably rapid reduction of parasitemia, starting almost immediately after administration [258, 259]. Fortunately the rapid parasite clearance induced by artemisinin drug treatment provides a simple pharmacodynamic measure that can be used in drug comparisons and assessment. Certainly, parasitological cure is the best end point measure of efficacy for patients with malaria. In this review, the available pharmacodynamic data of parasitemia reduction is evaluated with its associated PK result during the malaria treatment in human described as below.

5.4. Pharmacokinetic/Pharmacodynamic Evaluation of the Artemisinins

The pharmacokinetic/pharmacodynamic (PK/PD) results for artemisinin drugs in monotherapy may give us more comprehension in dosage regimen investigation. This section has analyzed the same subjects in one publication for the PK and PD analysis of artemisinin (QHS). However, for the other four drugs (AS, AE, AM, and DHA), the PK and PD with same drug, same administration route, and same dosage regimen are combined from two individual publications [37, 91, 200, 260-263].

Pharmacokinetics (PK), in general, shows an absorption phase of artemisinin drugs following oral or intramuscular administration. It then reaches peak concentration at 1-3 hours followed by a sharp decline in elimination phase. After multiple administrations, four drug concentrations (QHS, AS, AM, even DHA) has been reported to decline daily due to an auto-induction metabolism [95, 196-199]. Following oral administration, AS and DHA has short mean residence time (MRT) with 2.0 and 2.7 hr, respectively, and QHS has longer MRT with 7.4 hr. Due to prolonged absorption and accumulation in the injection sites, AE and AM have very long MRT at 13.9-42.9 hr in human treatment (table 17). For cases analysis, PK data of five artemisinin drugs (QHS, DHA, AE, AM and AS) associated with parasitological consequences in malaria patients are shown in table 17.

Pharmacodynamics (PD) is similar to PK profiles but measures efficacy parameters. The mean parasitemia-time curve following treatment with any antimalarial compounds presents a lag phase. The lag phase is then followed by a sharp decease in parasite counts (which presents a clearance phase), and is then slowly decreased to a very low parasitemia. This process is usually under the limitation of microscopic observation for both the dormant and terminal phases (figure 11, top). The artemisinin drugs affect these profiles in several ways. First, they appear to prevent the continuation of merogony at a later stage of parasite development than either quinine or mefloquine. This prevents or attenuates the occasional alarming sharp rise in parasitemia immediately following treatment described earlier (lag phase). Second, the decline in parasitemia is accelerated. This can be explained only by enhancement of clearance of erythrocytes infected with ring forms (clearance phase) [250, 264,]. After rapid termination, surviving and stage unaffected parasites have very low levels at a dormant status [265], which is a basis of the recrudescence (dormant and terminal phase). Different artemisinin drugs with different dosage regimens showed the different profiles of parasitemia-time (figure 11, bottom). Although the PK/PD publication is very limited, the possible PK and PD evaluations for individual drug with same regimens in monotherapy for human-malaria are described below.

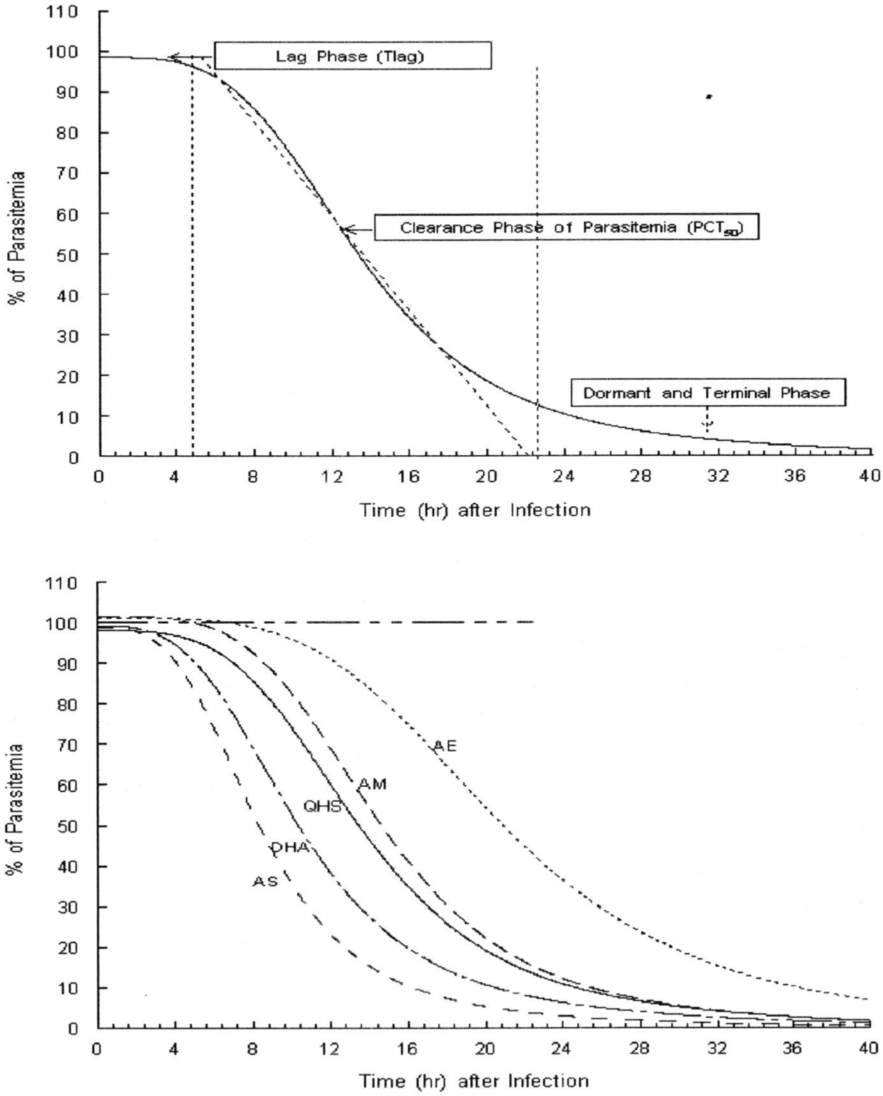

Figure 11. Standard parasite clearance curve in different stages (lag phase, clearance phase, dormant and terminal phase) and synchronicity of parasite development under antiparasitic drug received at 0 hour (top chart). The mean parasite clearance curves of AS (dashed line) at 100 mg first day and 50 mg b.i.d 2-6 days orally [91, 260]; DHA (dot and dashed line) at 200 mg first day and 100 mg 2-5 days orally [37, 160]; QHS (solid line) at 500 mg first day, 250 mg b.i.d 2-5 and 500 mg last day orally [197, 260]; AM (dashed line) at 3.2 mg/kg first day and 1.6 mg/kg 2-5 days intramuscularly [262, 263]; and AE (dot line) of 4.8 mg/kg at 0 hour and 1.6 mg/kg at 6 and then 2-5 days intramuscularly [22, 200] in malaria patients (bottom chart) (Table 17). The parasitemia at 0 hour was set as 100% of parasitemia.

Table 17. Pharmacokinetics/pharmacodynamic (PK/PD) parameters of AS (oral, 100 mg and even 50 mg b.i.d x 4), DHA (oral, 200 mg and even 100 mg x 4), AM (IM, 3.2 mg/kg and 1.6 mg x 4), and QHS (oral, 500 mg and 250 b.i.d x 4 and then 500 mg on D6) in human treatment with uncomplicated and severe/complicated malaria [22, 37, 91, 200, 260-263]

PK/PD Paremeters	AS	DHA	AM	AE	QHS
	(tablets)	(tablets)	(sesame oil)	(sesame oil)	(capsules)
Route of administration	Oral	Oral	IM	IM	Oral
First loading dosage	100 mg	200 mg	3.2 mg/kg	4.8 mg/kh	500 mg
Maintaining dosage	50 mg x 4	100 mg x 4	1.6 mg x 4	1.6 mg x 5	250 mg x 5
Refs	[91, 260]	[37, 261]	[262, 263]	[22, 200]	[197, 260]
PK parameters (Day 1)					
C_{max} (ng/ml)	1052 (DHA)	437.5	74.9	110.1	588.0
t_{max} (hr)	0.75	1.4	6.0	8.2	2.4
t_{lag} (hr)		0.2			0.45
$AUC_{0\text{-}24\ hr}$ (ng·h/ml)	1334 (DHA)	1329	1230	4702	2601
$t_{1/2}$ (absorption, hr)	0.36	0.67	1.88	3.2	1.21
$t_{1/2}$ (elimination, hr)	0.70	0.85	7.83	22.7	2.3
MRT (hr)	1.95	2.71	13.94	42.9	7.41
PD parameters (Day 1)*					
Time of lag phase (hr)	2.81	4.03	7.26	8.89	5.76
AUEC (%·h/µl)	921.2	1167.9	1613.4	2463.5	1464.4
PC_{50} (hr)	8.48	10.05	15.63	19.68	13.95
E_{max} (%) or MPC	0.0016	0.2132	0.0030	0.5504	0.0100
Curative rate (%)	81.3	76.0	86.7	48.0	74.3-75.2

*The data was fitted with WinNonlin (V5.0) by author.

PK = pharmacokinetics; PD = pharmacodynamics; MRT = Mean residence time; PC_{50} = Mean time for parasitemia to fall by half; AUEC = area under effect-time curve; QHS = Artemisinin; DHA = Dihydroartemisinin; AM = Artemether; AE = Arteether; AS = Artesunic acid; MPC = minimum parasiticidal concentration; IM = intramuscular.

5.4.1. Artesunate

Pharmacokinetic/pharmacodynamic profiles in plasma has been studied following AS oral administration in tablets of 100 mg/person dose on first day and then followed by 50 mg twice daily for 2-6 days (figure 12). The mean peak plasma concentration of DHA, a metabolite of AS, was reached at 1052 ng/ml and then declined with elimination half-life calculated at 0.75 hr (table 17). Also, the AS concentration declined daily during the 5 days of dosing [199]. Mean AUC of DHA was estimated at 1334 ng·h/ml, which was 6.4 times higher than that of its parent compound (AUC of 210 ng·h/ml), AS, in this clinical trial [91]. At same dosage regimen, the time of lag phase in the parasitemia curve was 2.81 hr, which was the shortest lag time compared with other 4 drugs (figure 11, bottom), indicating that the effect of AS tablets was very fast and efficient with 0.36 hr absorption half-life and 1052 ng/ml of Cmax [260]. Similarly, very rapid parasite clearance produced a mean time of 8.48 hr for clearance of half the parasitemia (PC_{50}), the lowest PC_{50} and the lowest area under effect-time curve (AUEC) with 921.2%·h/µl (table 17).

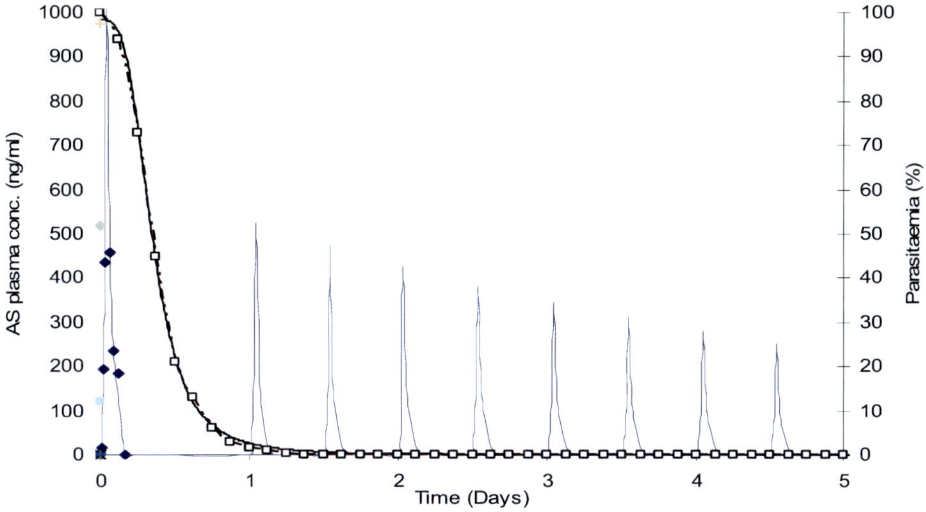

Figure 12. Pharmacokinetic/pharmacodynamic profiles are in plasma following artesunate (AS) oral administration of 100 mg/person dose on first day followed by 50 mg twice daily for 2-6 days by using tablets. DHA, a metabolite of AS, measured by HPLC-ECD (diamonds) and computer fitted curves (solid-line) [91], which was simulated by declining metabolism of AS in humans [199]. Mean parasite densities versus time measured by microscopy (empty squares) and computer fitting curve (dashed line) [260] are from malaria human trials. Relative PK/PD parameters are given in Table 17. The parasitemia was counted 100% at zero while the first dosing time.

After the computer fitting, the 0.0016% parasitemia of an E_{max} was estimated for the oral AS treatment in human (table 17) on the first day in (or for) computer modeling. The E_{max} was the principal pharmacodynamic parameter to determine the antimalarial response in maximum effect to the artemisinin derivatives, which had very steep concentration-effect relationships. The relationship may be caused by the time that blood concentrations exceed the minimum parasiticidal concentration (MPC), rather than the C_{max} or AUC [264]. For the data presented here, after 100 mg per patient of AS, the MPC was the lowest parasitemia remaining in blood when compared to other four artemisinin derivatives (figure 12).

5.4.2. Dihydroartemisinin

PK/PD profiles in plasma following DHA oral administration in tablets of 200 mg/person on day 1 and then 100 mg at day 2-5 are shown in figure 13. After 200 mg of DHA by oral dosing, the mean peak plasma concentration of DHA was reached at 437 ng/ml and then declined with elimination half-life calculated at 0.85 hr. Mean AUC of DHA was estimated at 1329 ng·h/ml. At 200 mg dosage regimen orally, the time of lag phase in the parasitemia curve was 4.03 hr. The lag time was longer than AS (2.81 hr) and still shorter than AM (7.26 hr), AE (8.89 hr) and QHS (5.76 hr) (table 17, figure 11, bottom), indicating that fast effect of DHA tablets was not as good as AS, but was more rapid than AM, AE and QHS regimens. In addition, the rapid parasite clearance resulted in a mean time of 10.05 hr of PC_{50} and the 1167.9 %·h/μl. of AUEC.

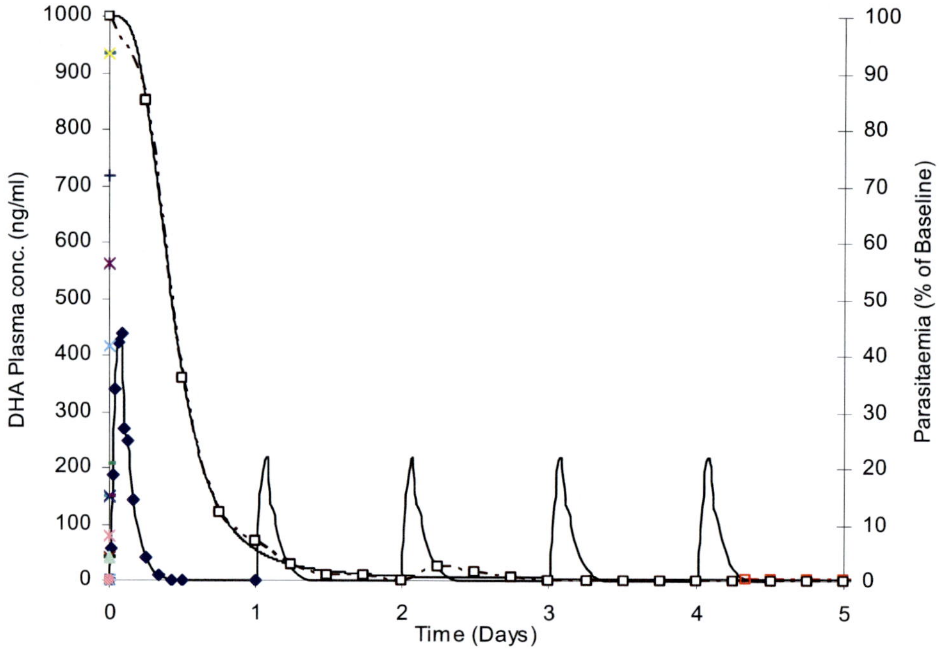

Figure 13. Pharmacokinetic/pharmacodynamic profiles are in plasma following dihydroartemisinin (DHA) oral administration of 200 mg/person on day 1 and then 100 mg daily at day 2-5 in tablets. DHA measured by HPLC-ECD (diamonds) and computer fitted curves (solid-line) [37, 261]. Mean parasite densities versus time measured by microscopy (empty squares) and computer fitting curve (dashed line) [261] are from malaria human trials. The parasitemia was counted 100% at zero while the first dosing time.

After first day computer modeling, the 0.213% parasitemia of an E_{max} was estimated for the oral DHA treatment in human. For the data presented here, after giving 200 mg per patient of DHA, more MPC remained in the blood when compared to the other three artemisinin derivatives (table 17). The absorption of DHA tablets with 0.67 hr half-life was 50% slower than the AS (0.36 hr) trial too, suggesting that the slow reduction of parasitemia may have resulted from the slow absorption. In addition, the AUCs of the two treatments (AS and DHA with double dose) were the same, only the C_{max} of AS dosing was two times higher than DHA treatment, indicating that the high peak concentration (C_{max}) may be another reason for the decrease of parasitemia in human [37, 261]. Compared with the AS study, DHA appeared to have very low bioavailability (< 50%). If calculated with an equal dose level, the C_{max} and AUC_{DHA} estimated from AS treatment was 4-fold and 2-fold, respectively, higher than the DHA dosage regimen. Our data demonstrated that the DHA tablet (Cotexin) in beagle dogs had only 24.4% obsolete bioavailability [160]. Rebound parasites (3%) on day 3 and one-fourth recrudescence rate (24%) were found in patients treated with DHA tablets in clinical work [37]. The 3% of rebound parasites was only found in DHA oral treatment in this comparison (figure 13).

5.4.3. Artemether

PK and PD profiles in plasma following AM intramuscular administration in sesame oil of 3.2 mg/kg on day 1 and then 1.6 mg/kg daily on day 2-5 can be seen in figure 14. The mean peak plasma concentration was reached at 74.9 ng/ml and then declined with elimination half-life calculated at 7.83 hr (table 17), indicating that this formulation had the lowest peak of drug concentration when compared to the other 4 artemisinin drugs. Mean AUC was estimated at 1230 ng·h/ml [262]. At the same dosage regimen the time of lag phase in the parasitemia curve was 7.26 hr, which was the second longest lag time compared with other 3 drugs except for AE, indicating that the effect of the AM intramuscular formulation had a very low and prolonged absorption from muscle injection sites [187]. Parasitemia counts in the beginning after dosing did not decrease due to the low peak concentration of AM, but increased markedly to 110% at 4 hours (parasitemia was counted 100% at zero while the first dosing time). That may be the reason why the lag time was longer at 7.26 hr with no parasites decrease after injection at hour 4. Similarly, there was very slow clearance to parasites produced at mean PC_{50} time of 15.6 hr, which was also the longest PC_{50} time compared to other 3 drugs (table 17). The highest AUEC of 1613.4 %·h/µl also revealed that the drug with the intramuscular regimen was not efficacious in reducing the parasitemia [263].

Although the intramuscular AM was not fast enough to kill parasites in patients, the long lasting exposure level of AM (7.83 hr elimination half-life) could reduce parasitemia at a good rate. The computer modeling estimated that the 0.003% parasitemia was the E_{max} in this clinical trial. The MPC (E_{max}) was only a little more than oral AS in the first day modeling, but much less than oral DHA, AE and QHS (table 17).

5.4.4. Arteether

PK and PD profiles in plasma following AE intramuscular administration in sesame oil of 4.8 mg/kg at 0 h and 1.6 mg/kg at 6 h on day 1 and then daily 1.6 mg from day 2-5 are illustrated in figure 15. The mean peak plasma concentration was reached at 110.1 ng/ml and then declined with elimination half-life calculated at 22.7 hr (table 17), indicating that this formulation has a low peak of drug concentration when compared to AS, DHA, and QHS. Mean AUC was estimated at 4702 ng·h/ml [200]. At the same dosage regimen the lag time in the parasitemia curve was 8.89 hr, which was the longest lag time compared with other 4 drugs, indicating that the effect of the AE intramuscular formulation had a very low and prolonged absorption from muscle injection sites [187]. Parasitemia counts in the beginning after dosing did not decrease due to the low peak concentration of AE, but increased markedly to 108% at 6 hours (100% parasitemia was counted at zero hour during the first dosing time). The increase may be the reason why the lag time is longer at 8.89 hr with no parasites killing after injection at 6 hours. Similarly, a very slow parasite clearance was produced at mean PC_{50} time of 19.68 hr, which was the longest PC_{50} time compared to other 4 drugs (table 17). The highest AUEC of 2463.5 %·h/µl revealed that the drug with the intramuscular regimen was not efficacious in reducing the parasitemia [263].

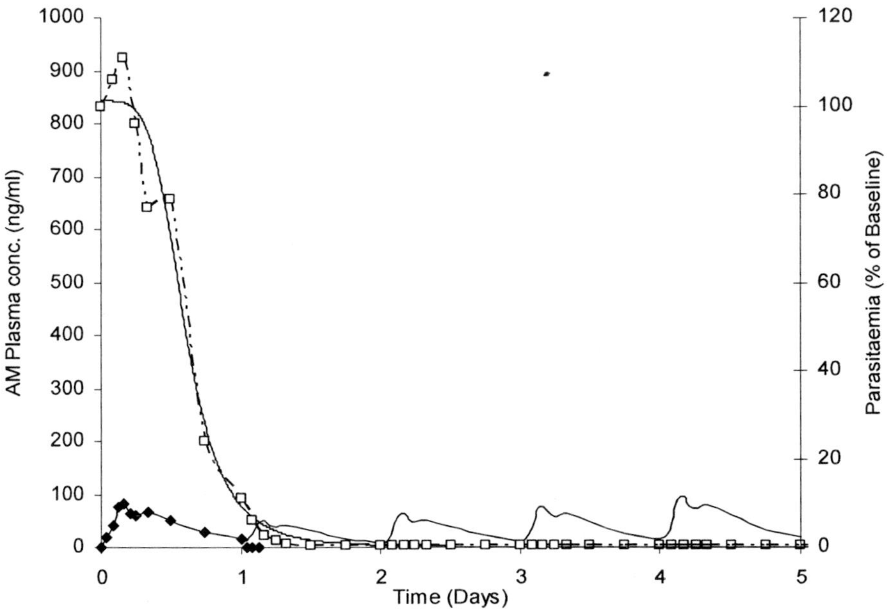

Figure 14. Pharmacokinetic/pharmacodynamic profiles are in plasma following artemether (AM) intramuscular administration of 3.2 mg/person on day 1 and then daily 1.6 mg at day 2-5 in sesame oil. AM measured by HPLC-ECD (diamonds) and computer fitted curves (solid-line) [262]. Mean parasite densities versus time measured by microscopy (empty squares) and computer fitting curve (dashed line) [263] are from malaria human trials. The parasitemia was counted 100% at zero while the first dosing time.

The intramuscular AE was neither able to exterminate parasites rapidly, nor to reduce parasitemia much in patients. The computer modeling estimated that the 0.550% parasitemia was the E_{max} in this clinical trial. In spite of two doses on day 1 (4.8 mg/kg at 0 hr and 1.6 mg/kg at 6 hr), the MPC was still the highest value compared to other four artemisinins (table 17).

5.4.5. Artemisinin

PK/PD evaluation in plasma following artemisinin (QHS) oral administration of 500 mg/person on first day followed by 250 mg twice daily for 4 days and then another 500 mg on 6th day is seen in figure 16. After 500 mg of QHS by oral dosing, the mean peak plasma concentration of QHS was reached at 588 ng/ml and then declined with elimination half-life calculated at 2.4 hr. Mean AUC of QHS was estimated at 2601 ng·h/ml, which was the highest AUC in comparison due to the highest oral dose taken. At 500 mg dosage regimen orally, the lag time in the parasitemia curve was 5.76 hr, which was longer than oral AS (2.81 hr) and DHA (4.03 hr) but was better than AM and AE trials (figure 11, bottom), indicating that fast effect of QHS capsules was not as good as oral AS and DHA even given the higher doses [197, 260, 266]. The patients treated with oral QHS showed a 13.95 hr of PC_{50} and the 1464.4 %·h/µl. of AUEC (table 17).

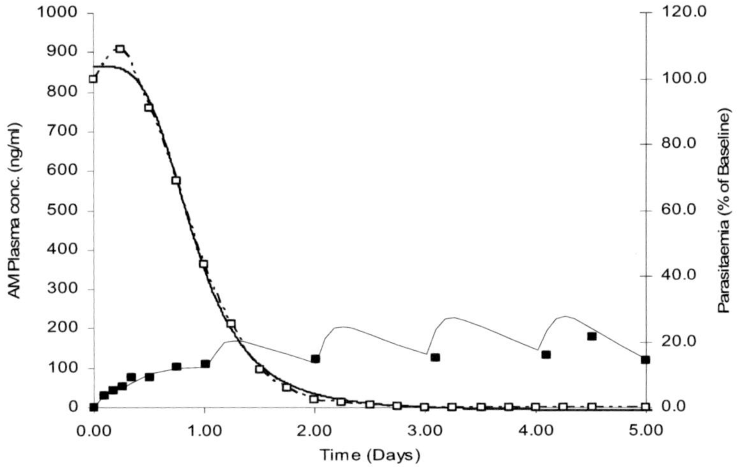

Figure 15. Pharmacokinetic/pharmacodynamic profiles are in plasma following arteether (AE) intramuscular administration of 4.8 mg/person at 0 hr and 1.6 mg/kg at 6 hr on day 1 and then daily 1.6 mg at day 2-5 in sesame oil. AE measured by HPLC-ECD (diamonds) and computer fitted curves (solid-line) [200]. Mean parasite densities versus time measured by microscopy (empty squares) and computer fitting curve (dashed line) [22, 200] are from malaria human trials. The parasitemia was counted 100% at zero while the first dosing time.

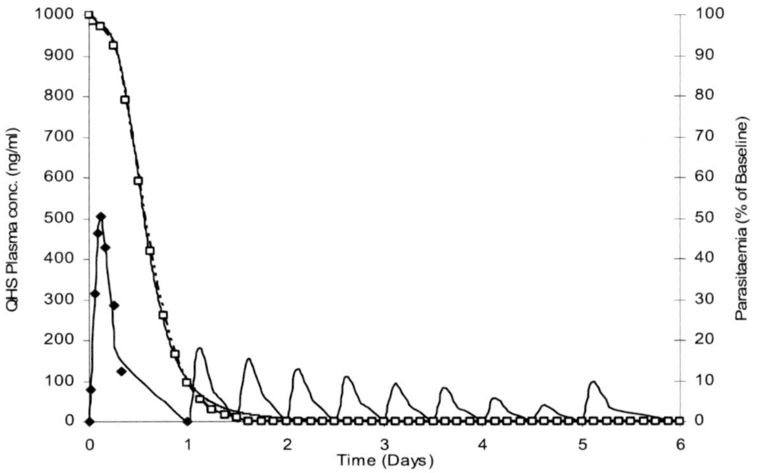

Figure 16. Pharmacokinetic/pharmacodynamic profiles are in plasma following artemisinin (QHS) oral administration of 500 mg/person on first day followed by 250 mg twice daily for 4 days and then another 500 mg on 6th day. QHS measured by HPLC-ECD (solid diamond) and computer fitted curves (solid-line), which was simulated by declining metabolism of QHS in humans [197, 266]. Mean parasite densities versus time measured by microscopy (empty squire) and computer fitting curve (dashed line) are from malaria human trials [260]. The parasitemia was counted 100% at zero while the first dosing time.

The absorption of QHS capsules with 1.21 hr half-life was slower than the absorptions of AS and DHA drugs, suggesting that the slow reduction of parasitemia may have resulted from the slow absorption. Compared with oral AS and DHA study, oral QHS appeared to have very low bioavailability of 30% [267, 268] and low antimalarial potency [1-4].

The relationships of PK and PD have been evaluated for the five-artemisinin drugs above, and the impressive inputs for each drug with the regimen could be summarized as follows:

1. Without intravenous PK/PD data, oral AS is the fastest killer in the malaria treatments out of the other four artemisinins. Oral AS can provide the highest peak concentration and very short exposure time (figure 12-15); the former as the role to eliminate parasites rapid (figure 11, bottom) and the latter to avoid fatal neurotoxicity (Section 3.5.) and to prevent resistance.
2. Although DHA has similar efficacy to AS in vitro [1-4], the agent does not have a rapid effect like that of AS even with double oral doses. The explanations include lower bioavailability [269, 270], slower absorption phase, and long lag time on effect activity. However, the principle reason is due to the lower peak concentration in the treated humans when compared to oral AS.
3. Intramuscular AM or AE reveals a low efficacy and slow parasite killing. Due to the sesame oil formulation, AM and AE have a very low and prolonged absorption from muscle injection sites [187]. In the beginning, parasitemia counts after dosing did not decrease due to the low and delayed peak concentrations (75-110 ng/ml) of AM and AE. The low peak concentration may be the reason why the lag time is longer for 7.2-8.9 hr without parasites killing after injection. Similarly, there is very slow clearance rate on parasites with mean PC_{50} time of 15.63-19.68 hr, which may have resulted in inadmissible failures in AE trials [200]. Although the drug exposure times of AM and AE are much longer than AS, DHA and QHS, the long exposure time did not assist efficacy. Instead, it induced neurotoxicity (Section 3.5.), therefore, the formulation would not be encouraged to use in humans to treat acute and severe malarias.
4. Oral artemisinin (QHS) does not show well in this PK/PD comparison probably due to the highest oral dose (500 mg/person). Although the high dose produced a higher plasma concentration (2601 ng·h/ml of AUC) and high peak concentration (588 ng/ml), the low relative antimalarial potency [1-4] and slow bioavailability [268] considerably limited the efficacy. It suggests that the artemisinin derivatives with lower antimalarial potency still can not produce rapid effects even at an increased dose level.

5.5. Rapid Efficacy Affected by Drug Peak Level and Antimalarial Potency

PK/PD evaluation indicates that the effect of parasitemia decrease appeared to be significantly slower (2.8-8.9 hours) than the decline of drugs, reflecting a sum mean of the lag phase time, stages effect time, and even body elimination time with the different compounds and dosage regimens, suggesting that PD effects are longer than PK outcomes. The elimination half lives in PK were in the range of 0.7-22.7 hr, whereas the PC_{50} in PD were in the range of 8.48-19.68 hr. In this evaluation, AS is pharmacokinetically and pharmacodynamically superior to other four artemisinins for the treatment of malaria, demonstrating the most rapid killing activities with greater E_{max} in the PD analysis after oral administration. AS showed the highest peak concentration, the fastest and most reliable oral absorption rate, and the most limited drug exposure time than other four artemisinins. Although AM and AE showed the longest half lives and the highest exposure level (high AUC values), they had the worst efficacy (the longest lag time, the greatest AUEC, and the longest PC_{50}) due to the slowest absorption rate and the lowest peak concentration (table 17). However, the inadmissible failure (48.0-86.8% curative rates) in those monotherapies led us to either re-assess their importance or seek alternative approaches (table 4):

1. In vitro, at dose range 10^{-7}-10^{-5} M (30 –3000 ng/ml), synchronous culture study shows that artemisinin is rapidly effective against both rings and schizonts, demonstrating 100% growth inhibition of these stages within 4-6 h. The inhibitory effects of AM are more gradual, requiring 8-10 hr of exposure time to achieve 70% growth inhibition of the ring and 40-50% inhibition of schizonts stages. DHA is found to be highly effective against all stages of the parasite, in most cases achieving 100% growth inhibition by 2-4 hr [5]. Concentration of 10^{-6}-10^{-5} M (280-2800 ng/ml) artemisinin shows a parasitical effect after only 3 hr of drug exposure, whereas 10^{-7} M (28 ng/ml) artemisinin requires 24 hr of exposure for a cidal effect [251]. It is clear that the low dose will increase the exposure time, and high dose will shorten the treatment period. Therefore, the low dose range cannot be selected for artemisinin drugs in human treatments in malaria because i) the artemisinins have very short half-lives, and ii) longer exposure time of artemisinins is principle factor to induce the fatal neurotoxicity.

In addition, in treating patients with severe and complicated malaria, where the ultimate survival of the patient is the key; low effective doses cannot be used without an undue delay in the necessary treatment time [252]. There is no evidence that rapid parasite killing with high sufficient doses is harmful and that the therapeutic blood drug concentration should be achieved as quickly as possible without danger of toxicity [247]. Therefore, the plasma concentration of the artemisinin derivatives in human against *P. falciparum* should at least be in the range of 10^{-6}-10^{-5} (300-3000 ng/ml) or even higher for AS or DHA as the more potent compounds. AE or AM should have higher plasma concentrations (more than that of AS or DHA). AL, being the lowest potency agent in regards to the first drug exposure [1-4], should have the highest plasma concentration.

2. Artemisinins reliably reduce initial malaria parasitemia by a factor of 10^4 per 48 hour. Therefore, asexual cycle and modeling studies suggest that six days of treatment should cure parasite burdens of up to 10^{12} parasites [271]. This model is difficult to reconcile with the high recrudescence rates (10%–15%) seen with artemisinin monotherapy and is also difficult to recognize with a higher potency agent (AS or DHA) and with higher concentrations. This poor efficacy of cure in the monotherapy, which is not due to resistance [272], is usually attributed to the

intrinsically lower peak concentration of artemisinins, which has been demonstrated in the above PK/PD evaluation.

The pharmacokinetic factors are not only focusing on the high peak concentration, but are also concentrating on tissue distribution in red blood cells of artemisinins [184]. More recently, the tissue distribution in rats and protein binding in human blood were conducted in WRAIR laboratory. Table 18 demonstrates the RBC/plasma ratios of five radiolabeled artemisinins in human whole blood at various concentrations [45, and our unpublished data]. For equal volumes of RBC and plasma, the fraction of the five artemisinins found in the RBC is lower than in the plasma in normal volunteer blood. The ratios are almost constant in human blood over a broad range of concentration. After correction for the 55:45 ratios of plasma and RBC volumes, the RBC/plasma ratios are 0.23 for ^{14}C-AE, 0.28 for ^{14}C-AM, 0.44 for ^{14}C-AL, 0.52 for ^{14}C-DHA, and 0.71 for ^{14}C-AS, indicating that the radioactivity remained in human RBC is the highest for AS and the lowest for AE.

The big advantage of DHA and AS is its readiness of entering human red blood cell (0.52 and 0.71 ratio of RBC/plasma, respectively) compared to AE and AM (0.23 and 0.28 ratio of RBC/plasma, respectively). It means that to reach same targets (RBC) the drug peak concentrations for AE and AM should be required to be two to three times higher than that of DHA and AS. In addition, the binding affinities are high for AE and AM radiolabels with 1945 and 1673 ng/ml of 50% bound concentration in human plasma (BC_{50}). Conversely, the binding affinities are low for AS and DHA radioactivities with 143 and 162 ng/ml of BC_{50}, indicating the free drug concentration can be much higher in human plasma with AS or DHA than that with AE and AM.

Table 18. The bound ratios of human red blood cells (RBC) and plasma with ^{14}C-AE, ^{14}C-AM, ^{14}C-AL, ^{14}C-DQHS, and ^{14}C-AS in human whole blood from low to high concentration with incubated dialysis method at 37°C [165]

Concentration (MW)	^{14}C-AE (312.4)	^{14}C-AM (298.4)	^{14}C-AL (418.5)	^{14}C-DHA (284.9)	^{14}C-AS (384.4)
0.125 nM	0.20 ± 0.01	0.28 ± 0.01	0.43 ± 0.01	0.52 ± 0.03	0.72 ± 0.05
0.25 nM	0.24 ± 0.03	0.27 ± 0.01	0.44 ± 0.02	0.53 ± 0.04	0.71 ± 0.03
0.5 nM	0.22 ± 0.02	0.28 ± 0.01	0.47 ± 0.02	0.52 ± 0.05	0.73 ± 0.05
1 nM	0.23 ± 0.02	0.27 ± 0.02	0.43 ± 0.03	0.51 ± 0.03	0.74 ± 0.04
2 nM	0.22 ± 0.01	0.26 ± 0.01	0.45 ± 0.02	0.50 ± 0.03	0.74 ± 0.06
4 nM	0.23 ± 0.01	0.29 ± 0.02	0.45 ± 0.01	0.51 ± 0.04	0.69 ± 0.06
8 nM	0.24 ± 0.03	0.27 ± 0.02	0.45 ± 0.02	0.53 ± 0.03	0.64 ± 0.04
16 nM	0.25 ± 0.03	0.29 ± 0.03	0.44 ± 0.02	0.51 ± 0.04	0.59 ± 0.08
Mean value	0.23 ± 0.02	0.28 ± 0.02	0.44 ± 0.02	0.52 ± 0.04	0.71 ± 0.08

All values represent mean ± SD for n = 4 individual samples, AE = arteether, AM = artemether, AL = artelinic acid, DHA = dihydroartemisinin; MW = molecular weight.

3. Although DHA tablets and AM intramuscular formulation have a similar AUC compared to AS tablets (table 17), their efficacies are much lower than that of AS tablets (figure 11, bottom). The initial killing of parasites do not appear to be done very well by the two drug regimens because they do not have enough high peak

concentration to cover all red blood cells. The uptake of DHA in infected erythrocytes has been shown to be 300 times higher than in the uninfected erythrocytes, and the maximum uptake of the drug occurs after 1-2 hr [265]. In this case, as we discussed above, the plasma concentration of the artemisinin derivatives in human against *P. falciparum* should be much more than the range of 10^{-6}-10^{-5} (300-3000 ng/ml) for the first drug exposure in order to cover all RBC targets [251, 252]. In the report above, compared to oral AS, the other 4 artemisinins with oral and intramuscular formulations have a lower peak level, could not stop the parasite and cover all RBC in the initial several hours having greatly extended the lag and PC_{50} times.

4. High peak concentration (C_{max}) is also more important than high drug concentration (AUC) to cure malaria because sufficient drug is needed to cover all RBCs (including infected cells) in order to kill as many parasites as possible in the initial dosing. AUC concentration is counted during this period of time and very often lacks the necessary high peak concentrations. For example, in the AE clinical trial, the AUCs are higher than other four artemisinin drugs (table 17), but it has lower C_{max} value that results in poor efficacy. Therefore, the high concentration (AUC) without high peak level is not able to cover all RBCs; this could have given rise to some untreated RBCs, including infected cells. The untreated RBCs may be the reason for recrudescence in all monotherapy approaches with artemisinins. In addition, QHS is a low antimalarial potency agent [1-4]. Even though oral doses 5-fold higher than AS have been given to patients in trials, QHS still demonstrates poor efficacy because its peak concentration is only a half of that of AS, suggesting that any artemisinin drug with lower antimalarial potency should not be used in malaria treatment.

In conclusion, the rapid efficacy of artemisinins is principally dependent on drug peak concentration (C_{max}) in the first drug exposure and drug relative antimalarial potency. The relative antimalarial potency is maintained by the capability for killing various stages of parasites, rapid oral absorption, high peak concentration, plasma protein binding, drug distribution in targets (RBCs), and membrane permeability of RBCs in infected subjects. Other factors of the pharmacokinetic parameters, such as drug exposure level (AUC) and drug exposure time (half-life), tend to be of minor significance when considering efficacy.

6. How to Maintain Rapid Efficacy and Avoid Lethal Toxicities

6.1. Deserting Some of the Artemisins

Artemisinin compounds have impressive parasiticidal properties in vitro, rapidly arresting parasite metabolism in concentrations within the lower nanomolar range and killing parasites more quickly than other antimalarial drugs [264]. These compounds have variously been formulated for oral, rectal, and parenteral administrations. AE was developed under the sponsorship of the World Health Organization despite lacking clear advantages over AM, for which a much larger clinical experience already exists; AE is no longer being investigated as an antimalarial agent because AE is not better than AM either in efficacy or in pharmacokinetic profiles in our PK/PD analysis (table 17) with a more slow absorption from muscle [22, 200] and therapeutic efficacy summary of the clinical trials (table 4). However, locally formulated intramuscular products are used in India (α and β arteether) and the Netherlands (β-arteether, Artemotil). Data from India showed that α and β–AE dissolved in peanut oil have good efficacy in uncomplicated and even severe malaria with 6.7-14.0% recrudescence (re-infection) and 8.5% mortality in the patients with severe malaria [39-43, 273-274]. Although pharmacokinetic results of α and β-AE are not available from humans, some animal studies (rats and monkeys) demonstrated that the C_{max} of α and β-AE with peanut oil could reach levels up to 160-360 ng/ml [275-277] suggesting that the C_{max} profile is better than β-AE alone dissolved in sesame oil with a C_{max} in the range of 78-161 ng/ml in rats and monkeys after first dosing (figure 2, 3, 6).

Artemisinin (QHS) itself is a highly crystalline compound that does not dissolve in oil or water; thus, QHS can only be given by the oral route. This may be the reason that the oral efficacy of QHS in humans is poor [260] and that the oral efficacy of QHS is also inferior with regards to pharmacokinetic benefit [197, 266]. Since humans were last reported to use QHS tablets in 1998 [278], no recent reports have been found for using QHS to treat malaria. For these derivatives, the sodium salts of AS and AL are used for parenteral administration. AL (a water soluble derivative) was at one time under development by the Walter Read Army Institute of Research. Although AL has not been further developed since 2003 (principally due to a 3-fold higher toxicity than AS [66, 179]), various formulations and combinations of AS with other antimalarials are under active development.

That these three artemisinins (AE, QHS, and AL) are paid less attention today with respect to further development is not a surprise. AE clinical trials with sesame oil in humans [200] have been pharmacokinetically inferior to other artemisinins demonstrated (table 17). In addition, QHS and AL have shown poor efficacy due to the lower relative antimalarial potency [1-4] – not to mention suffering the moderate toxicity of AL [66]. These results suggest that only AS, AM, and DHA are suitable for further advanced development and treatment in humans with the advent of artemisinin-based combination therapy for uncomplicated malaria or using monotherapy for severe and complicated malaria.

6.2. Artemisinin-Based Combination Therapy (ACT) for Uncomplicated Malaria

Artemisinin-based combination therapies (ACTs) hold considerable promise for both increased efficacy and for retardation in the rate of development of parasite resistance. Recently, WHO has endorsed ACTs as the "policy standard" for all malaria infections in areas where *P. falciparum* is the predominant infecting species [128]. ACT has been shown to improve cure rates, decrease malaria transmission and decrease antimalarial resistance on the north-west border of Thailand [126]. Also, enhanced cure rates and decreased gametocyte carriage has been confirmed in clinical trials in Africa as well [279-280].

Due to the rapid parasite clearance of artemisinin drugs in treating early cases of uncomplicated malaria, ACTs may both prevent the progression of malaria to severe disease and reduce severe cases as well as mortality. AM-Lumefantrine is the first registered, fixed, ACT treatment, which constitutes about 70% of all current clinically-used ACTs [129]. It is highly effective when given orally twice a day for three days (6-dose) with a small amount of fat [130, 131]. In the PK/PD evaluation above, intramuscular AM did not show exciting efficacy, pointing to pharmacokinetic disadvantages in humans. How could the AM reveal successful therapy after oral administration in the combination with lumefantrine?

A pharmacokinetic study exhibited that the oral administration of AM has greater pharmacokinetic advantage than that of intramuscular AM in humans. The antimalarial activity of AM following oral or intramuscular administration in the plasma of 15 adults with acute uncomplicated *P. falciparum* malaria was measured by bioassay. The peak concentrations (C_{max}) in plasma following oral administration were higher in patients in the acute phase (median, 541.8 ng/ml of DHA) than in patients in the convalescent phase (median, 271.6 ng/ml of DHA). Antimalarial activity in terms of the peak concentration in plasma (541.8 ng/ml) after oral administration was a median of 16 times higher than that after intramuscular administration (34.4 ng/ml). The ratio of the area under the plasma concentration-time curve during the first 24 h (AUC_{0-24}) after oral administration of AM to the AUC_{0-24} after intramuscular administration was a median of 3.3. In the acute phase, the time to C_{max} was significantly shorter after oral administration (median, 1 h) than after intramuscular administration (median, 8 h). Intramuscular AM is absorbed very slowly in patients with acute malaria [281]. Similar studies also reported that the oral AM produced C_{max} from 406 to 818 ng/ml that are 5.5-11.2 folds higher than that of intramuscular AM [29, 46, 172, 282, 283].

Another commonly used ACT treatment, AS-mefloquine, has been distributed widely since 1994 as the first-line treatment in South-East Asian countries such as Thailand and Cambodia and remains highly effective for uncomplicated falciparum malaria. Under the WHO system of efficacy assessment, more than 95% of patients will remain free of malaria 28 days after such treatment (E2) [134, 135]. In uncomplicated malaria, when artemisinins are used orally, most pharmacokinetic information is now available for AS. In present report, the PK/PD evaluation demonstrated that oral AS is pharmacokinetically and pharmacodynamically superior to the other four artemisinins for the treatment of malaria. The absolute bioavailability of antimalarial activity after a single dose of oral AS in uncomplicated adult malaria is about 60% [91, 173]. Peak concentration (C_{max}) of DHA after oral AS can easily reach between 519 and 1309 ng/ml in many clinical trials [91, 173, 254, 269, 270, 284]. If the values of DHA and AS are included, the total C_{max} (624-1522 ng/ml) are significantly higher than that after oral AM (406-818 ng/ml) and that after oral DHA (466-1143 ng/ml) [269, 270, 282, 285, 286]. Although absolute bioavailability studies for oral AM and DHA are not possible given lack of intravenous formulations, pharmacodynamic activity (parasite clearance) after oral dosing of these derivatives is satisfactory but less than that of oral AS. Therefore, only four ACTs with AM and AS (without DHA) were recommended currently by a WHO Expert Consultative Group in 2001; there are AM-lumefantrine (Coartem), AS-mefloquine (Artequin), AS-amodiaquine, and AS-sulfadoxine/pyrimethamine [127].

In addition, oral formulation of AS and AM result in a great conversion of drugs to DHA in malaria patients. Actually, oral AS and AM are the prodrug of DHA with ratios of 1.4-8.6 for DHA/AM and 6.4-9.7 for DHA/AS (table 8) [161-173]. Following GI absorption (first-pass effects) and conversion (hydrolysis) of AS and AM, the concentration of DHA has a very large variability, from 248 to 8840 ng·h/ml (AUC values) in individual patients [161]. Four patients who were not cured by the oral AM regimen used in this study and had significantly lower plasma concentrations of DHA, the metabolite of AM [25]. Using same dose amount as AM, a much lower AUC (834 ng·h/ml) was detected in the four patients compared to the AUC (3684 ng·h/ml) in the other 46 patients. The low level of DHA present is likely responsible for the treatment failures.

However, these combinations still have some dosing difficulties. The AM-lumefantrine should ideally be given with food (preferably containing fat) to ensure adequate absorption and thus efficacy. In the initial study, the 4-dose AM-lumefantrine regimen showed a relatively high rate of late treatment failure (E1) [132]. In one study, the 6-dose AM-lumefantrine regimen was associated with a 28% treatment failure at 14 days in an area with high-grade mefloquine resistance (E3) [133]. Another commonly used ACT treatment, AS-mefloquine, has been used in South-East Asian countries such as Thailand and Cambodia quite widely since 1994 and remains highly effective for uncomplicated falciparum malaria. However, the failure rate of AS-mefloquine combination was up to 13% in Thailand and Cambodia [136], and the neuropsychiatric effects of mefloquine as well as its relative expense are problematic [137].

6.3. Injectable AS for Severe and Complicated Malaria

Peak concentration (C_{max}) is more important than plasma concentration (AUC) in producing the improved efficacy of antimalarial drugs that has been confirmed in the above PK/PD evaluation. Moreover, it is the antimalarial activity with high killing capability in xblood in the first few hours following the first administration of a parenteral drug that is critical from a therapeutic standpoint, particularly in patients with severe malaria, in whom mortality can reach between 15% and 20%, despite appropriate antimalarial and supportive treatment [138].

When the peak concentration reaches 1052 ng/ml of DHA in plasma after a single 100 mg oral dose of AS [91, 260], it obtains the best efficacy in uncomplicated malaria compared to the other four-artemisinin drugs (figure 11 and table 17), and there is a total molecular number of DHA of 2.11 x 10^{12}/ml in plasma. This should be 0.87 x 10^{12}/ml in RBC (hematocrit =0.41), with the DHA molecular number at 94.5 in each erythrocyte in healthy subjects including other artemisinin derivatives that are mainly bound with RBC membranes [287]. This calculation is according to the data of DHA ratio of RBC/human plasma (table 18) and protein binding capacity of DHA at 1000 ng/ml (figure 17) in humans [288].

We know that the uptake of DHA in infected erythrocytes has been shown to be 300 times more than the uninfected erythrocytes *in vitro* [265], this is because the malaria parasite *P. falciparum* induces some unselective cation conductance in the RBC membrane that changes the permeability [289]. An in-patient who has 1% of erythrocyte infected malaria, with all drugs at C_{max} of 1052 ng/ml on average, the amount entering infected RBCs would be only 100 times higher than uninfected RBCs. In 5% or 20% RBC infected patients; the uptake of DHA in infected RBCs would be only 5 or 20 times higher than that in uninfected RBCs. Although we do not know the degree of DHA uptake by RBCs in malarial human, it is suggested that the high concentration (1052 ng/ml) in malaria patients is still not sufficient to distribute the drug to every erythrocyte (infected and uninfected) in each patient (from 1-20% infected RBC). Therefore, it is clear that the peak level at 1000 ng/ml in plasma is far from enough to cure the severe malaria with a hyperparasitemia. In this estimation, the minimum peak concentration for hyperparasitemia (> 5%) will be at least at 10,000-15,000 ng/ml.

Fortunately, the intravenous AS can provide sufficiently high peak concentration in the patients with a fast exposure time. In current clinical trials, the C_{max} was shown to be from 112 - 16149 ng/ml resulting from a dose of 120 mg/person or 2.4 mg/kg in various malaria including severe malaria [91, 173, 270, 290, 291]. Although those dose regimens are still not enough to cure severe and complicated malaria 100% of the time [91, 173, 270, 290, 291], there is now convincing evidence that for those who do develop severe malaria, intravenous AS will reduce the risk of death by approximately one-third [145, 146]. It is also encouraging is that intravenous AS is also safer and easier to use than injectable quinine [138].

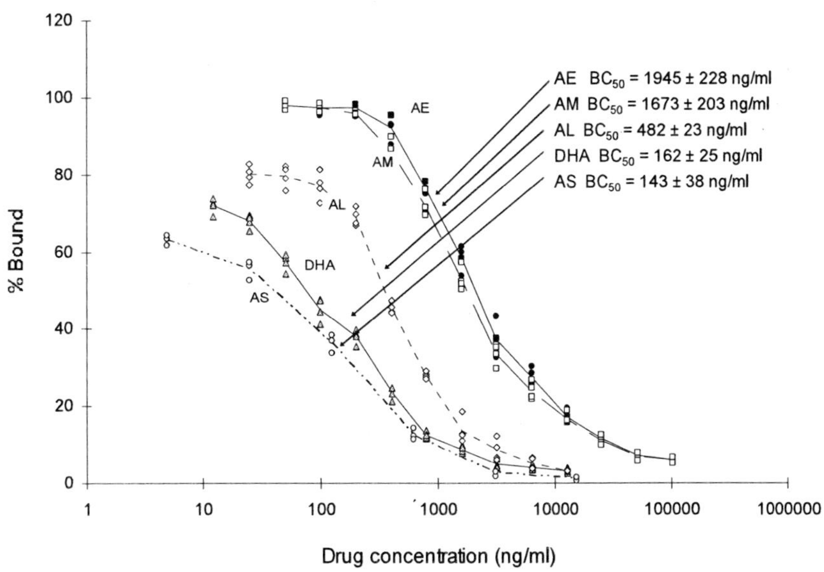

Figure 17. Comparison of 50% bound concentration (BC_{50}) of artemether (AM), arteether (AE), artelinic acid (AL), artesunate (AS) and dihydroartemisinin (DQHS) at varied concentration in human plasma samples by microdialysis equilibrium method at 37°C for 6 hours (n = 4).

Recently, there was a milestone clinical trial in the treatment development for severe malaria. Previous trials using intramuscular AM demonstrated less toxicity but no clear mortality benefit over quinine [141], most likely due to the erratic absorption of the intramuscularly administered oil-based preparation of AM [144]. More recent trials have used intravenous AS, a water-soluble derivative with a more favorable pharmacokinetic profile. The SEAQUAMAT trial, a multicentre randomized trial conducted in Bangladesh, Myanmar,

Indonesia and India, recently reported a 34.7% reduction in mortality associated with intravenous AS compared with intravenous quinine [145, 146].

In this trial, AS with 5% $NaHCO_3$ buffer (Artesunate for Injection, Guilin) administered intravenously effectively clears parasites at or above 1 mg/kg administered daily or twice on the first day. Regimens using 2.4 mg/kg clear parasites and resolve fever more quickly than intravenous quinine with fewer side effects. Comparative studies to parenteral quinine demonstrated statistically significant reductions in parasite clearance times, yet most studies have not shown significant differences in coma resolution times. Clinical side effects in these efficacy trials have been rare but include rash (hives or a red rash) and possibly a higher incidence of blackwater fever. Minor side effects and laboratory abnormalities are often impossible to distinguish from the full array of pathophysiologic effects of severe malaria [145]. In SEAQUAMAT, intravenous AS was again well tolerated. There was a statistically ($p = 0.009$) significant reduction in hypoglycemia post study entry, which is a known side effect of quinine and quinidine. There were no differences in the incidence of hemodynamic shock, convulsions, dialysis or mechanical ventilation. There was a higher non-statistical rate of hemoglobinuria and neurological sequelae in the AS group among survivors, which may reflect the survival of severe cerebral cases who may have died in the quinine group. No other significant adverse events were attributed to AS [145, 146].

This is the largest trial ever performed in severe malaria and the first to demonstrate conclusively a mortality reduction over standard quinine therapy. This is good news for malaria-endemic areas in South-East Asia. The burden of malaria in this region is far worse than previously thought, with over 120 million cases each year in south/south-east Asia. The World Health Organization now advocates the use of ACT for uncomplicated malaria [137], a move that is likely to reduce the number of people who develop the severe disease. In making the case for WHO and the international physician community to accept injectable AS in the role of the preferred treatment for severe malaria, two proposals are offered here:

1) The monotherapy of intravenous AS should still be used.

To treat severe malaria, the monotherapy of injectable AS is needed in the first couple days in order to rapidly rescue lives and possibly reduce mortality. The TropNetEurop is recommending using intravenous AS to cure the patients with severe malaria [147] because they have been encouraged by the large and successful SEAQUAMAT trials in Asian. Unfortunately, there is currently no product available that is produced under good manufacturing practice (GMP) conditions.

Patients with malaria in rural areas may be obtunded or be experiencing bouts of vomiting, making them unable to take oral medications and leading to significant delay in treatment if facilities for parenteral treatment are unavailable. In such circumstances, the intravenous or rectal route of administration is attractive because rural healthcare workers can be trained to identify moderate and severe malaria and administer intravenous or rectal drugs before transfer of patients to hospital; of course, this assumes that the intravenous or rectal route of administration is culturally acceptable in these areas.

There are some cases, highlighted especially in patients with uncomplicated hyperparasitemic falciparum malaria (> 4% infected RBC), who are at risk of severe malaria and treatment failure. These infections require a three to five day course of treatment with oral agents. The only alternative is parenteral quinine, which is less effective (145, 146), more expensive, and less well tolerated [140]. In addition, in the second and third trimesters of pregnancy, injectable AS is also a better drug for uncomplicated malaria, but it needs to be given for long term oral treatment course with a dose adjustment because of the altered kinetics in pregnant women [112, 207]. Physicians would like to prescribe appropriate antimalarial therapy without the need for oral tablets but this is unlikely to be possible in the near future, especially for injectable AS [148, 149]. They also hope that some manufacturers will continue to supply injectable AS alone to be used in specific circumstances.

2) Loading dose of intravenous AS for severe and complicated malaria should be pursued.

All cases of falciparum malaria are potentially severe and life threatening, especially when managed inappropriately. A major reason for progression from mild through complicated to severe disease is missed or delayed diagnosis. Once diagnosed, the priority for treatment of complicated and severe disease is the parenteral administration of adequate, safe doses of an appropriate antimalarial, in the setting of the highest possible level of clinical care. Supportive management of complications such as coma, convulsions, metabolic acidosis, hypoglycemia, fluid and electrolyte disturbances, renal failure, secondary infections, bleeding disorders and anemia is also important. The most recent advance in decreasing mortality has been the use of intravenous AS instead of injection quinine [145. 146], which may very well revolutionize the management of severe disease [148]. However, recrudescence is still relatively high with monotherapy of intravenous AS alone [292]. Since recrudescence is not due to parasite resistance [78], one possible explanation of this parasitological failure may be a low peak concentration after first loading dose with the intravenous AS.

Currently, the therapeutic dosages of injectable AS to treat severe and complicated malaria are in the range of 2-2.4 mg/kg alone. The dose was designed in accordance with prior experience of physicians concerned with neurotoxicity, to reduce dose-dependent hemotoxicity, to prevent a submaximal antimalarial effect, and to keep a minimum curative rate (> 90%) during over twenty years of treatments [12, 161]. However, as this report describes in previous sections, this regimen will only produce 112 - 16149 ng/ml of C_{max} with great variability, which is a lower peak concentration than needed for patients with hyperparasitemia (ie. the C_{max} in the malaria patients with a high variability). In theory, the patients with severe malaria require 10,000-15,000 ng/ml peak concentration to cover each RBC, including infected cells, because the infected cell can concentrate 300-fold more DHA than normal RBC during the first 1-2 hr after dosing. The large variability in pharmacokinetics and pharmacodynamics by using AS should also be considered.

In an individual patient, several factors determine the profile of drug pharmacodynamics and pharmacokinetics. The stage and synchronicity of the infecting parasite population and the multiplication rate of sequestered mature stages (schizonts) determine the initial parasitemia time profile after drug administration [293]. If the patient is admitted to hospital at a time when a significant proportion of the parasites are undergoing schizogony, then parasitemia will rise following antimalarial drug treatment as schizonts rupture and release merozoites, which then invade new erythrocytes to produce circulating ring stages. These stages can be seen by the microscopist and counted, whereas the sequestered stages are not seen and therefore are not counted. The implication is that parasitemia will fall. If the majority of the parasites in the blood are young rings, and a drug which has little effect on the ring stage is used in treatment, then parasitemia will plateau and fall later as a result of sequestration [9, 293].

The overall individual parasitemia profile thus represents a hybrid of these different processes, and a population of patients provides a series of very different parasitemia profiles. As a result there is considerable inter-individual variance in parasite clearance profiles, although it is reasonable to assume that the distribution of parasite stages should be random in a patient population as there is no particular reason why a patient should present one level of parasite development – and not another – in the hospital. Thus, even before attempting to assess the effect of the drug in vivo, there is considerable inter-patient variance in the pharmacodynamic variables [68]. This means that the intravenous dose should be increased to a higher level (4-8 mg/kg) than current use for the loading dose. However, the question remains: is this intravenous dose safe for treatment of severe and complicated malaria?

Compared to oral AS, the injectable AS is superior in pharmacokinetics and pharmacodynamics to the oral AS and other four artemisinins in treating patients with severe malaria; injectable AS shows the highest peak concentration, the fastest effective time, rapid elimination, and a very short exposure moment compared to oral AS (table 5) [44]. As discussed in Section 3, the drug exposure time of artemisinins is the principle factor responsible for induction of neurotoxicity in animal species. Therefore, the active metabolites (DHA), the drug distributed in CNS, and/or the drug exposure level play relatively less important roles than the drug exposure time. The water-soluble artemisinins, AS in particular, have very short half-lives and produce limited exposure time in animal species and humans, indicating that once-daily oral or intravenous administration of AS is relatively safe. In fact, the animal experiments demonstrated that no neurotoxicity (pathologically or behaviourally) has been observed in animal species following intravenous administration at any repeated doses up to maximum tolerated doses (MTD). The MTD of AS was 240 mg/kg following intravenous injection daily in rats for 3 days, but no neurotoxicity was detected in these animals [66]. In another study, intravenous AS had no effect on neurotoxic scores at 120 mg/kg in sodium carbonate daily for 7 days (our unpublished data). After one intramuscular injection, a high dose of 420 mg/kg of AS did not produce any neuronal necrosis in the rats. Also, up to 200 mg/kg of AS used orally daily for 5-7 days did not exhibit neuronal changes or any specific clinical signs [56]. Therefore, the 4-8 mg/kg dose level with intravenous formulation should be safe with regards to neurotoxicity [152] and also safe with regards to hemotoxicity [16, 179]. One study used a high dose of oral AS, up to 6 mg/kg, with the AS being extremely well tolerated; to date, there is no convincing evidence that dose as high as this of oral AS have any significant toxicity [68]. In our current Phase I clinical trials, the 2-8 mg/kg doses have been exceedingly well tolerated following both single and multiple intravenous injections in volunteers with our new formulation (our unpublished data). In malaria patients, this dose offers a satisfactory margin of safety and would be unlikely to produce a submaximal antimalarial effect.

Angus et al., in order to characterize the *in vivo* dose-response relationship for AS (and thus, rationalize dosing), 47 adult patients with acute uncomplicated falciparum malaria and parasitemia >1% were randomized to receive a single oral dose of AS varying between 0 and 250 mg together with a curative dose of oral mefloquine. Acceleration of parasite clearance was used as the pharmacodynamic variable. An inhibitory sigmoidal maximum effect (E_{max}) pharmacodynamic model typical of a dose-response curve was fitted to the relationship between dose and shortening of parasite clearance time (PCT). The E_{max} was estimated as 28.6 h, and the 50% effective concentration was 1.6 mg/kg of body weight. These results imply that there is no reduction in PCTs with the use of single oral doses of artesunate higher than 2 mg/kg, effectively reflecting the average lower limit of the maximally effective dose [68]. It is suggested that the 2 mg/kg is a maximum effective dose in those selected patients. However, the author also pointed out that this dosage of 2 mg/kg would be the lowest to give maximum effects in an "average" patient. When taking into account the considerable variance between individuals in both pharmacokinetics and pharmacodynamics [68, 161, 294], a larger dose would be required to ensure that a maximum effect was obtained in all patients. Therefore, the loading dose of injection AS is reasonable to increase to another higher level (4-8 mg/kg) for the consideration of WHO experts and investigators in the further development and treatment.

After the first drug exposure to reduce parasitemia below 1%, the maintaining dose could be significantly cut or switch (sequentially) to another slower acting and low dose antimalarial agents (not artemisinins) in order to protect AS from recrudescence or resistance and to optimize antimalarial therapy in severe and complicated malaria [295]. Because these artemisinins have excellent intrinsic activity, which produce reductions in asexual parasite biomass of up to 10,000-fold per cycle, these drugs still need to be present in therapeutic concentrations during four asexual life cycles, or 8 days [271]. Previous studies have shown that once-daily administration with the artemisinin derivatives provides equivalent cure rates relative to more frequent administration [296, 297]. This suggests that exposure of the infecting parasite population to therapeutic concentrations of drug twice each life cycle is sufficient for maximum effect [293].

7. Conclusion

Artemisinins have been used empirically in the treatment of malaria for twenty years with excellent efficacy and favotable toxicity during which time their mechanism of action and pharmacokinetic properties have gradually cleared. Empiric judgments of efficacy and optimal administration have been influenced by their undoubtedly impressive parasite clearance kinetics, which are superior to other commonly used antimalarials. Among the artemisinins, the pharmacodynamic and pharmacokinetic profiles of intravenous and oral AS are relatively more superior to the other four major artemisinin derivatives used with various dosing regimens.

The principal mechanisms that result in neurotoxicity and reproductive toxicity are currently understood. The artemisinin's exposure time has an imperative role in the induction of neurotoxicity in animal species. Other factors in the commonly measured pharmacokinetic parameters, such as drug distribution in the brain, toxicity of active metabolite (DHA), or drug exposure level, tend to have minor importance and influence. Neurotoxicity could be avoided simply by a reduction in drug exposure time. In regards to reprotoxicity, the high peak concentration is the major reason resulting in select embryotoxicity in animals, and this is only in the days of marked sensitivity corresponding to the period of yolk sac hematopoiesis, which occurs during GD 9–14 in rats or GD 15 to week 6 in humans. Reproductive toxicity ideally should be avoided by limiting the exposure of artemisinins in these sensitive days (in humans this would be during the first trimester). This time frame is the critical period for induction of embryo damage and resorption, and represents a risk period if trying to protect pregnant women from malaria with treatment using artemisinin derivatives, especially via intravenous route. There is general agreement though that the artemisinin derivatives should not be withheld at any stage of pregnancy in cases of severe and complicated malaria, especially if the life of the mother is felt to be at risk. It is generally considered and supportable that oral regimens of artemisinins are safer than parenteral administrations in pregnant patients if this is a viable option.

This report has also observed that the rapid efficacy of artemisinins is principally at the mercy of drug peak concentration (C_{max}) in the first drug exposure and drug relative antimalarial potency. Other factors in the pharmacokinetic parameters, such as drug exposure level (AUC) and drug exposure time (half-life), tend to have minor significance in efficacy. Some artemisinins (AE, AL, and QHS) that can not produce higher peak concentration with existing regimens or possess less antimalarial potency have been deserted in current development and treatment programs. The fundamental and reliable measures of efficacy in cure and mortality rates for uncomplicated and severe malaria demonstrated that current artemisinins (AS, AM, and DHA), either as combination as ACTs or monotherapy, provide a clear-cut advantage over other antimalarials in some geographical locations. The most recent advance was the large severe malaria study that found a remarkable decrease in mortality (34.7%) using intravenous AS, as opposed to injection quinine. While artemisinins are poorly efficacious at curing malaria as monotherapy, this shortage has been overcome by combinations known as ACTs (AM-lumefantrine, AS-mefloquine, AS-amodiaquine, and AS-sulfadoxine/pyrimethamine) and will be overcome with injection AS because it will be used in combination or preferably, sequentially with a slower acting antimalarial drug, such as mefloquine. In any case, previous arguments for the long-term benefits of combination or sequential therapies in preventing the resistance and recrudescence still stand. When attempting fast parasite killing and with increasing awareness of variance between individuals in both pharmacokinetics and pharmacodynamics, monotherapy and larger loading dose of injection AS may be required to ensure that maximum effect is obtained in all patients with severe and complicated malaria.

Acknowledgment

This study was supported by the United States Army Research and Materiel Command. The opinions or assertions contained herein are the private views of the author and are not to be construed as official, or as reflecting true views of the Department of the Army or the Department of Defense.

References

[1] Xie, HL; Gerena, L; Kyle, DE; Milhous, WK; Zhang, J; Li, QG. Development and validation of flow cytometric measurement for parasitemia in cultures of *P. falciparum* vitally stained with YOYO-1. *Parasitology*, 2006 (submitted)

[2] Bustos, MDG; Gay, F; Diquet, B. In vitro tests on Philippine isolates of Plasmodium falciparum against four standard antimalarials and four qinghaosu derivatives. *Bull. World Health Organization*, 1994, 72, 729-735.

[3] Basco, LK; Bras, JLe. In vitro activity of artemisinin derivatives against African isolates and clones of Plasmodium falciparum. *Am. J. Trop. Med Hyg.* 1993, 49, 301-307.

[4] China Cooperative Research Group on Qinghaosu and Its Derivatives as Antimalarials. Antimalarial efficacy and mode of action of qinghaosu and its derivatives in experimental models. *J. Trad. Chinese Med*, 1982, 2, 17-24.

[5] Skinner, TS; Manning, LS; Johnston, WA; Davis, TME. In vitro stage-specific sensitivity of Plasmodium falciparum to quinine and artemisinin drugs. *Int. J. Parasit.* 1996, 26, 519-525.

[6] China Cooperative Research Group on Qinghaosu and Its Derivatives as Antimalarials. The chemistry and synthesis of qinghaosu derivatives. *J. Trad. Chinese Med.* 1982, 2, 9-16.

[7] Gu, HM; Warhurst, DC; Peters, W. Rapid action of Qinghaosu and related drugs on incorporation of ^{3}H-isoleucine by Plasmodium falciparum in vitro. *Biochem. Pharmacol.* 1983, 32: 2463-2466.

[8] Caillard, VA; Beaute-Lafitte, A; Chabaud, AG; Landau, I. Plasmodium vinckei petteri: identification of the stages sensitive to arteether. *Exp. Parasit.* 1992, 75, 449-456.

[9] ter Kuile, FT; White, NJ; Holloway, P; Pasvol, G; Krishna, S. Plasmodium falciparum: In vitro Studies of the pharmacodynamic properties of drugs used for the treatment of severe malaria. *Exp. Parasit.* 1993, 76, 85-95.

[10] Dutta, GP; Bajpai, R; Vishwakarma, RA. Blood schizontocidal activity of artemisinin and arteether against Plasmodium berghei. *J. Parasit.* 1987, 11, 253-257.

[11] Dutta, GP; Bajpai, R; Vishwakarma, RA. Comparison of antimalarial efficacy of artemisinin and arteether against Plasmodium cynomolgi B infection in monkeys. *Trans. R. Soc. Trop. Med. Hug.* 1989, 83, 56-57.

[12] Barradell, LB; Fitton, A. Artesunate, A review of its pharmacology and therapeutic efficacy in the treatment of malaria. *Drugs.* 1996, 50: 714-741.

[13] Geary, TG; Divo, AA; Jensen, JB. Stage specific actions of antimalarial drugs on Plasmodium falciparum in culture. *Am. J. Trop. Med. Hyg.* 1989, 40: 240-244.

[14] Woerdenbag, HJ; Pras, N; Uden, W; Wallaart, TE; Beekman, AC; Lugt, CB. Progress in the research of artemisinin-related antimalarials: an update. *Pharm. World Sci.* 16, 169-180.

[15] Tripathi, R; Puri, SK;. Dutta, GP. Sodium beta-artelinate - a new potential gametocytocide. *Exp. Parasit*, 1996, 82, 251-254.

[16] Navaratnam, V; Mansor, SM; Sit, NW; Grace, J; Li, QG; Olliaro, P. Pharmacokinetics of artemisinin-type compounds. *Clin. Pharmacokinet.* 2000, 39, 255-270.

[17] Shmuklarsky, MJ; Klayman, DL; Milhous, W.K; Rossan, RN; Ager AL; Tang, Jr. DB; Heiffer, MH; Canfield, CJ; Schuster, BG. Comparison of ß-artemether and ß-arteether against malaria parasites in vivo and in vitro., *Am. J. Trop. Med. Hyg.*, 1993, 48, 377-384.

[18] Lin, AJ; Klayman, DL; Milhous, WK. Antimalarial activity of new water-soluble dihydroartemisinin derivatives. *J. Med. Chem*, 1987, 30, 2147-2150.

[19] Tripathi, R; Dutta, GP; Vishwakarma, RA. Comparison of antimalarial efficacy of α, ß, and α/ß arteether against Plasmodium cynomolgi B infection in monkeys. *Am. J. Trop. Med. Hyg.* 1991, 44, 560-563.

[20] Maeno, Y; Brown, AE; Smith, CD; Tegoshi, T; Toyoshima, T; Ockenhouse, CF; Corcoran, KD; Ngampochjana, M; Kyle, DE; Webster HK, et al.: A nonhuman primate model for human cerebral malaria: effects of artesunate (qinghaosu derivative) on rhesus monkeys experimentally infected with plasmodium coatneyi. *Am. J. Trop. Med. Hyg.* 1993. 49, 726-734.

[21] Looareesuwan, S; Wilairatana, P. The rational use of qinghaosu and its derivatives: what is the future of new compounds? *Med. Trop.* 1998, 58 (Suppl 3), 89S-92S.

[22] Looareesuwan, S; Oosterhuis, B; Schilizzi, BM; Sollie, FA; Wilairatana, P; Krudsood, S; Lugt, CB; Peeters, PA; Peggins, JO. Dose-finding and efficacy study for i.m. artemotil (beta-arteether) and comparison with i.m. artemether in acute uncomplicated P. falciparum malaria. *Br. J. Clin. Pharm.* 2002, 53, 492-500.

[23] van Hensbroek, MB; Onyiorah, E; Jaffar, S; Schneider, G; Palmer, A; Frenkel, J; Enwere, G; Forck, S; Nusmeijer, A; Bennett, S; Greenwood, B; Kwiatkowski, D. A trial of artemether or quinine in children with cerebral malaria. *N. Engl. J. Med.* 1996, 335, 69-75.

[24] Tran, TH; Day, NP; Nguyen, HP; Nguyen, TH; Tran, TH; Pham, PL; Dinh, XS; Ly, VC; Ha, V; Waller, D; Peto, TE; White, NJ. A controlled trial of artemether or quinine in Vietnamese adults with severe falciparum malaria. *N. Engl. J. Med.* 1996, 335, 76-83.

[25] Karbwang, J; Na-Bangchang, K; Thanavibul, A; Molunto, P. Plasma concentrations of artemether and its major plasma metabolite, dihydroartemisinin, following a 5-day regimen of oral artemether, in patients with uncomplicated falciparum malaria. *Ann. Trop. Med. Parasit.* 1998, 92, 31-36.

[26] Looareesuwan, S; Wilairatana, P; Viravan, C; Vanijanonta, S; Pitisutitithum, P; Kyle, DE. Open randomized trial of oral artemether alone and a sequential combination with mefloquine for acute uncomplicated falciparum malaria. *Am. J. Trop. Med. Hyg.* 1997, 56, 613-617.

[27] Mohamed, SS; Khalid, SA; Ward, SA; Wan, TSM; Tang, HPO; Zheng, M; Haynes, RK; Edwards, G, Simultaneous determination of artemether and its major metabolite dihydroartemisinin in plasma by gas chromatography-mass spectrometry-selected ion monitoring. *J. Chromatograph.* 1999, B 731, 251-260

[28] Murphy, S; English, M; Waruiru, C; Mwangi, I; Amukoye, E; Crawley, J; Newton, C; Winstanley, P; Peshu, N; Marsh, K. An open randomized trial of artemether versus quinine in the treatment of cerebral malaria in African children. *Trans. R. Soc. Trop. Med. Hyg.* 1996, 90, 298-301.

[29] Na-Bangchang, K; Karbwang, J; Thomas, CG; Thanavibul, A; Sukontason, K; Ward, SA; Edwards, G. Pharmacokinetics of artemether after oral administration to health Thai males and patients with acute, uncomplicated falciparum malaria. *Br. J. Clin. Pharm.* 1994, 37, 249-253.

[30] Salako, LA; Walker, O; Sowunmi, A; Omokhodion, SJ; Adio, R; Oduola, AM. Artemether in moderately severe and cerebral malaria in Nigerian children. *Trans. R. Soc. Trop. Med. Hyg.* 1994, 88 Suppl 1, S13-5.

[31] Sowunmi, A; Oduola, AMJ. Efficacy of artemether in severe falciparum malaria in African children. *Acta Tropica.* 1996, 61, 57-63.

[32] Walter, O; Salako, LA; Omokhodion, SI; Sowunmi, A. An open randomized comparative study of intramuscular artemether and intravenous quinine in cerebral malaria in children. *Trans. R. Soc. Trop. Med. Hyg.* 1993, 87, 564-566.

[33] de Vries, PJ; Dien, TK. Clinical pharmacology and therapeutic potential of artemisinin and its derivatives in the treatment of malaria. *Drugs.* 1996, 52, 818-836.

[34] Looareesuwan, S; Wilairatana, P; Vanijanonta, S; Pitisuttithum, P; Ratanapong, Y; Andrial, M. Monotherapy with sodium artesunate for uncomplicated falciparum malaria in Thailand: a comparison of 5- and 7-day regimens. *Acta Trop.* 1997, 67, 197-205.

[35] Li, GQ; Wang, XH; Guo, XB; Fu, LC; Jian, HX; Chen, PQ; Li, GQ. Dose finding of dihydroartemisinin in treatment of falciparum malaria. *Southeast Asian J. Trop. Med. Pub. Health.* 1999, 30, 17-19.

[36] Looareesuwan, S; Wilairatana, P; Vanijanonta, S; Pitisuttithum, P; Viravan, C. Treatment of acute, uncomplicated, falciparum malaria with oral dihydroartemisinin. *Ann. Trop. Med. Parasit.* 1996. 90, 21-28.

[37] Wilairatana, P; Chanthavanich, P; Singhasivanon, P; Treeprasertsuk, S; Krudsood, S; Chalermrut, K; Phisalaphong, C; Kraisintu, K; Looareesuwan, S. A comparison of three different dihydroartemisinin formulations for the treatment of acute uncomplicated falciparum malaria in Thailand. *Intern. J. Parasit.* 1998, 28, 1213-1218.

[38] Xu, C; Ding, Y; Qi, Z. Efficacy of dihydroartemisinin in treatment of 37 malaria cases. *Zhonghua Nei Ke Za Zhi.* 1997, 36, 187-189.

[39] Mishra, SK; Asthana, OP; Mohanty, S; Patnaik, JK; Das, BS; Srivastava, JS; Satpathy, SK; Dash, S; Rath, PK; Varghese, K. Effectiveness of alpha, beta-arteether in acute falciparum malaria. *Trans. R. Soc. Trop. Med. Hyg.* 1995, 89, 299-301.

[40] Mohanty, S; Mishra, SK; Satpathy, SK; Dash, S; Patnaik, J. Alpha, beta-arteether for the treatment of complicated falciparum malaria. *Trans. R. Soc. Trop. Med. Hyg.* 1997, 91, 328-330.

[41] Mohapatr, PK; Khan, AM; Prakash, A; Mahanta, J; Srivastava, VK. Effect of arteether alpha/beta on uncomplicated falciparum malaria cases in Upper Assam. *Indian J. Med. Res* 1996, 104, 284-287.

[42] Singh N, Shukla MM, Asthana OP, Sharma VP, 1998. Effectiveness of alpha-beta arteether in clearing Plasmodium falciparum parasitemia in central India (Madhya Pradesh). *Southeast Asian J. Trop. Med. Pub. Health.* 29: 225-227.

[43] Valecha, N; Gupta, S; Usha, D; Biswas, S; Sharma, A; Adak, T; Asthana, OP; Sharma, VP. Efficacy of alpha, beta-arteether in acute uncomplicated *P. Falciparum* malaria. *Inter. J. Clin. Pharm. Res.* 1997, 17, 11-15.

[44] Li, QG; Peggins, JO; Fleckenstein, L; Masonic, K; Heiffer, MH; Brewer, TG. Bioavailability and pharmacokinetics of dihydroartemisinin, arteether, artemether, artesunic acid and artelinic acid in rats. *J. Pharm. and Pharm.* 1998, 50, 173-182.

[45] Li, QG; Peggins, JO; Lin, AJ; Masonic, K; Trotman KM; Brewer, TG. Pharmacology and toxicology of artelinic acid: Preclinical investigation on pharmacokinetics, metabolism, protein and RBC binding, acute and anorectic toxicities. *Tran. Roy. Soc. Trop. Med. Hyg.* 1998, 92, 332-340.

[46] Teja-Isavadharm, P; Nosten, F; Kyle, DE; Luxemburger, C; Ter Kuile, F; Peggins, JO; Brewer, TG; White, NJ. Comparative bioavailability of oral, rectal, and intramuscular artemether in healthy subjects: use of simultaneous measurement by high performance liquid chromatography and bioassay. *Br. J. Clin. Pharmac.* 1996, 42, 599-604.

[47] Zhao, KC; Song, ZY. Pharmacokinetics of dihydroqinhaosu given orally to rabbits and dogs. *Yao Hsueh Hsueh Pao.* 1990, 25, 147-149.

[48] Benakis, A; Schopfer, C; Paris, M; Plessas, ChT; Karayannakos, PE; Dondas, I; Kotsarelis, D; Plessas, ST; Skalkeas, G. Pharmacokinetics of arteether in dog. *Eur. J. Drug Metab. Pharmacokin.* 1991, 16, 325-328.

[49] Titulaer, HA; Eling, WM; Zuidema, J. Pharmacokinetic and pharmacodynamic aspects of artelinic acid in rodents. *J. Pharm. Pharmacol.* 1993, 45, 830-835.

[50] van Vianen, PH; Klayman, DL; Lin, AJ; Lugt, CB; van Engen, AL; van der Kaay, HJ; Mons, B. Plasmodium berghei: the antimalarial action of artemisinin and sodium artelinate in vivo and in vitro, studied by flow cytometry. *Exp. Parasitol.* 1990, 70, 115-123.

[51] Grace, JM; Skanchy, DJ; Aguilar, AJ. Metabolism of artelinic acid to dihydroqinhaosu by human liver cytochrome P4503A. *Xenobiotica.* 1999, 29: 703-717.

[52] Brewer, TG; Grate, SJ; Peggins, JO; Weina, PJ; Petras, JM; Levine, BS; Heiffer, MH; Schuster, BG. Fatal neurotoxicity of arteether and artemether. *Am. J. Trop. Med. Hyg.* 1994, 51, 251-259.

[53] Genovese, RF; Petras, JM; Brewer, TG. Arteether neurotoxicity in the absence of deficits in behavioural performance in rats. *Ann. Trop. Med. Parasitol.* 1995, 89, 447-449.

[54] Kamchonwongpaisan, S; McKeever, P; Hossler, P; Ziffer, H; Meshnick, SR. Artemisinin neurotoxicity: Neuropathology in rats and mechanistic studies in vitro. *Am. J. Trop. Med. Hyg.* 1997, 56, 7-12.

[55] Petras, JM; Kyle, DE; Ngampochjana, M; Young, GD; Bauman, RA; Webster, HK; Corcoran, JD; Peggins, JO; Vane, MA; Brewer, TG. Arteether: Risks of two-week administration in macaca mulatta. *Am. J. Trop. Med. Hyg.* 1997, 57, 390-396.

[56] Dayan, AD. Neurotoxicity and artemisinin compounds do the observations in animals justify limitation of clinical use? *Med. Trop.* 58, 32S-37S.

[57] Brewer, TG; Peggins, JO; Grate, SJ; Petras, JM; Levine, BS; Weina, PJ; Swearengen, J; Heiffer, MH; Schuster, BG. Neurotoxicity in animals due to arteether and artemether. *Trans. R Soc. Trop. Med. Hyg.* 1994, 88 (Suppl, 1), 33-36.

[58] Davidson, DE. Role of arteether in the treatment of malaria and plans for further development. *Trans. R Soc. Trop. Med. Hyg.* 1994, 88 (Suppl, 1): S51-52.

[59] Genovese, RF; Newman, DB; Li, QG; Peggins, JO; Brewer, TG. Dose-dependent brainstem neuropathology following repeated arteether administration in rats. *Brain Res. Bull.* 1998, 45, 199-202.

[60] Meshnick, SR. Artemisinin: mechanisms of action, resistance and toxicity. *Int. J. Parasitol.* 2002, 32, 1655-1660.

[61] Si, YZ; Li, QG; Mog, SR; Upadhyay, R; Wong, E; Xie, LH; Weina, PJ. Toxicokinetics and neurotoxicity evaluation following oral administration of artelinic acid in rats. *Am. J. Trol. Med. Hyg.* 2000, 67, 255.

[62] Nontprasert, A; Pukrittayakamee, S; Nosten-Bertrand, M; Vanijanonta, S; White, NJ. Studies of the neurotoxicity of oral artemisinin derivatives in mice. *Am. J. Trop. Med. Hyg.* 2000, 62, 409-412.

[63] Nontprasert, A; Pukrittayakamee, S; Prakongpan, S; Supanaranond, W; Looareesuwan, S; White, NJ. Assessment of the neurotoxicity of oral dihydroartemisinin in mice. *Trans. R. Soc. Trop. Med. Hyg.* 2002, 96, 99-101.

[64] Nontprasert, A; Nosten-Bertrand, M; Pukrittayakamee, S; Vanijanonta, S; Angus, BJ; White, NJ. Assessment of the neurotoxicity of parenteral artemisinin derivatives in mice. *Am. J. Trop. Med. Hyg.* 1998, 59, 519-522.

[65] Classen, W; Altmann, B; Gretener, P; Souppart, C; Skelton-Stroud, P; Krinke, G. Differental effects of orally versus parenterally administered qinghaosu derivatives artemether in dogs. *Exp. Toxic. Pathol.* 1999, 51, 507-516.

[66] Li,QG; Xie, LH; Johnson, TO; Si, YZ; Haeberle, AS; Weina, PJ. Toxicity evaluation of artesunate and artelinate in *Plasmodium berghei*-infected and uninfected rats. *Trans. R. Soc. Trop. Med. Hyg.* 2006 Jul 19; [Epub ahead of print]

[67] Karbwang, J; Na-Bangchang, K; Wattanakoon, Y; Thanavibul, A; Harinasuta, T. Artemether 5 versus 7 day regimen for severe falciparum malaria. *Southeast Asian J. Trop. Med. Public. Health.* 1994, 25, 702-706.

[68] Angus, BJ; Thaiaporn, I; Chanthapadith, K; Suputtamongkol, Y; White, NJ. Oral artesunate dose-response relationship in acute falciparum malaria. *Antimicrob Agents Chemother.* 2002, 46, 778-782.

[69] Wilairatana, P; Krudsood, S; Treeprasertsuk, S; Chalermrut, K; Looareesuwan, S. The future outlook of antimalarial drugs and recent work on the treatment of malaria. *Arch. Med. Res.* 2002, 33, 416-421.

[70] Price, R; van Vugt, M; Phaipun, L; Luxemburger, C; Simpson, J; McGready, R; ter Kuile, F; Kham, A; Chongsuphajaisiddhi, T; White, NJ; Nosten, F. Adverse effects in patients with acute falciparum malaria treated with artemisinin derivatives. *Am. J. Trop. Med. Hyg.* 1999, 60, 547-555.

[71] Hien, TT. An overview of the clinical use of artemisinin and its derivatives in the treatment of falciparum malaria in Viet Nam. *Trans. R. Soc. Trop. Med. Hyg.* 1994, 88 Suppl 1, S7-8.

[72] Kar, K; Shankar, G; Bajpai, R; Dutta, GP; Vishwakarma, RA. Artemisinin: a potent antimalarial agent, general pharmacological properties. *Ind. J. Parasitol.* 1988, 12, 209-212.

[73] Li, GQ; Guo, XB; Fu, LC; Jian, HX; Wang, XH. Clinical trials of artemisinin and its derivatives in the treatment of malaria in China. *Trans. Royal Soc. Trop. Med. Hyg.* 1994, 88 (Suppl. 1), S1/5-6.

[74] Meshinick, S.R; Taylor, TE; Kamchonwongpaisan, S. Artemisinin and the antimalarial endoperroxides: from herbal remedy to targeted chemotherapy. *Microbil. Rev.* 1996, 60, 301-315.

[75] Myint, PT; Shwe, T. The efficacy of artemether (qinghaosu) in Plasmodium falciparum and P. vivax in Burma. *Southeast Asian J. Trop. Med. Public Health.* 1986, 17, 19-22.

[76] Myint, PT; Shwe, T. A controlled clinical trial of artemether (qinghaosu derivative) versus quinine in complicated and severe falciparum malaria. *Trans. R. Soc. Trop. Med. Hyg.* 1987, 81, 559-561.

[77] Afolabi, BB; Okoromah, CN. Intramuscular arteether for treating severe malaria. *Cochrane Database Syst. Rev.* 2004. 18, CD004391.

[78] Yeates RA. Artemotil Artecef. *Curr. Opin. Investig. Drugs.* 2002. 3, 545-549.

[79] White, NJ. Artemisinin: current status. *Trans. Royal Soc. Trop. Med. Hyg.* 1994, 88 (Suppl. 1), S1/3-4.

[80] Miller, LG; Planosian, CB. Ataxia and slurred speech after artesunate treatment for falciparum malaria. *New Engl. J. Med.* 1997, 336, 1328.

[81] Causer, LM; Filler, S; Wilson, M; et al. Evaluation of reported malaria chemoprophylatic failure among travelers in a US university exchange program, 2000. *Clin. Infect. Dis.* 2004, 39, 1583-1588.

[82] Keystone, JS. The sound of hoof beats does not always mean that it is a zebra. *Clin. Infect. Dis.* 2004, 39, 1589-1590.

[83] Franco-Paredes, C; Dismukes, R; Nicholls, D; Kozarsky, PE. Neurotoxicity due to antimalarial therapy associated with misdiagnosis of malaria [letter]. *Clin. Infect. Dis.* 2005, 40, 1710-1711.

[84] Newton, PN; Day, NPJ; White, NJ. Misattribution of central nervous system dysfunction to artesunate. *Clin. Infect. Dis.* 2005, 41, 1687-1688.

[85] Gachot, B; Eliaszewicz, M; Dupont, B. Artesunate and cerebellar dysfunction in falciparum malaria. *N. Engl. J. Med.* 1997, 337, 792-793.

[86] Miller, LG; Panosian, CB. Artesunate and cerebellar dysfunction in falciparum malaria-reply. *N. Engl. J. Med.* 1997, 337, 793.

[87] Ribeiro, IR; Olliaro, P. Safety of artemisinin and its derivatives. A systematic review of published and unpublished clinical trials. *Med. Trop. (Mars)*, 1998, 58 (Suppl 3); S50-53.

[88] Toovey, S; Jamieson, A. Audiometric changes associated with the treatment of uncomplicated falciparum malaria with co-artemether. *Trans. R. Soc. Trop. Med. Hyg.* 2004, 98, 261-269.

[89] Toovey, S. Effects of weight, age, and time on artemether-lumefantrine associated ototoxicity and evidence of irreversibility. *Travel Med. Infect. Dis.* 2006 (in press)

[90] Hutagalung, R; Htoo, H; Nwee, P; Arunkamomkiri, J; Zwang, J; Carrara, VI; Ashley, E; Singhasivanon, P; White, NJ; Nosten, F. A case-control auditory evaluation of patients treated with artemether-lumefantrine. *Am. J. Trop. Med. Hyg.* 2006, 74, 211-214.

[91] Newton, P; Suputtamongkol, Y; Teja-Isavadharm, P; Pukrittayakamee, S; Navaratnam, V; Bates, I; White, N. Antimalarial bioavailability and disposition of artesunate in acute falciparum malaria. *Antimicrob Agents Chemother.* 2000, 44, 972-977.
[92] Karbwang, J; Na-Bangchang, K; Thanavibul, A; Bunnag, D; Chongsuphajaisiddhi, T; Harinasuta, T. Comparison of oral artesunate and quinine plus tetracycline in acute uncomplicated falciparum malaria. *Bull. World Health Organization* 1994, 72, 233-238.
[93] Kager, PA; Schultz, MJ; Zijlstra, EE; van Berg, B; van Boxtel, Ch.J. Arteether administration in humans: preliminary studies of pharmacokinetics, safety and tolerance. *Trans. R. Soc. Trop. Med. Hyg.* 1994, 88 (suppl 1), 53-54.
[94] Hoffman, SL. Artemether in severe malaria – still to many deaths. *New Engl. J. Med.* 1996, 335, 124-125.
[95] Park, BK; O'Neill, PN; Maggs, JL; Pirmohamed, M. Safety assessment of peroxide antimalarials: clinical and chemical perspectives. *Br. J. Clin. Pharmacol.* 1998, 46, 521-529.
[96] China Cooperative Research Group on qinghaosu and its derivatives as antimalarials. Studies on the toxicity of qinghaosu and its derivatives. *J. Tradit. Chin. Med.* 1982, 2, 31-38.
[97] Chen, LJ; Wang, MY; Sun, WK; Liu, MZ. Embryotoxicity and teratogenicity studies on artemether in mice, rats and rabbits. *Zhongguo Yao Li Xue Bao.* 1984, 5, 118-122.
[98] Li, ZL. Teratogenicity of sodium artesunate. *Zhong Yao Tong Bao*, 1988, 13, 42–44, 63–64.
[99] Si, YZ; Zeng, Q; Zhang, J; Johnson, TO; Xie, LH; Weina, PJ; Milhous, WK; Li, QG. Evaluation of the embryonic toxicity of artesunate in rats. *Am. J. Trop. Med. Hyg.* 2004, 71, 260.
[100] Xu, JH; Zhang, YP. Contragestational effects of dihydroartemisinin and artesunate. *Yao Xue Xue Bao.* 1996, 31, 657-661.
[101] Clark, RL; White, TE; Clode, SA; Gaunt, I; Winstanley, P; Ward, SA. Developmental toxicity of artesunate and an artesunate combination in the rat and rabbit. *Birth Defects Res. B. Dev. Reprod. Toxicol.* 2004, 71, 380-394.
[102] Longo, M; Zanoncelli, S; Torre, PD; Riflettuto, M; Cocco, F; Pesenti, M; Giusti, A; Colombo, P; Brughera, M; Mazue, G; Navaratman, V; Gomes, M; Olliaro, P. In vivo and in vitro investigations of the effects of the antimalarial drug dihydroartemisinin (DHA) on rat embryos. *Reprod Toxicol.* 2006 Aug 14; [Epub ahead of print]
[103] Ejiofor, JI; Kwanashie, HO; Anuka, JA. Some Pregnancy-Related Effects of Artemether in Laboratory Animals. *Pharmacology.* 2006, 77, 166-170.
[104] Longo, M; Zanoncelli, S; Manera, D; Brughera, M; Colombo, P; Lansen, J; Mazue, G; Gomes, M; Taylor, WR; Olliaro, P. Effects of the antimalarial drug dihydroartemisinin (DHA) on rat embryos in vitro. *Reprod. Toxicol.* 2006, 21, 83-93.
[105] Chen, HH; Zhou, HJ; Wu ,GD; Lou, XE. Inhibitory effects of artesunate on angiogenesis and on expressions of vascular endothelial growth factor and VEGF receptor KDR/flk-1. *Pharmacology.* 2004, 71, 1-9.
[106] Lou, XE; Zhou, HJ. Effects of artesunate on progesterone estrogen content and decidua in rats. *Yao Xue Xue Bao.* 2001, 36, 254-257.

[107] Lou, XE; Zhou, HJ; Huang, HB. Lipid-peroxidantion damage of embryo and placenta induced by artesunate in rats. *Zhejiang Da Xue Xue Bao Yi Xue Ban*. 2003, 32, 41-45.

[108] World Health Organization. Assessment of the safety of artemisinin compounds in pregnancy. Report of two informal consultations convened by WHO in 2002 (RBM and TDR). WHO/CDS/MAL/2003.1094.

[109] Li, GQ; Guo, XB; Jin, R; Wang, ZC; Jian, HX; Li, ZY. Clinical trials on qinghaosu and its derivatives: *Guangzhou College of Traditional Chinese Medicine*, 1990.

[110] Wang, TY. Follow-up observation on the therapeutic effects and remote reactions of artemisinin (Qinghaosu) and artemether in treating malaria in pregnant woman. *J. Tradit. Chin. Med.* 1989, 9, 28-30.

[111] Deen, JL; von Seidlein, L; Pinder, M; Walraven, GE; Greenwood, BM. The safety of the combination artesunate and pyrimethamine-sulfadoxine given during pregnancy. *Trans. R. Soc. Trop. Med. Hyg.* 2001, 95, 424-428.

[112] McGready, R; Cho, T; Keo, NK; Thwai, KL; Villegas, L; Looareesuwan, S; White, NJ; Nosten, F. Artemisinin antimalarials in pregnancy: a prospective treatment study of 539 episodes of multidrug-resistant Plasmodium falciparum. *Clin. Infect. Dis*. 2001, 33, 2009-2016.

[113] Adam, I; Ali, DM; Abdalla, MA. Artesunate plus sulfadoxine-pyrimethamine in the treatment of uncomplicated Plasmodium falciparum malaria during pregnancy in eastern Sudan. *Trans. R. Soc. Trop. Med. Hyg.* 2006 Jan 24 (ahead of print)

[114] Bounyasong, S. Randomized trial of artesunate and mefloquine in comparison with quinine sulfate to treat P. falciparum malaria pregnant women. *J. Med. Assoc. Thai.* 2001, 84, 1289-1299.

[115] McGready, R; Brockman, A; Cho, T; Cho, D; van Vugt, M; Luxemburger, C; Chongsuphajaisiddhi, T; White, NJ; Nosten, F. Randomized comparison of mefloquine-artesunate versus quinine in the treatment of multidrug-resistant falciparum malaria in pregnancy. *Trans. R. Soc. Trop. Med. Hyg.* 2000, 94, 689-693.

[116] McGready, R; Cho, T; Samuel; Villegas, L; Brockman, A; van Vugt, M; Looareesuwan, S; White, NJ; Nosten, F. Randomized comparison of quinine-clindamycin versus artesunate in the treatment of falciparum malaria in pregnancy. *Trans. R. Soc. Trop. Med. Hyg.* 2001, 95, 651-656.

[117] McGready, R; Keo, NK; Villegas, L; White, NJ; Looareesuwan, S; Nosten, F. Artesunate-atovaquone-proguanil rescue treatment of multidrug-resistant Plasmodium falciparum malaria in pregnancy: a preliminary report. *Trans. R. Soc. Trop. Med. Hyg.* 2003, 97, 592-594.

[118] McGready, R; Stepniewska, K; Edstein, MD; Cho, T; Gilveray, G; Looareesuwan, S; White, NJ; Nosten, F. The pharmacokinetics of atovaquone and proguanil in pregnant women with acute falciparum malaria. *Eur. J. Clin. Pharmacol.* 2003, 59, 545-552.

[119] McGready, R; Ashley, EA; Moo, E; Cho, T; Barends, M; Hutagalung, R; Looareesuwan, S; White, NJ; Nosten, F. A randomized comparison of artesunate-atovaquone-proguanil versus quinine in treatment for uncomplicated falciparum malaria during pregnancy. *J. Infect. Dis*. 2005, 192, 846-853.

[120] Orton, L; Garner, P. Drugs for treating uncomplicated malaria in pregnant women. *Cochrane Database Syst. Rev*. 2005, 20, CD004912.

[121] Brabin, BJ; Ramagosa, C; Abdelgalil, S; Menendez, C; Verhoeff, FH; McGready, R; Fletcher, KA; Owens, S; d'Alessandro, U; Nosten, F; Fischer, PR; Ordi, J; The sick placenta: the role of malaria. *Placenta.* 2004, 25, 359-378.

[122] Price, RN. Artemisinin drugs: novel antimalarial agents. Expert Opin. Investig. *Drugs.* 2000, 9, 1815–1827.

[123] White, NJ; Olliaro, P. Artemisinin and derivatives in the treatment of uncomplicated malaria. *Med. Trop. (Mars.)* 1998, 58 (Suppl.3), 54–56.

[124] White, NJ. Antimalarial drug resistance and combination chemotherapy. *Philos. Trans. R. Soc. Lond. B. Biol. Sci.* 1999, 354, 739–749.

[125] White, NJ. Delaying antimalarial drug resistance with combination chemotherapy. *Parasitologia.* 1999, 41, 301–308.

[126] Nosten, F; vanVugt, M; Price, RN; Luxemburger, C; Thway, KL; Brockman, A; McGready, R; ter Kuile, F; Looareesuwan, S; White, NJ. Effects of artesunate-mefloquine combination on incidence of Plasmodium falciparum malaria and mefloquine resistance in western Thailand: a prospective study. *Lancet.* 2000, 356, 297–302.

[127] World Health Organization. Antimalarial Drug Combination Therapy: *Report of a Technical Consultation.* 2001, WHO, Geneva.

[128] Roll Back Malaria. The RBM partnership's global response; a programmatic strategy 2004–2008. Available at: http://rbm.who.int/partnership/ board/meetings/docs/ strategy_rev.pdf (accessed November 2004).

[129] Haynes, RK. From artemisinin to new artemisinin antimalarials: biosynthesis, extraction, old and new derivatives, stereochemistry and medicinal chemistry requirements. *Curr. Top Med. Chem.* 2006, 6, 509-537.

[130] White, NJ; van Vugt, M; Ezzet, F. Clinical pharmacokinetics and pharmacodynamics of artemether lumefantrine. *Clin. Pharmacokinet.* 1999, 37, 105–125.

[131] van Vugt, M; Looareesuwan, S; Wilairatana, P; McGready, R; Villegas, L; Gathmann, I; Mull, R; Brockman, A; White, NJ; Nosten, F. Artemether-lumefantrine for the treatment of multidrug-resistant falciparum malaria. *Trans. R. Soc. Trop. Med. Hyg.* 2000, 94, 545–548.

[132] Omari, AA; Gamble, C; Garner, P. Artemether-lumefantrine for uncomplicated malaria: a systematic review. *Trop. Med. Int. Health.* 2004, 9, 192-199.

[133] Poravuth, Y; Socheat, D; Fandeur, T; et al. Efficacy and safety of six dose regimen of Coartem® in the treatment of acute uncomplicated falciparum malaria in Cambodia 2002. In: Gay F, editor. Proceedings of Mekong Malaria Symposium, 2002, Siem Reap, Angkor Wat, Kingdom of Cambodia. (Mekong Malaria Forum, RMCP-EC): 54.

[134] Hien, TT; Dolecek, C; Mai, PP; et al. Dihydroartemisinin-piperaquine against multidrug-resistant Plasmodium falciparum malaria in Vietnam: randomized clinical trial. *Lancet.* 2004, 363, 18-22.

[135] Guthmann, JP; Cohuet, S; Rigutto, C; Fortes, F; Saraiva, N; Kiguli, J; Kyomuhendo, J; Francis, M; Noel, F; Mulemba, M; Balkan, S. High efficacy of two artemisinin-based combinations (artesunate + amodiaquine and artemether + lumefantrine) in Caala, Central Angola. *Am. J. Trop. Med. Hyg.* 2006, 75, 143-145.

[136] Khim, N; Bouchier, C; Ekala, MT; Incardona, S; Lim ,P; Legrand, E; Jambou, R; Doung, S; Puijalon, OM; Fandeur, T. Countrywide survey shows very high prevalence of Plasmodium falciparum multilocus resistance genotypes in Cambodia. *Antimicrob. Agents Chemother.* 2005, 49, 3147-3152.

[137] Davis, TM; Karunajeewa, HA; Ilett, KF. Artemisinin-based combination therapies for uncomplicated malaria. *Med. J. Aust.* 2005, 21, 182, 181-185.

[138] Anstey, NM; Price, RN; White, NJ. Improving the availability of artesunate for treatment of severe malaria. Artesunate reduces mortality and should now be the treatment of choice in severe malaria in adults: good news for countries in our region, but registration in Australia must wait. *Med. J. Aust.* 2006, 184, 3-4.

[139] Malik, EM; Mohamed, TA; Elmardi, KA; Mowien, RM; Elhassan, AH; Elamin, SB; Mannan, AA; Ahmed, ES. From chloroquine to artemisinin-based combination therapy: The Sudanese experience. *Malar. J.* 2006, 5, 65.

[140] Luxemburger, C; Nosten, F; Raimond, SD; Chongsuphajaisiddhi, T; White, NJ. Oral artesunate in the treatment of uncomplicated hyperparasitemic falciparum malaria. *Am. J. Trop. Med. Hyg.* 1995, 53, 522-525.

[141] Artemether-Quinine Meta-analysis Study Group. A meta-analysis using individual patient data of trials comparing artemether with quinine in the treatment of severe falciparum malaria. *Trans. R. Soc. Trop. Med. Hyg.* 2001, 95, 637-650.

[142] Whitty, CJ; Ansah, E; Reyburn, H. Treating severe malaria. *BMJ.* 2005, 330, 317-318.

[143] Davis, TM; Phuong, HL; Ilett, KF; et al. Pharmacokinetics and pharmacodynamics of intravenous artesunate in severe falciparum malaria. *Antimicrob. Agents Chemother.* 2001, 45, 181-186.

[144] Hien, TT; Davis, TM; Chuong, LV; et al. Comparative pharmacokinetics of intramuscular artesunate and artemether in patients with severe falciparum malaria. *Antimicrob. Agents Chemother.* 2004, 48, 4234-4239.

[145] Dondorp, A; Nosten, F; Stepniewska, K; Day, N; White, N. South East Asian Quinine Artesunate Malaria Trial (SEAQUAMAT) group. Artesunate versus quinine for treatment of severe falciparum malaria: a randomised trial. *Lancet.* 2005, 366, 717-725.

[146] Ashley, EA; White, NJ. Artemisinin-based combinations. *Curr. Opin. Infect. Dis.* 2005, 18, 531-536.

[147] Jelinek, T. Intravenous artesunate recommended for patients with severe malaria: position statement from TropNetEurop. *Euro Surveill.* 2005, 10, E051124.5.

[148] Pasvol, G. The treatment of complicated and severe malaria. *Br. Med. Bull.* 2006, 75-76, 29-47.

[149] Nosten, F; Ashley, E; McGready, R; Price, R. We still need artesunate monotherapy. *BMJ.* 2006, 333, 45.

[150] Weina, PJ; Haeberle, AS; Lowe, MC; Cantilena, L; Milhous, WK. Intravenous artesunate: New product for the treatment of severe and complicated malaria. *Am. J. Trop. Med. Hyg.* 2005, 73, 32.

[151] Gordi, T; Lepist, EI. Artemisinin derivatives: toxic for laboratory animals, safe for humans? *Toxicol. Lett.* 2004, 147, 99-107.

[152] Li, QG; Mog, SR; Si, YZ; Kyle, DE; Gettayacamin, M; Milhous, WK. Neurotoxicity and efficacy of arteether related to its exposure times and exposure levels in rodents. *Am. J. Trop. Med. Hyg.* 2002, 66, 516-525.

[153] McLean, WG; Ward, SA. In vitro neurotoxicity of artemisinin derivatives. *Med. Trop. (Mars).* 1998, 58(3 Suppl), 28-31.

[154] Fishwick , J; McLean, WG; Edwards, G; Ward, SA. The toxicity of artemisinin and related compounds on neuronal and glial cells in culture. *Chem. Biol. Interact.* 1995, 96, 263-271.

[155] Li, QG; Brewer, TG; Peggins, JO. Anorectic toxicity of dihydroartemisinin, arteether and artemether in rats following multiple intramuscular doses. *International. J. Toxicol.* 1998, 17, 663-676.

[156] Wesche, DL; DeCoster, MA; Tortella, FC; Brewer, TG. Neurotoxicity of artemisinin analogs in vitro. *Antimicrob Agents Chemother.* 1994, 38, 1813-1819.

[157] Benakis, A; Binh, TQ; Keundjian, A; Scheiwe, MW. Pharmacokinetics/ Pharmacodynamics findings after repeated administration of ARTESUNATE thermostable suppositories (RECTOCAPS) in Vietnamese patients with uncomplicated malaria. *Eur. J. Drug. Metab. Pharmacokinet.* 2006, 31, 41-45.

[158] Batty, KT; Le, AT; Ilett, KF; Nguyen, PT; Powell, SM; Nguyen, CH; Truong ,XM; Vuong, VC; Huynh, VT; Tran,QB; Nguyen, VM; Davis, TM. A pharmacokinetic and pharmacodynamic study of artesunate for vivax malaria. *Am. J. Trop. Med. Hyg.* 1998, 59, 823-827.

[159] Li, QG; Bossone, CA; Ohrt, C; Chung, H; Harris, D; Harre, J; Lee, P; Kathcart, AK; Brueckner, RP. Early signs and biomarkers of the neurotoxicity: toxicokinetic and toxicodynamic evaluation following 15-mg/kg arteether daily intramuscular injections for two weeks in beagle dogs. *Am. J. Trol. Med. Hyg.* 2000, 62, 142.

[160] Li, QG; Carpenter, C; Trotman, C; Kathcart, AK; Donahue, R; Milhous, WK. Pharmacokinetic comparison of artesunate and dihydroartemisinin in beagle dogs. *Am. J. Trol. Med. Hyg.* 1999, 61: 274.

[161] Kyle, DE; Teja-Isavadharm, P; Li, Q; Leo, K. Pharmacokinetics and pharmacodynamics of qinghaosu derivatives: how do they impact on the choice of drug and the dosage regimens? *Med. Trop. (Mars).* 1998, 58(3 Suppl), 38-44.

[162] Karbwang, J; Na-Bangchang, K; Tin, T; Sukontason, K; Rimchala, W; Harinasuta, T. Pharmacokinetics of intramuscular artemether in patients with severe falciparum malaria with or without acute renal failure. *Br. J. Clin. Pharmacol.* 1998, 45, 597-600.

[163] van Agtmael, MA; Van Der Graaf, CA; Dien, TK; Koopmans, RP; van Boxtel, CJ. The contribution of the enzymes CYP2D6 and CYP2C19 in the demethylation of artemether in healthy subjects. *Eur. J. Drug Metab. Pharmacokinet.* 1998, 23, 429-436.

[164] Karbwang, J; Na-Bangchang, K; Congpuong, K; Thanavibul, A; Wattanakoon, Y; Molunto, P. Pharmacokinetics of oral artemether in Thai patients with uncomplicated falciparum malaria. *Fundam. Clin. Pharmacol.* 1998, 12, 242-244.

[165] Mordi, MN; Mansor, SM; Navaratnam, V; Wernsdorfer, WH. Single dose pharmacokinetics of oral artemether in healthy Malaysian volunteers. *Br. J. Clin. Pharmacol.* 1997, 43, 363-365.

[166] Thomas, CG; Ward, SA; Edwards, G. Selective determination, in plasma, of artemether and its major metabolite, dihydroartemisinin, by high-performance liquid chromatography with ultraviolet detection. *J. Chromatogr.* 1992, 583, 131-136.

[167] van Agtmael, MA; Butter, JJ; Portier, EJ; van Boxtel, CJ. Validation of an improved reversed-phase high-performance liquid chromatography assay with reductive electrochemical detection for the determination of artemisinin derivatives in man. *Ther. Drug Monit.* 1998, 20, 109-116.

[168] van Agtmael, MA; Gupta, V; van der Wosten, TH; Rutten, JP; van Boxtel, CJ. Grapefruit juice increases the bioavailability of artemether. *Eur. J. Clin. Pharmacol.* 1999, 55, 405-410.

[169] Navaratnam, V; Mansor, SM; Chin, LK; Mordi, MN; Asokan, M; Nair, NK. Determination of artemether and dihydroartemisinin in blood plasma by high-performance liquid chromatography for application in clinical pharmacological studies. *J. Chromatogr. B. Biomed. Appl.* 1995, 669, 289-294.

[170] Karbwang, J; Na-Bangchang, K; Molunto, P; Banmairuroi, V; Congpuong, K. Determination of artemether and its major metabolite, dihydroartemisinin, in plasma using high-performance liquid chromatography with electrochemical detection. *J. Chromatogr. B. Biomed. Sci. Appl.* 1997, 690, 259-265.

[171] van Agtmael, MA; Gupta, V; van der Graaf, CA; van Boxtel, CJ. The effect of grapefruit juice on the time-dependent decline of artemether plasma levels in healthy subjects. *Clin. Pharmacol. Ther.* 1999, 66, 408-414.

[172] Tan-ariya, P; Na-Bangchang, K; Ubalee, R; Thanavibul, A; Thipawangkosol, P; Karbwang, J. Pharmacokinetic interactions of artemether and pyrimethamine in healthy male Thais. *Southeast Asian J. Trop. Med. Public Health.* 1998, 29, 18-23.

[173] Batty, KT; Thu, LT; Davis, TM; Ilett, KF; Mai, TX; Hung, NC; Tien, NP; Powell, SM; Thien, HV; Binh, TQ; Kim, NV. A pharmacokinetic and pharmacodynamic study of intravenous vs oral artesunate in uncomplicated falciparum malaria. *Br. J. Clin. Pharmacol.* 1998, 45, 123-129.

[174] Benakis, A; Paris, M; Loutan, L; Plessas, CT; Plessas, ST. Pharmacokinetics of artemisinin and artesunate after oral administration in healthy volunteers. *Am. J. Trop. Med. Hyg.* 1997, 56, 17-23.

[175] Navaratnam, V; Mansor, SM; Mordi, MN; Akbar, A; Abdullah, MN. Comparative pharmacokinetic study of oral and rectal formulations of artesunic acid in healthy volunteers. *Eur. J. Clin. Pharmacol.* 1998, 54, 411-414.

[176] Navaratnam, V; Mordi, MN; Mansor, SM. Simultaneous determination of artesunic acid and dihydroartemisinin in blood plasma by high-performance liquid chromatography for application in clinical pharmacological studies. *J. Chromatogr. B. Biomed. Sci. Appl.* 1997, 692, 157-162.

[177] Genovese, RF; Newman, DB; Brewer, TG. Behavioral and neural toxicity of the artemisinin antimalarial, arteether, but not artesunate and artelinate, in rats. *Pharmacol. Biochem. Behav.* 2000, 67, 37-44.

[178] Li, Q; Xie, LH; Si, Y; Wong, E; Upadhyay, R; Yanez, D; Weina, PJ. Toxicokinetics and hydrolysis of artelinate and artesunate in malaria-infected rats. *Int. J. Toxicol.* 2005, 24, 241-250.

[179] Xie, LH; Johnson, TO; Weina, PJ; Si, Y; Haeberle, A; Upadhyay, R; Wong, E; Li, Q. Risk assessment and therapeutic indices of artesunate and artelinate in Plasmodium berghei-infected and uninfected rats. *Int. J. Toxicol.* 2005, 24, 251-264.

[180] China Cooperative Research Group on Qinghaosu and Its Derivatives as Antimalarials. Metabolism and pharmacokinetics of qinghaosu and its derivatives. *J. Tradit. Chin. Med,* 1982, 2, 25-30.

[181] Niu, XY; Ho, LY; Ren, ZH; Song, ZY. Metabolic fate of Qinghaosu in rats; a new TLC densitometric method for its determination in biological material. *Eur. J. Drug Metab. Pharmacokinet.* 1985, 10, 55-59.

[182] Zhao, KC; Song, ZY. Distribution and excretion of artesunate in rats. *Proc. Chin. Acad. Med. Sci. Peking Union Med. Coll.* 1989, 4, 186-188.

[183] Jiang, JR; Zou, CD; Shu, HL; Zeng, YL. Assessment of absorption and distribution of artemether in rats using a thin layer chromatography scanning technique. *Zhongguo Yao Li Xue Bao.* 1989, 10, 431-434.

[184] Li, QG; Xie, LH; Haeberle, A; Zhang, J; Weina, PJ. The evaluation of radiolabeled artesunate on tissue distribution in rats and protein binding in humans. (accepted May 23, 2006, ASTMH, in press)

[185] Kearney, BP; Aweeka, FT. The penetration of anti-infectives into the central nervous system. *Neurol Clin.* 1999, 17, 883-900.

[186] Davis, TM; Binh, TQ; Ilett, KF; Batty, KT; Phuong, HL; Chiswell, GM; Phuong, VD; Agus, C. Penetration of dihydroartemisinin into cerebrospinal fluid after administration of intravenous artesunate in severe falciparum malaria. *Antimicrob. Agents Chemother.* 2003, 47, 368-370.

[187] Li, QG; Brueckner, RP; Peggins, JO; Trotman, KM; Brewer, TG. Arteether toxicokinetics and pharmacokinetics in rats after 25 mg/kg/day single and multiple doses. *Eur. J. Drug Metab. Pharmacokinet.* 1999, 24, 213-223.

[188] Kager, PA; Schultz, MJ; Zijlstra, EE; van den Berg, B; van Boxtel, CJ. Arteether administration in humans: preliminary studies of pharmacokinetics, safety and tolerance. *Trans R. Soc. Trop. Med. Hyg.* 1994, 88 Suppl 1, S53-S54.

[189] Brewer, TG; Genovese, RF; Newman, DB; Li, Q. Factors relating to neurotoxicity of artemisinin antimalarial drugs "listening to arteether". *Med. Trop. (Mars).* 1998, 58(3 Suppl), 22-27.

[190] Rowland, M; Tozer, TN. Clinical Pharmacokinetics: Concepts and applications, Malcolm Rowland and Thomas N. Tozer (Ed.), Willianms and Wilkins, Baltimore, 1995, USA, 83.

[191] Mayer, PR. Absorption, metabolism, and other factors that influence drug exposure in toxicology studies. *Toxicol. Pathol.* 1995, 23, 165-169.

[192] Shargel, L; Yu, ABC. Applied Biopharmaceutics and Pharmacokinetics, Leon Shargel and Andrew B.C (Ed.), YU. *Appleton and Lange,* 1993, Norwalk, CN, 353.

[193] Li, QG; Peggens, JO; Brown, LD; Brewer, TG. Pharmacokinetics and hydrolysis of sodium artelinate in dogs. *AM. J. Trop. Med. Hyg.* 1994, 51, 260.

[194] Noker, P; Lin, TT. Toxicity dose range study of 14 days oral administration of artelinic acid in dogs. Contract Research Reports, Southern Research Institute, Birmingham, USA, 2000. (Contract Report, unpublished data)

[195] Li, QG; Xie, LH; Peggins, JO. Pharmacokinetics and tolerant dose range studies of AL and AS following daily intramuscular dosing for 7 days in rats. *Am. J. Trol. Med. Hyg.* 2001, 65, 214.

[196] Ashton, M; Hai, TN; Sy, ND. Artemisinin pharmacokinetics is time-dependent during repeated oral administration in healthy male adults. *Drug Metab. Dispos.* 2998. 26, 2601-2605.

[197] Ashton, M; Sy, ND; Gordi, T; Hai, TN. Thach, DC; Huong, NV; Johansson, M; Coeng, LD. Evidence for time-dependence artemisinin kinetics in adults with uncomplicated malaria. *Pharm. Pharmacol. Lett.* 1996. 6, 127-130.

[198] van Agtmael, MA; Xiungquing, J; Koopmans, RP; Degen, P; Royce, CM. van Boxtel, CJ. Multiple dose pharmacokinetics of artemether in Chinese patients treated for falciparum malaria. *Acta Pharmacol. Ther. Latinoam.* 1996, 46, 244.

[199] Khanh, NX; de Vries, PJ; Ha, LD; van Boxtel, CJ; Koopmans, R; Kager, PA. Declining concentrations of dihydroartemisinin in plasma during 5-day oral treatment with artesunate for falciparum malaria. *Antimicro. Agent Chemtherap.* 1999, 43, 690-692.

[200] Li, Q; Lugt, CB; Looareesuwan, S; Krudsood, S; Wilairatana, P; Vannaphan, S; Chalearmrult, K; Milhous, WK. Pharmacokinetic investigation on the therapeutic potential of artemotil (beta-arteether) in Thai patients with severe Plasmodium falciparum malaria. *Am. J. Trop. Med. Hyg.* 2004, 71, 723-731.

[201] Klaassen, CD; Rozman, K. Chapter 3, Absorption, distribution, and excretion of toxicants, In. Casarett and Doull's Toxicology, The Basic Science of Poisons, Mary O. Amdur, John Doull, and Cortis D (Ed.). 1993, Klaassen. McGraw-Hill, Inc. Press. 53.

[202] Li, QG; Milhous, WK; Weina, PJ. Regimen strategy to decrease artemisinin agents related failure and recrudescence in severe and complicated malaria treatment. *Medicine and Health in the Tropics* (Marseille-France) 2005, Abstract Book, 131.

[203] Geyer, HJ; Scheuntert, I; Rapp, K; Kettrup, A; Korte, F; Greim, H; Rozman, K. Correlation between acute toxicity of 2,3,7,8-tetrachlorodibenzo-p-dioxin (TCDD) and total body fat content in mammals. *Toxicology.* 1990, 65, 97-107.

[204] Kimbrough, RD. How toxic is 2,3,7,8-tetrachlorodibenzodioxin to humans? *J. Toxicol. Environ. Health.* 1990, 30, 261-271.

[205] Culotta, E; Koshland, DE Jr. DNA repair works it works its way to the top. *Science.* 1994, 266, 1926-1929.

[206] Dawes, M; Chowienczyk, PJ. Drugs in pregnancy. Pharmacokinetics in pregnancy. *Best Pract. Res. Clin. Obstet. Gynaecol.* 2001. 15, 819-826.

[207] McGready, R; Stepniewska, K; Ward, SA; Cho, T; Gilveray, G; Looareesuwan, S; White, NJ; Nosten, F. Pharmacokinetics of dihydroartemisinin following oral artesunate treatment of pregnant women with acute uncomplicated falciparum malaria. *Eur. J. Clin. Pharmacol.* 2006. 62, 367-371.

[208] Clyde, DF. Clinical problems associated with the use of primaquine as a tissue schizontocidal and gametocytocidal drug. *Bull. World Health Organ.* 1981, 59, 391-395.

[209] Salako, LA. Pharmacokinetics of antimalarial drugs: their therapeutic and toxicological implications. *Ann. Ist. Super Sanita.* 1985. 21, 315-325. .

[210] Nosten, F; McGready, R; d'Alessandro, U; Bonell, A; Verhoeff, F; Menendez, C; Mutabingwa, T; Brabin, B. Antimalarial Drugs in Pregnancy: *Current Drug Safety*, Volume 1, Number 1, January 2006, pp. 1-15(15)

[211] Colwell, EJ; Hickman, RL; Kosakal, S. Tetracycline treatment of chloroquine-resistant falciparum malaria in Thailand. *JAMA.* 1972. 220, 684-686.

[212] Cohlan, SQ; Bevelander, G; Tiamsic, T. Growth inhibition of prematures receiving tetracycline. *Am. J. Dis. Child.* 1963. 105, 453-461.

[213] Manson, JD. Tetracyclines and the teeth. *Lancet.* 1966. 1(7446), 1104.

[214] Krejci, L; Brettschneider, I. Congenital cataract due to tetracycline. *Ophthal. Paediat. Genet.* 1983. 3, 59-60.

[215] Schiffer, MA. Fatty liver associated with administration of tetracycline in pregnant and nonpregnant women. *Am. J. Obstet. Gynecol.* 1966. 96, 326-332.

[216] Allen, ES; Brown, WE. Hepatic toxicity of tetracycline in pregnancy. *Am. J. Obstet. Gynecol.* 1966, 95, 12-18.

[217] Fakeye, TO; Fehintola, FA; Ademowo, OG; Walker, O. Therapeutic monitoring of chloroquine in pregnant women with malaria. *West Afr. J. Med.* 2002, 21, 286-287.

[218] Massele, AY; Kilewo, C; Aden Abdi, Y; Tomson, G; Diwan, VK; Ericsson, O; Rimoy, G; Gustafsson, LL. Chloroquine blood concentrations and malaria prophylaxis in Tanzanian women during the second and third trimesters of pregnancy. *Eur. J. Clin. Pharmacol.* 1997. 52, 299-305.

[219] Na Bangchang, K; Davis, TM; Looareesuwan, S; White, NJ; Bunnag, D; Karbwang, J. Mefloquine pharmacokinetics in pregnant women with acute falciparum malaria. *Trans. R. Soc. Trop. Med. Hyg.* 1994. 88, 321-323.

[220] McGready, R; Stepniewska, K; Seaton, E; Cho, T; Cho, D; Ginsberg, A; Edstein, MD; Ashley, E; Looareesuwan, S; White, NJ; Nosten, F. Pregnancy and use of oral contraceptives reduces the biotransformation of proguanil to cycloguanil. *Eur. J. Clin. Pharmacol.* 2003. 59, 553-557.

[221] Na-Bangchang, K; Manyando, C; Ruengweerayut, R; Kioy, D; Mulenga, M; Miller, GB; Konsil, J. The pharmacokinetics and pharmacodynamics of atovaquone and proguanil for the treatment of uncomplicated falciparum malaria in third-trimester pregnant women. *Eur. J. Clin. Pharmacol.* 2005. 61, 573-582.

[222] Menendez C. Malaria during pregnancy. *Curr. Mol. Med.* 2006. 6, 269-273.

[223] Akintonwa, A; Meyer, MC; Yau, MK. Placental transfer of chloroquine in pregnant rabbits. *Res. Commun. Chem. Pathol. Pharmacol.* 1983. 40, 443-455.

[224] Si, YZ; Xie, LH; Young-Sun, Y; Melendez, V; Weina, P; Milhouse, WK; Li, QG. Pharmacokinetic comparison of artesunate in rats following Intravenous, intramuscular and subcutaneous administration. *Experimental Biology.* 2004 (Annual Meeting of ASPET) in Washington, DC, April 17-21, 2004.

[225] Si, YZ; Li, QG; Haeberle, A; Milhouse, WK; Weina, P. [14C] artesunate tissue distribution in pregnant rats following a single intravenous dose with whole-body autoradiography. *Am. J. Trop. Med. Hyg.* 2006, 75 (5), 18.

[226] Potchoiba, MJ; West, M; Nocerini, MR. Quantitative comparison of autoradioluminographic and radiometric tissue distribution studies using carbon-14 labeled xenobiotics. *Drug Metab. Dispos.* 1998. 26, 272-277.

[227] Schweitzer, A; Fahr, A; Niederberger, W. A simple method for the quantitation of 14C-whole-body autoradiograms. *Int. J. Rad. Appl. Instrum. [A]* 1987. 38, 329-333.

[228] Solon, EG; Kraus, L. Quantitative whole-body autoradiography in the pharmaceutical industry. Survey results on design, methods, and regulatory compliance. *J. Pharmacol. Toxicol. Methods.* 2001. 46, 73-81.

[229] Chen, HH; Zhou, HJ; Wang, WQ; Wu, GD. Antimalarial dihydroartemisinin also inhibits angiogenesis. *Cancer Chemother. Pharmacol.* 2004. 53, 423-432.

[230] Anfosso, L; Efferth, T; Albini, A; Pfeffer, U. Microarray expression profiles of angiogenesis-related genes predict tumor cell response to artemisinins. *Pharmacogenomics J.* 2006. 6, 269-278.

[231] Efferth, T. Mechanistic perspectives for 1,2,4-trioxanes in anti-cancer therapy. *Drug Resist. Updat.* 2005. 8, 85-97.

[232] Dell'Eva, R; Pfeffer, U; Vene, R; Anfosso, L; Forlani, A; Albini, A; Efferth, T. Inhibition of angiogenesis in vivo and growth of Kaposi's sarcoma xenograft tumors by the anti-malarial artesunate. *Biochem. Pharmacol.* 2004. 68, 2359-2366.

[233] Huan-huan, C; Li-Li, Y; Shang-Bin, L. Artesunate reduces chicken chorioallantoic membrane neovascularisation and exhibits antiangiogenic and apoptotic activity on human microvascular dermal endothelial cell. *Cancer Lett.* 2004. 211, 163-173.

[234] Chen, HH; Zhou, HJ. Inhibitory effects of artesunate on angiogenesis. *Yao Xue Xue Bao.* 2004. 39, 29-33.

[235] Chen, HH; Zhou, HJ; Fang, X. Inhibition of human cancer cell line growth and human umbilical vein endothelial cell angiogenesis by artemisinin derivatives in vitro. *Pharmacol. Res.* 2003. 48, 231-236.

[236] Zon, LI. Developmental biology of hematopoiesis. *Blood.* 1995. 8, 2876–2891.

[237] Choe, H; Hansen, JM; Harris, C. Spatial and temporal ontogenesis of glutathione peroxidase, and glutathione disulfide reductase during development of the prenatal rat. *J. Biochem. Mol. Toxicol.* 2001, 15, 197–206.

[238] Phillips-Howard, PA; Wood, D. The safety of antimalarial drugs in pregnancy. *Drug Saf.* 1996. 14, 131-145.

[239] Adam, I; Ali, DM; Abdalla, MA. Artesunate plus sulfadoxine-pyrimethamine in the treatment of uncomplicated Plasmodium falciparum malaria during pregnancy in eastern Sudan. *Trans. R. Soc. Trop. Med. Hyg.* 2006. 100, 632-635.

[240] Steketee, RW; Wirima, JJ; Campbell, CC. Developing effective strategies for malaria prevention programs for pregnant African women. *Am. J. Trop. Med. Hyg.* 1996. 55(1 Suppl), 95-100.

[241] Steketee, RW; Nahlen, BL; Parise, ME; Menendez, C. The burden of malaria in pregnancy in malaria-endemic areas. *Am. J. Trop. Med. Hyg.* 2001. 64(1-2 Suppl), 28-35.

[242] Newman, RD; Parise, ME; Slutsker, L; Nahlen, B; Steketee, RW. Safety, efficacy and determinants of effectiveness of antimalarial drugs during pregnancy: implications for prevention programmes in Plasmodium falciparum-endemic sub-Saharan Africa. *Trop. Med. Int. Health.* 2003. 8, 488-506.

[243] Kumar, N; Zheng, H. Stage-specific gametocytocidal effect in vitro of the antimalaria drug qinghaosu on *Plasmodium falciparum*. *Parasitol. Res.* 1990. 76, 214-218.

[244] Mehra, N; Bhasin, VK. In vitro gametocytocidal activity of artemisinin and its derivatives on *Plasmodium falciparum*. *Jpn. J. Med. Sci. Biol.* 1993. 46, 37-43.

[245] Dutta, GP; Mohan, A; Tripathi, R. Study of the gametocytocidal/sporontocidal action of qinghaosu (artemisinin) by electron microscopy. *J. Parasitol.* 1990. 76, 849-852.

[246] Ding, Y; Qi, Z; et al.: Efficacy of dihydroartemisinin in treatment of 37 malaria cases. *Chin. J. Intern. Med.* 1997. 36, 187-189.

[247] White, NJ. Antimalarial pharmacokinetics and treatment regimens. *Br. J. Clin. Pharmacol.* 1992. 34, 1-10.

[248] Klayman, DL. An antimalarial drug from China. *Science.* 1985. 228, 1049-1055.

[249] Hien, TT; White, NJ. Qinghaosu. *Lancet.* 1993. 341, 603-608.

[250] Thu, LTA; Davis, TME; Binh, TQ; van Phuong, N; Anh, TK. Delayed parasite clearance in a Splenectomized patients with falciparum malaria who was treated with artemisinin derivatives. *Clin. Infect. Dis.* 1997. 25, 923-925.

[251] Alin, MH; Bjorkman, A. Concentration and time dependence of artemisinin efficacy against Plasmodium falciparum in vitro. *Am. J. Trop. Med. Hyg.* 1994. 50, 771-776.

[252] White, NJ; Krishna, S. Treatment of malaria: some considerations and limitations of the current methods of assessment. *Trans. Roy .Soc. Trop. Med. Hug.* 1989. 83, 767-777.

[253] Sharma, P; Swarup, D; Saxena, GN; Bhandari, S; Sharma, UB; Tuteja, R. An open study to evaluate the efficacy of artemether in severe falciparum malaria. *J. Assoc. Physicians India.* 1999. 47, 883-885.

[254] Suputtamongkol, Y; Newton, PN; Angus, B; Teja-Isavadharm, P; Keeratithakul, D; Rasameesoraj, M; Pukrittayakamee, S; White, NJ. A comparison of oral artesunate and artemether antimalarial bioactivities in acute falciparum malaria. *Br. J. Clin. Pharmacol.* 2001. 52, 655-661.

[255] Marsh, K; Forster, D; Waruiru, C; Mwangi, I; Winstanley, M; Marsh, V; Newton, C; Winstanley, P; Warn, P; Peshu, N. et al. Indicators of life-threatening malaria in African children. *N. Engl. J. Med.* 1995. 332, 1399-1404.

[256] Looareesuwan, S. Overview of clinical studies on artemisinin derivatives in Thailand. *Trans. Roy. Soc. Trop. Med. Hyg.* 1994. 88 (Suppl 1), 9-11.

[257] Ambroise-Thomas, P. Intra-muscular artemether in the treatment of severe malaria: synthesis of current results. *Med. Trop. (Mars).* 1997. 57, 289-293..

[258] Bhatt, KM; Samia, BM; Bhatt, SM; Wasunna, KM. Efficacy and safety of an artesunate/mefloquine combination, (artequin) in the treatment of uncomplicated P. falciparum malaria in Kenya. *East Afr. Med. J.* 2006. 83, 236-242.

[259] Kaiwa, S; Kano, S; Suzuki , M. Morphologic effects of artemether on Plasmodium falciparum in Aotus trivirgatus. *Am. J. Trop. Med. Hyg.* 1993. 49, 812-818.

[260] Hassan, Alin M; Ashton, M; Kihamia, CM; Mtey, GJ; Bjorkman, A. Multiple dose pharmacokinetics of oral artemisinin and comparison of its efficacy with that of oral artesunate in falciparum malaria patients. *Trans. R. Soc. Trop. Med. Hyg.* 1996. 90, 61-65.

[261] Na-Bangchang, K; Tippawangkosol, P; Thanavibul, A; Ubalee, R; Karbwang, J. Pharmacokinetic and pharmacodynamic interactions of mefloquine and dihydroartemisinin. *Int. J. Clin. Pharmacol. Res.* 1999. 19, 9-17.

[262] Titulaer, HAC; Zuidema, J; Lugt, CB. Formulation and pharmacokinetics of artemisinin and its derivatives. *Intern. J. Pharmaceui*. 1991. 69, 83-92.

[263] Murphy, S; Watkins, WM; Bray, PG; Lowe, B; Winstanley, PA; Peshu, N; Marsh, K. Parasite viability during treatment of severe falciparum malaria: differential effects of artemether and quinine. *Am. J. Trop. Med. Hyg*. 1995. 53, 303-305.

[264] White, NJ. Clinical pharmacokinetics and pharmacodynamics of artemisinin and derivatives. *Trans. R. Soc. Trop. Med. Hyg*. 1994. 88(Suppl 1), S41–S43.

[265] Gu, H.M; Warhurst, DC; Peters, W. Uptake of [3H]-dihydroartemisinin by erythrocytes infected with plasmodium falciparum in-vitro. *Trans. R. Soc. Trop. Med. Hyg*. 1984. 78, 265-270.

[266] Ashton, M; Hai, TN; Sy, ND; Huong, DX; Van Huong, N; Nieu, NT; Cong, LD. Artemisinin pharmacokinetics is time-dependent during repeated oral administration in healthy male adults. *Drug Metab. Dispos*. 1998. 26, 25-27.

[267] Zhao, KC; Song, ZY. Pharmacokinetics of dihydroqinghaosu in human volunteers and comparison with qinghaosu. *Yao Xue Xue Bao*. 1993, 28, 342-346.

[268] Koopmans, R; Ha, LD; Duc, DD; Dien, TK; Kager, PA; Khanh, NX; van Boxtel, CJ; De Vries, PJ. The pharmacokinetics of artemisinin after administration of two different suppositories to healthy Vietnamese subjects. *Am. J. Trop. Med. Hyg*. 1999. 60, 244-247.

[269] Na-Bangchang, K; Krudsood, S; Silachamroon, U; Molunto, P; Tasanor, O; Chalermrut, K; Tangpukdee, N; Matangkasombut, O; Kano, S; Looareesuwan, S. The pharmacokinetics of oral dihydroartemisinin and artesunate in healthy Thai volunteers. *Southeast Asian J. Trop. Med. Public Health*. 2004. 35, 575-582.

[270] Binh, TQ; Ilett, KF; Batty, KT; Davis, TM; Hung, NC; Powell, SM; Thu, LT; Thien, HV; Phuong, HL; Phuong, VD. Oral bioavailability of dihydroartemisinin in Vietnamese volunteers and in patients with falciparum malaria. *Br. J. Clin. Pharmacol*. 2001. 51, 541-546.

[271] White, NJ. Antimalarial drug resistance. *J. Clin. Invest*. 2004. 113, 1084-1092.

[272] Ittarat, W; Pickard, AL; Rattanasinganchan, P; Wilairatana, P; Looareesuwan, S; Emery, K; Low, J; Udomsangpetch, R; Meshnick, SR. Recrudescence in artesunate-treated patients with falciparum malaria is dependent on parasite burden not on parasite factors. *Am. J. Trop. Med. Hyg*. 2003. 68, 147-152.

[273] Pareek, A; Nandy, A; Kochar, D; Patel, KH; Mishra, SK; Mathur, PC. Efficacy and safety of beta-arteether and alpha/beta-arteether for treatment of acute Plasmodium falciparum malaria. *Am. J. Trop. Med. Hyg*. 2006. 75, 139-142.

[274] Asthana, OP; Srivastava, JS; Pandey, TK; Vishwanathan, KA; Dev, V; Mahapatra, KM; Nayak, NC; Balsara, AB; Mandal, OP; Gupta, N; Mishra, SK; Mohanty, S; Sathpathy, S; Das, BS; Patnaik, JK; Sathpathy, SK; Dash, B. Multicentric clinical trials for safety and efficacy evaluation of alpha;beta arteether in complicated P. falciparum malaria. *J. Assoc. Physicians India*. 2001. 49, 1155-1160.

[275] Rajanikanth, M; Madhusudanan, KP; Gupta, RC. An HPLC-MS method for simultaneous estimation of alpha,beta-arteether and its metabolite dihydroartemisinin, in rat plasma for application to pharmacokinetic study. *Biomed. Chromatogr*. 2003. 17, 440-446.

[276] Sabarinath, S; Rajanikanth, M; Madhusudanan, KP; Gupta, RC. A sensitive and selective liquid chromatographic/electrospray ionization tandem mass spectrometric assay for the simultaneous quantification of alpha-,beta-arteether and its metabolite dihydroartemisinin in plasma, useful for pharmacokinetic studies. *J. Mass Spectrom.* 2003. 38, 732-742.

[277] Rajanikanth, M; Madhusudanan, KP; Gupta, RC. Liquid chromatographic-mass spectrometric method for the determination of alpha-, beta-arteether in rat serum. *J. Chromatogr. B. Analyt. Technol. Biomed. Life Sci.* 2003. 783, 391-399.

[278] Ashton, M; Nguyen, DS; Nguyen, VH; Gordi, T; Trinh, NH; Dinh, XH; Nguyen, TN; Le, DC. Artemisinin kinetics and dynamics during oral and rectal treatment of uncomplicated malaria. *Clin. Pharmacol. Ther.* 1998. 63, 482-493.

[279] von Seidlein, L; Milligan, P; Pinder, M; Bojang, K; Anyalebechi, C; Gosling, R; Coleman, R; Ude, JI; Sadiq, A; Duraisingh, M; Warhurst, D; Alloueche, A; Targett, G; McAdam, K; Greenwood, B; Walraven, G; Olliaro, P; Doherty, T. Efficacy of artesunate plus pyrimethamine-sulphadoxine for uncomplicated malaria in Gambian children: a double-blind, randomised, controlled trial. *Lancet.* 2000. 355, 352-357.

[280] Adjuik, M; Babiker, A; Garner, P; Olliaro, P; Taylor, W; White, N. International Artemisinin Study Group. Artesunate combinations for treatment of malaria: meta-analysis. *Lancet.* 2004. 363, 9-17.

[281] Silamut, K; Newton, PN; Teja-Isavadharm, P; Suputtamongkol, Y; Siriyanonda, D; Rasameesoraj, M; Pukrittayakamee, S; White, NJ. Artemether bioavailability after oral or intramuscular administration in uncomplicated falciparum malaria. *Antimicrob. Agents Chemother.* 2003. 47, 3795-3798.

[282] Le, NH; Na-Bangchang, K; Le, TD; Thrinh, KA; Karbwang, J. Pharmacokinetics of a single oral dose of dihydroartemisinin in Vietnamese healthy volunteers. *Southeast Asian J. Trop. Med. Public Health.* 1999. 30, 11-16.

[283] Karbwang, J; Na-Bangchang, K; Congpuong, K; Molunto, P; Thanavibul, A. Pharmacokinetics and bioavailability of oral and intramuscular artemether. *Eur. J. Clin. Pharmacol.* 1997. 52, 307-310.

[284] Chanthap, L; Tsuyuoka, R; Na-Bangchang, K; Nivanna, N; Suksom, D; Sovannarith, T; Socheat, D. Investigation of bioavailability, pharmacokinetics and safety of new pediatric formulations of artesunate and mefloquine. *Southeast Asian J. Trop. Med. Public Health.* 2005. 36, 34-43.

[285] Newton, PN; van Vugt, M; Teja-Isavadharm, P; Siriyanonda, D; Rasameesoroj, M; Teerapong, P; Ruangveerayuth, R; Slight, T; Nosten, F; Suputtamongkol, Y; Looareesuwan, S; White, NJ. Comparison of oral artesunate and dihydroartemisinin antimalarial bioavailabilities in acute falciparum malaria. *Antimicrob Agents Chemother.* 2002. 46, 1125-1127.

[286] Na-Bangchang, K; Thanavibul, A; Tippawangkosol, P; Karbwang, J. Pharmacokinetics of the four combination regimens of dihydroartemisinin/mefloquine in acute uncomplicated falciparum malaria. *Southeast Asian J. Trop. Med. Public Health.* 2005. 36, 23-33.

[287] Asawamahasakda, W; Benakis, A; Meshnick, SR. The interaction of artemisinin with red cell membranes. *J. Lab. Clin. Med.* 1994. 123, 757-762.

[288] Li, QG; Xie, LH; Barcus, M; Wellington, S; Brueckner, RP; Weina, P. Binding evaluation of new artemisinin analogs to plasma proteins and red blood cell of human and animal species in vitro and in vivo. (*unpublished data*)

[289] Brand, VB; Sandu, CD; Duranton, C; Tanneur, V; Lang, KS; Huber, SM; Lang, F. Dependence of Plasmodium falciparum in vitro growth on the cation permeability of the human host erythrocyte. *Cell Physiol. Biochem*. 2003. 13, 347-356.

[290] Nealon, C; Dzeing, A; Muller-Romer, U; Planche, T; Sinou, V; Kombila, M; Kremsner, PG; Parzy, D; Krishna, S. Intramuscular bioavailability and clinical efficacy of artesunate in gabonese children with severe malaria. *Antimicrob Agents Chemother*. 2002. 46, 3933-3939.

[291] Ilett, KF; Batty, KT; Powell, SM; Binh, TQ; Thu le, TA; Phuong, HL; Hung, NC; Davis, TM. The pharmacokinetic properties of intramuscular artesunate and rectal dihydroartemisinin in uncomplicated falciparum malaria. *Br. J. Clin. Pharmacol*. 2002. 53, 23-30.

[292] Rehwagen, C. WHO ultimatum on artemisinin monotherapy is showing results. *BMJ*. 2006. 332(7551), 1176.

[293] White, NJ. Assessment of the pharmacodynamic properties of antimalarial drugs in vivo. *Antimicrob. Agents Chemother*. 1997. 41, 1413–1422.

[294] Newton, PN; Barnes, KI; Smith, PJ; Evans, AC; Chierakul, W; Ruangveerayuth, R; White, NJ. The pharmacokinetics of intravenous artesunate in adults with severe falciparum malaria. *Eur. J. Clin. Pharmacol*. 2006. 62, 1003-1009.

[295] White, NJ; Nosten, F; Looareesuwan, S; Watkins, WM; Marsh, K; Snow, RW; Kokwaro, G; Ouma, J; Hien, TT; Molyneux, ME; Taylor, T; Newbold, CI; Ruebush II, TK; Danis, M; Greenwood, BM; Anderson, RM; Olliaro, P. Averting a malaria disaster. *Lancet*. 1999. 353, 1965–1967.

[296] Bunnag, D; Viravan, C; Looareesuwan, S; Karbwang, J; Harinasuta, T. Double blind randomised clinical trial of oral artesunate at once or twice daily dose in falciparum malaria. *Southeast Asian J. Trop. Med. Public Health* 1991. 22, 539–543.

[297] Luxemburger, C; ter Kuile, FO; Nosten, F; Dolan, G; Bradol, JH; Phaipun, L; Chongsuphajaisiddhi, T; White, NJ. Single day mefloquine- artesunate combination in the treatment of multi-drug resistant falciparum malaria. *Trans. R. Soc. Trop. Med. Hyg*. 1994. 88, 213–217.

In: Drug Toxicity: New Research
Editor: Cam E. Vellotis, pp.187-222
ISBN 978-1-60456-320-7

Chapter 6

Nephrotoxicity of Nonsteroidal Anti-Inflammatory Drugs: Focus on Selective Cyclooxygenase-2 (COX-2) Inhibitors

Steven G. Coca[1] and Mark A. Perazella[2*]
[1]Section of Nephrology, Department of Medicine,
Yale University School of Medicine
[2]Renal Fellowship Program, Acute Dialysis Services
Section of Nephrology, Department of Medicine
Yale University School of Medicine

Abstract

Traditional (non-selective) NSAIDs cause nephrotoxicity through inhibition of cyclooxygenase (COX) activity and prostaglandin formation in the kidney. Patients with prostaglandin-dependent disease states are the group at most risk for this adverse effect. It has become apparent that the COX-2 enzyme isoform is constitutively expressed and upregulated in the human kidney during states of renal stress. COX-2 derived prostaglandins importantly modulate renal blood flow and glomerular filtration rate as well as sodium, potassium and water excretion by the kidney. As a result, clinical renal syndromes induced by the selective COX-2 inhibitors are quite similar to those described with the traditional NSAIDs, suggesting that COX-2 derived prostaglandins are important in maintaining normal renal function. Inhibition of prostaglandins causes a reduction in renal blood flow and acute renal failure in patients with predisposing conditions. These include true volume depletion from nausea/vomiting, diarrhea and excessive diuretic therapy. Effective volume depletion from clinical disease states such as heart failure, cirrhosis, and nephrotic syndrome as well as diseases such as chronic

* Mark A. Perazella, , MD, FACP. Associate Professor of Medicine, Director, Renal Fellowship Program, Director, Acute Dialysis Services, Section of Nephrology, Department of Medicine, Yale University School of Medicine,FMP 107 333 Cedar Street, New Haven, CT 06520-8029

kidney disease and renal artery stenosis also portend risk of acute renal failure from prostaglandin inhibition.

Prostaglandins also modulate renal potassium excretion through stimulation of the renin-angiotensin-aldosterone system. Inhibition of prostaglandins can result in hyperkalemia when co-existent conditions such as renal failure, diabetes mellitus and therapy with certain medications (ACE inhibitors, angiotensin receptor blockers, potassium-sparing diuretics) are also present. The classic syndrome of hyporeninemic hypoaldosteronism with a type-4 renal tubular acidosis (RTA) picture (hyperkalemic metabolic acidosis) can be observed when selective COX-2 inhibitor therapy is superimposed. Inhibition of prostaglandins is associated with decreased renal sodium and water excretion and all NSAIDs, including the selective COX-2 inhibitors cause some degree of sodium retention. All patients suffer from this effect, but only patients with certain clinical conditions develop obvious edema, hypertension or heart failure. Patients with underlying hypertension (especially those on antihypertensive medications), heart disease and other salt-retentive disease states (cirrhosis, nephrosis, renal failure) are at highest risk for these complications. Hypertension is a particularly important complication of these drugs as small changes in blood pressure are associated with increased cardiovascular events. Hyponatremia from impaired water excretion also complicates therapy.

Less commonly, acute interstitial nephritis (with or without a glomerulopathy) has been described with these drugs. To reduce adverse renal effects from NSAIDs, including all of available the selective COX-2 inhibitors, identification of patients with renal risk should be undertaken. Defining patient risk profiles based on level of kidney function (stage of chronic kidney disease) as well as on the presence of certain co-morbidities (hypertension, heart failure, diabetes mellitus, liver disease/cirrhosis, electrolyte imbalance, old age, certain medications) is one simple approach that can be taken. Based on the renal risk, recommendations for therapy and monitoring can be utilized in a rational fashion.

Key words: cyclooxygenase (COX), selective COX-2 inhibitors, nonsteroidal anti-inflammatory drugs (NSAIDs), acute renal failure, hyponatremia, hyperkalemia, hypertension, edema, acute interstitial nephritis.

Introduction

Nonsteroidal anti-inflammatory drugs (NSAIDs) have been prescribed for several decades to reduce fever, pain and inflammation. In addition to prescription NSAIDs, the general population consumes a large number of over-the-counter NSAIDs. Over 60 million people ingest these medications on a regular basis. The price paid for these beneficial therapeutic effects include gastrointestinal (GI) complications and, to a lesser extent, adverse kidney effects. In response to this problem, a new class of selective NSAIDs was designed, based on the discovery of two cyclooxygenase (COX) isoforms (COX-1, COX-2), to reduce drug-related toxicity [1,2]. The selective COX-2 inhibitors, celecoxib and rofecoxib, were introduced into clinical practice for this purpose in 1999 [3,4]. These new drugs have documented therapeutic efficacy while also significantly reducing GI toxicity and platelet dysfunction [3,4].

In addition to improved GI safety, a reduction in traditional (non-selective) NSAID-associated adverse renal effects was another goal of this new pharmacological class of selective COX-2 inhibitors. Based on data that suggested that COX-2 is not constitutively expressed, but can be rapidly induced in response to inflammatory stimuli, it was speculated that the functions of the COX isoforms were mutually exclusive. The paradigm that COX-1 maintains the normal physiologic functions of the kidney and that COX-2 is involved primarily in inflammatory processes was attractive. Furthermore, compartmentalization of the COX isoforms in the kidney would reduce NSAID-associated nephrotoxicity. However, the original paradigm describing the biologic activity of COX-1 and COX-2 is not completely accurate. While it is true that COX-2 is induced at sites of inflammation and plays a major role in the production of prostaglandin (PG) E_2 and other arachidonic acid metabolites produced at inflammatory sites, COX-1 may also contribute to inflammatory responses (1,2). Importantly, a critical role of COX-2 in physiological processes, and namely in the maintenance of renal function has come to light. Cyclooxygenase-2 dependent renal physiological effects are inferred from observations that demonstrate constitutive expression and upregulation of this isoform in the kidney. As such, COX-2 enzyme may have an important role in the synthesis of prostanoids integral to the regulation of renal perfusion, salt and water handling and renin release.

Prostaglandins in the Kidneys

Prostaglandin Synthesis

Prostaglandins (PG) are the major products of COX enzyme metabolism [5-7]. These prostanoids are produced throughout the body and act locally in an autocrine and paracrine fashion [5-7]. Synthesis of prostaglandins commences with liberation of the second messenger, arachidonic acid from cell membrane phospholipids in a reaction mediated by the enzyme phospholipase A_2. A number of factors trigger the activation of phospholipase A_2, serving to modulate subsequent prostaglandin production through the provision of arachidonic acid substrate. Arachidonic acid is then bound by prostaglandin endoperoxide synthase, a complex of cyclooxygenase and peroxidase, which subsequently catalyzes the redox reaction. Further regulation of prostaglandin synthesis occurs through expression and activation of COX enzyme. A short-lived, unstable intermediary cyclic endoperoxide called PGG_2-PGH_2 is synthesized and rapidly metabolized to more stable prostaglandins by cell specific enzymes [5-7]. Following synthesis, prostaglandins promptly exit the cell via facilitated diffusion to bind prostaglandin receptors found on parent or neighbouring cells, thereby modulating cellular functions [5-7]. Figure 1 demonstrates the pathway of prostaglandin synthesis within cells and local action at the cell level.

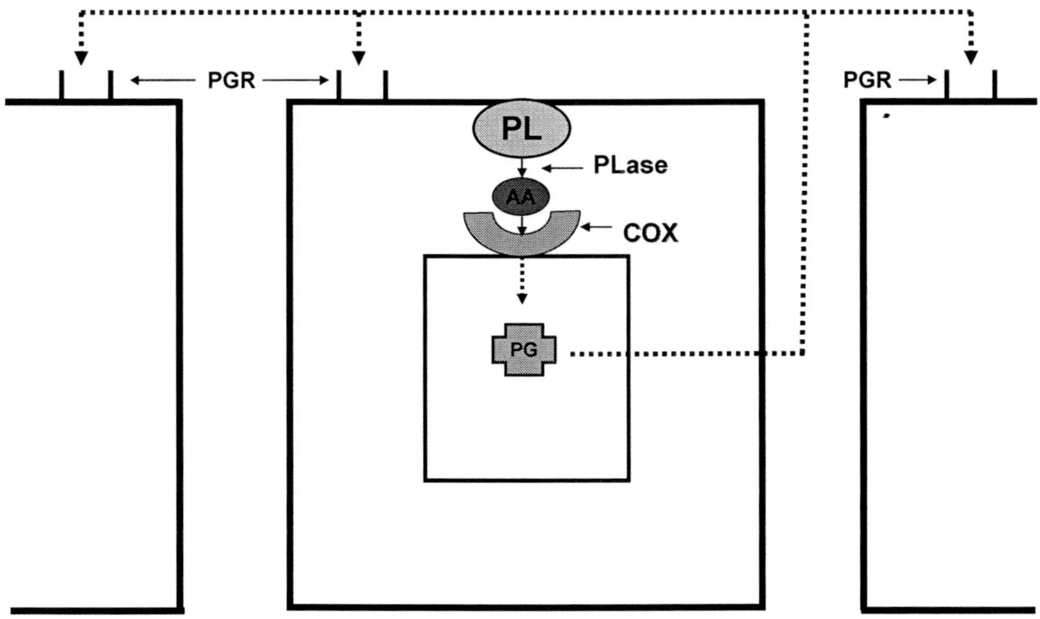

Figure 1. The pathway of prostaglandin synthesis within cells and local action at the cellular level

Cyclooxygenase Function

Synthesis of prostaglandins from the arachidonic acid substrate is catalyzed by one of two isomers of cyclooxygenase, COX-1 or COX-2. These enzymes are approximately 65% identical in their amino acid sequence and nearly identical at their catalytic site [2,7]. Conservation of their structures at the catalytic site allows these isoforms to carry out similar enzymatic functions and produce similar prostaglandins. Downstream cell-specific enzymes further modify these prostaglandins to form their final prostaglandin product (TXA_2, PGE_2, PGI_2, PGD_2, $PGF_{2\alpha}$, etc). Cyclooxygenase-1 is a 22-kilobase gene located on human chromosome 9, while the 8-kilobase COX-2 gene resides on chromosome 1 [2,7]. The COX isoforms can also be distinguished by their respective patterns of gene transcription. The COX-2 DNA sequence identifies it as an "inducible" gene that is expressed chiefly in response to a variety of stimuli. The COX-2 gene has a number of sites that links its transcription to the presence of appropriate protein triggers such as cytokines, growth factors or hormones [2,7]. In contrast, the gene sequence of COX-1 lacks the sites that are required to facilitate rapid protein transcription in response to stimuli, consistent with a gene that expresses its constitutive product protein without any prerequisite signal. It is more likely that provision of arachidonic acid substrate influences COX-1 enzyme activity and subsequent prostaglandin production.

The above-noted differences in gene regulation between the cyclooxygenase isomers provide a molecular basis for their purported roles as "constitutive" (COX-1) and "inducible" (COX-2) enzymes. In general, these labels accurately describe the synthesis of cyclooxygenase in most tissues, where COX-1, but not COX-2 is expressed in appreciable levels at baseline [2,7,8]. A prime example of COX-1 predominance is the GI tract, in particular the stomach mucosa. In contrast, abundant expression of COX-2 is demonstrated in macrophages and other cell types in response to inflammatory mediators [2,7,8]. It is these characteristics of the COX isoforms that initially suggested that inflammation, fever and pain could be targeted while homeostatic cellular functions could be spared. As will be discussed later, this paradigm is flawed by the fact that COX-2 is also constitutively expressed and upregulated in the kidney and importantly modulates renal physiology [2,9-11,12]. Table 1 lists the differences between the two COX enzyme isoforms.

Table 1. Characteristics of COX-1 and COX-2 Enzymes

COX-1 Enzyme	COX-2 Enzyme
Chromosome 9	Chromosome 1
22 kilobase gene	8 kilobase gene
Constitutive	Inducible
Tissue Expression	Tissue Expression
GI Tract	Macrophages
Kidney	Synoviocytes
Brain	Cartilage
Vasculature	Kidney
Platelets	Brain
Unchanged by Glucocorticoids	Blocked by Glucocorticoids
Instantaneous Inhibition by NSAIDs	Time-Dependent Inhibition by NSAIDs

Abbreviations: COX, cyclooxygenase; NSAIDs, nonsteroidal anti-inflammatory drugs; GI, gastrointestinal

Prostaglandins in Renal Physiology

In healthy individuals with normal intravascular volume status, prostaglandin synthesis is of minimal or no importance in the kidney. As such, prostaglandins are not primary regulators of renal function. Rather, these eicosanoids locally modulate the effects of both systemic and locally produced vasoconstrictor hormones, contribute to sodium and water balance, and play a protective role in the renal medulla [6]. A variety of prostaglandins are synthesized within distinct anatomic locations in the kidney, including PGI_2, PGE_2, thromboxane A_2 (TXA_2), and $PGF_{2\alpha}$ (Table 2). In general, PGI_2 and PGE_2 are the predominant mediators of physiologic activity in the kidney. PGI_2 is most abundantly produced in the renal cortex by cortical arterioles and glomeruli, whereas PGE_2 is synthesized in juxtamedullary glomeruli, in medullary interstitial cells, and in the medullary portion of the collecting duct [5,7,13-15]. However, there exists considerable overlap of prostaglandin synthesis at these renal sites. Functionally, PGI_2 and PGE_2 induce vasodilatation in interlobular arteries, afferent and efferent arterioles, and glomeruli. Prostaglandin-mediated vasodilatation increases renal perfusion in inner cortical and medullary regions and increases sodium excretion through post-glomerular perfusion [5,7,13-15].

Table 2. Renal Sites of Prostaglandin Action

Eicosanoid	Site	Action
PGI_2	Glomeruli, arterioles	Vasodilatation Maintain GFR
	Loop of Henle Juxtaglomerular apparatus macula densa)	Renin Release, TG feedback
PGE_2	Glomeruli, arterioles	Vasodilatation, Maintain GFR
	Loop of Henle	Renin Release Excretion of NaCl and H_20
	Juxtaglomerular apparatus (macula densa)	TG feedback
TXA_2	Glomerular podocytes and Mesangial cells	Vasoconstriction
$PGF_{2\alpha}$	Medullary interstitial cells and Tubular cells	Excretion of NaCl and H_2O

Abbreviations: GFR, glomerular filtration rate; TG, tubuloglomerular

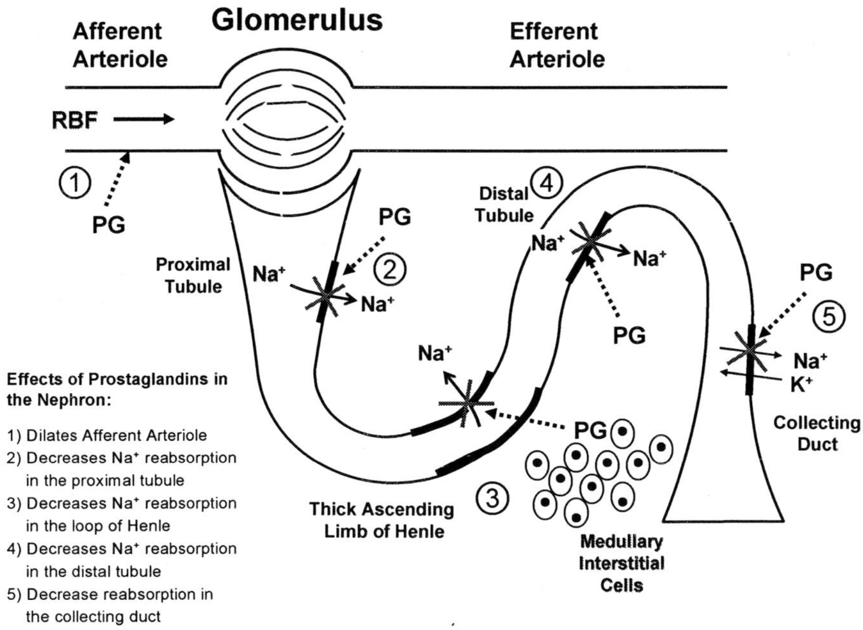

Figure 2. Site of prostaglandin action in the nephron to reduce sodium chloride reabsorption

In the loop of Henle and distal nephron (Figure 2), PGE_2 decreases cellular transport of sodium chloride in thick ascending limb cells, distal tubular and collecting duct cells, respectively [5,7,13-15]. An increase in renal sodium excretion and a decrease in medullary tonicity are the direct results of PGE_2 action in these nephron segments [5,7,13-15]. PGE_2 and PGI_2 also stimulate renin secretion in the juxtaglomerular apparatus. Renin cleaves both circulating and local angiotensinogen into angiotensin I, which is then converted to angiotensin II. Subsequently, this hormone stimulates adrenal aldosterone release, enhancing sodium retention and potassium excretion in the distal nephron. Finally, PGE_2 and PGI_2 also inhibit cAMP synthesis and interfere with the action of antidiuretic hormone (ADH) to increase water absorption by reducing aquaporin channels in the apical membrane [5,7,13-

15]. This promotes a water diuresis and helps maintain normal serum osmolality and sodium concentration.

Prostaglandins in Pathophysiologic States

Prostaglandins have their major role in the preservation of renal function when pathologic states supervene and compromise physiologic processes in the kidney. The development of intravascular volume depletion, as seen with vomiting, diarrhea and diuretic therapy, stimulates COX enzyme activity and prostaglandin synthesis to optimize renal blood flow (RBF) and maintain normal glomerular filtration rate [5,6,14]. In addition, effective decreases in RBF as seen with congestive heart failure (CHF), cirrhosis and nephrotic syndrome also enhance compensatory prostaglandin production [5,6,14]. PGI_2 and PGE_2 antagonize the local effects of circulating angiotensin II, endothelin, vasopressin and catecholamines that would normally maintain systemic blood pressure at the expense of the renal circulation [5,6,14]. Specifically, these eicosanoids preserve glomerular filtration rate (GFR) by antagonizing afferent arteriolar vasoconstriction and blunting mesangial and podocyte contraction induced by these endogenous vasopressors [5-7].

Prostaglandin production is also increased in chronic kidney disease (CKD) [16]. Upregulation of prostaglandin synthesis in CKD is induced by intrarenal mechanisms activated to increase perfusion of remnant nephrons [16]. Studies examining the effect of prostaglandins on remnant renal function substantiate the prostaglandin dependence of CKD [13,16-18]. As a result, impairment of prostaglandin production in this setting is associated with acute reductions in RBF and GFR, resulting in hemodynamic acute renal failure (ARF).

Renal prostaglandins also importantly modulate salt and water homeostasis. In response to volume overload and salt loading, prostaglandin inhibition of tubular sodium chloride (NaCl) reabsorption increases salt excretion [5,6,14]. This effect modulates the blood pressure raising effect as well the tendency to form edema that would occur with sodium retention in disease states (underlying hypertension, cirrhosis, nephrosis, CKD) dependent on prostaglandin function in the kidney. Antagonism of vasopressin effect on water channels by these autacoids also facilitates excretion of a water load in patients with nonosmotic-induced elevations in vasopressin associated with cirrhosis and nephrosis [5,6,14]. In addition, the regulation of medullary blood flow by PGE_2 contributes to the kidney's ability to modify renal solute excretion [5,6,14]. Taken together, these modulating effects ensure the kidney's regulation of salt and water through their appropriate retention or excretion. Ultimately, intravascular volume status and plasma osmolality are maintained in a more physiologic state.

Traditional NSAID-Associated Nephrotoxicity

To better understand selective COX-2 inhibitor nephrotoxicity, the adverse effects of traditional NSAIDs on the kidney will be reviewed. While disruption of COX enzyme by NSAIDs produces therapeutic drug effects, inhibition of COX enzyme function produces kidney dysfunction. Several well-described clinical syndromes of NSAID-associated nephrotoxicity have been noted (Table 3). They include hemodynamic acute renal failure, disorders of sodium balance (edema and hypertension), disturbances in water homeostasis (hyponatremia) and abnormal renal potassium handling (hyperkalemia, type-4 RTA). Other adverse renal effects include acute interstitial nephritis with or without an associated glomerulopathy. These nephrotoxic effects will be briefly reviewed in the following sections.

Table 3. NSAID-Associated Renal Syndromes

- Acute Renal Failure
- Disorders of Sodium Balance
    - Edema
    - Hypertension
    - Diuretic Resistance
- Disorders of Water Balance
    - Hyponatremia
- Disorders of Potassium Homeostasis
    - Hyperkalemia
    - Metabolic Acidosis
- Acute Interstitial Nephritis
- Nephrotic Syndrome
    - Minimal Change Disease
    - Membranous Glomerulonephritis
- Acute Papillary Necrosis
- Chronic Tubulointerstitial Nephritis
    - Analgesic Nephropathy
    - Chronic Papillary Sclerosis

Abbreviations: NSAIDs, nonsteroidal anti-inflammatory drugs

Renal Blood Flow/Glomerular Filtration Rate

Hemodynamic ARF

It has been estimated that anywhere from 1 to 5% of patients who ingest NSAIDs will develop some form of nephrotoxicity [19]. Some calculations approximate that 500,000 persons are likely to develop some form of NSAID-associated adverse renal impairment. Administration of NSAIDs to patients with prostaglandin-dependent disease states has been shown to consistently precipitate ARF [5,6,14,17]. As outlined previously, patients with states of vasoconstrictor excess depend on renal prostaglandin synthesis to ensure sufficient renal perfusion. In the absence of the counterbalancing effects of prostaglandins, unopposed vasoconstriction induced by NSAIDs leads to a decrease in RBF and a decline in GFR [5,6,14] (Figure 3). Similarly, in patients with underlying CKD, NSAID administration can precipitate reversible ARF [13,16-22]. Since NSAIDs are highly protein bound, hypoalbuminemia also portends risk for renal impairment. Increased concentrations of free drug in the circulation, due to loss of sufficient protein binding of the NSAID, account for the adverse renal effect [6]. Although NSAID-associated ARF is probably both dose- and duration-dependent, even small doses given for short courses may induce renal impairment in patients with multiple risk factors.

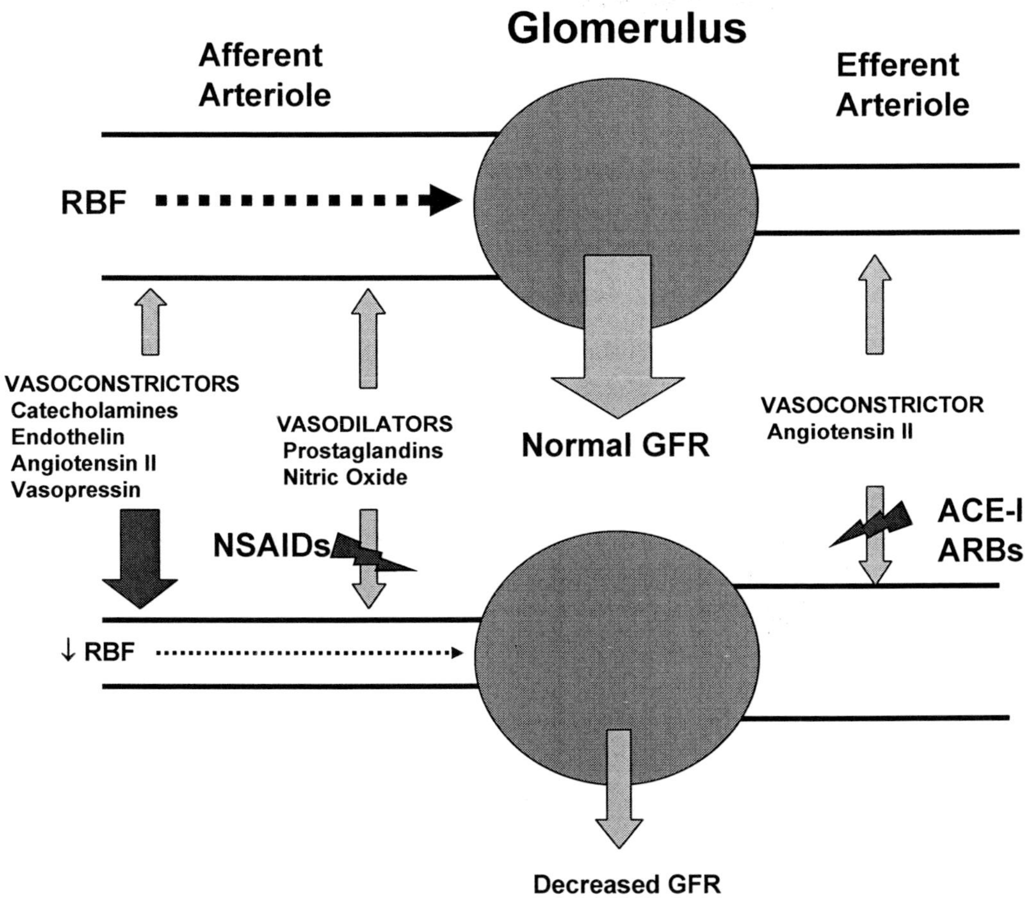

Figure 3. Effect of NSAIDs to induce vasoconstriction with an associated decrease in RBF and GFR in patients dependent on prostaglandins to maintain renal prefusion

Exposure to NSAIDs has been noted to double the risk of hospitalization for ARF in patients with CKD [23]. Similar rates of ARF with NSAIDs have been described in the elderly, those with cardiac disease and patients receiving ACE inhibitors. Several studies in patients in the general population documented adjusted relative risks of clinical ARF of two to four-fold higher in NSAID users versus nonusers [24-26]. Patients with a history of heart failure and hypertension, as well as those treated with diuretics exhibited the greatest risk (adjusted relative risk = 11.6) when treated with an NSAID [26]. The effect also appeared to be dose-related with ARF occurring with higher NSAID dose. Hospitalized patients have even greater risk, as a higher percentage of the cases of drug-induced ARF that develop in the hospital are due to NSAID therapy [27]. In general, renal failure reverses within 2 to 5 days following discontinuation of the NSAID [5,6]. However, restoration of baseline renal function may be prolonged in high-risk patients [5,6]. Rarely, acute dialytic intervention may be required for severe uremia, CHF or life-threatening electrolyte and acid-base disturbances.

Sodium Balance

Edema

Edema formation and volume overload may also complicate treatment with NSAIDs as they blunt the natriuretic effect of prostaglandins on the nephron. Sodium retention and mild lower extremity edema are frequently observed (25%) following therapy with these drugs [28]. Patients with underlying sodium avid states, such as cirrhosis and CHF, are particularly at risk to suffer from the sodium-retaining properties of NSAIDs. As a result, severe and symptomatic edema, such as CHF and anasarca may develop in some patients [28]. Two separate studies in elderly patients demonstrate that NSAIDs were associated with an increased risk for the development of volume overload and CHF [29,30]. One of these publications was a large cohort study in over 10, 500 patients [29]. A doubling of the risk for hospitalization with CHF was observed in patients taking diuretics and NSAIDs as compared with those ingesting diuretics alone [29]. A case control study similarly documented a twofold risk for first admission to the hospital with CHF in patients treated with NSAIDs as compared with patients who did not receive these drugs [30]. In this study, the effect was related to higher drug dosage and longer drug half-life. The presence of underlying heart disease significantly increased risk for CHF in NSAID treated patients as noted by an odds ratio for CHF admission of 10.5 in these patients [30]. An extreme example of this NSAID effect includes the case of a 70-year old patient who developed anasarca characterized by a fluid gain of 15 kg during a 17-day course of ibuprofen [31].

In addition to sodium retention with edema formation, NSAIDs also attenuate the natriuretic and aquaretic effects of diuretics. In fact, diuretic resistance has been noted to complicate therapy with these drugs, especially in patients with underlying salt-retentive states [28]. The underlying mechanism of diuretic resistance is due to multiple NSAID effects including 1) inhibition of the increase in renal blood flow that attends diuretic therapy, decreasing the filtered load of sodium available for excretion [32], 2) inhibition of natriuretic prostaglandin formation in the thick ascending limb of Henle typically stimulated by loop diuretics [33], 3) competition of NSAIDs with diuretic drugs at the tubular secretory level, thereby reducing the amount of drug reaching its site of action, and 4) enhanced ADH effect with resultant water retention [34].

Hypertension

Since sodium retention is associated with increases in blood pressure, the inhibitory effect of NSAIDs on prostaglandin-induced natriuresis raises concerns that normal blood pressure regulation might be impaired by these drugs. In fact, development of new onset hypertension and exacerbation of previously controlled hypertension has been observed in patients treated with NSAIDs [28,35,36]. In a study performed in approximately 20,000 elderly Medicaid enrollees, NSAID therapy within 2 months of study initiation was associated with a two-fold risk of requiring antihypertensive therapy [35]. Average increases in mean arterial pressure of 5 to 10 mmHg were noted in patients treated with NSAIDs [36-38]. This effect was most marked in hypertensive patients on blood pressure lowering medications, while normotensive patients did not develop hypertension. It appears that certain drugs are more likely to lose efficacy in lowering blood pressure when NSAIDs are administered. These include β-adrenergic blockers, ACE inhibitors, and as noted above, diuretics. In contrast, direct vasodilators such as the calcium channel blockers continue to maintain efficacy despite NSAID therapy. Patients with low renin hypertension, such as blacks and the elderly also appear more susceptible to the hypertensive effects of these drugs. The mechanism of NSAID-associated hypertension is largely related to the sodium retention that occurs, but there is likely a contribution from vasoconstriction of resistance vessels induced by inhibition of local vasodilatory prostaglandins (PGE_2, prostacyclin) in the endothelium of vessels. The effect of NSAIDs on blood pressure is a particularly vexing problem since an estimated 12 million Americans receive concurrent therapy with antihypertensive drugs and NSAIDs [28].

Water Balance

Hyponatremia

Mild to moderate levels of hyponatremia may also develop in patients treated with NSAIDs [5,6]. This disturbance in water balance results from two major effects. First, prostaglandin deficiency induced by NSAIDs magnifies the medullary interstitial osmotic gradient and leads to greater resorption of water in the distal nephron via aquaporins, which are apical membrane water channels in collecting duct cells. Second, since prostaglandins normally blunt the antidiuretic effects of vasopressin, suppression of prostaglandin synthesis with NSAIDs allows increased entry of water into tubular cells of the collecting duct. PGE2 has been shown to reduce water reabsorption by retrieving aquaporin-2 from the apical membrane. A recent study demonstrated that indomethacin increased the shuttling of aquaporin-2 to the apical plasma membrane of collecting duct cells [39]. This effect was unrelated to changes in ADH levels and likely was a direct effect of indomethacin on adenylyl cyclase complex. These effects impair solute-free water excretion and can lead to total body water excess and hyponatremia [5,6].

Potassium Homeostasis

Hyperkalemia

Hyperkalemia is another potential complication of treatment with NSAIDs [5,6,40,41]. NSAIDs can result in the development of potentially life-threatening hyperkalemia when prescribed to patients with underlying renal insufficiency or to those ingesting other potassium-altering medications [40,41]. These medications include the widely prescribed ACE inhibitors, ARBs, aldosterone antagonists (spironolactone, eplerenone), trimethoprim, heparin, and calcineurin inhibitors. The initial description of hyperkalemia associated with an NSAID, which also provided insight into the mechanism of disturbed potassium homeostasis, was published by Tan and colleagues [41]. The patient, who had underlying proteinuric kidney disease, developed severe hyperkalemia (serum K^+ = 6.2 mEq/L) and a reduction in baseline urinary prostaglandin excretion (PGE_2 = 598 ng/24 hours decreased to PGE_2 < 10 ng/24 hours) following therapy with indomethacin. These effects developed in association with a decline in plasma renin activity, plasma aldosterone concentration and urinary aldosterone excretion, consistent with drug-induced hyporeninemic hypoaldosteronism. All of these parameters reversed to normal following discontinuation of indomethacin. A series of five cases of hyperkalemia was also published further incriminating NSAIDs as a cause of disturbed renal potassium excretion and hyperkalemia [43]. Serum potassium concentrations increased in all patients (baseline serum creatinine concentrations in the 1.0 to 2.2 mg/dl range) treated with indomethacin and declined following drug discontinuation. It appears that this cation disorder develops from NSAID-induced reductions in the synthesis of renin and aldosterone, inducing a state of hyporeninemic hypoaldosteronism [5,6,40,41]. Since aldosterone stimulates renal potassium excretion via the creation of a favorable electrochemical gradient for potassium transport into the urinary space, it is not surprising that reduced aldosterone production by NSAIDs is the most prominent cause of hyperkalemia [41]. NSAID-associated reductions in the delivery of NaCl and water to the distal tubule also contribute to hyperkalemia. Decreased delivery of NaCl and water limits potassium secretion by diminishing the intraluminal sodium available for sodium-potassium exchange and reducing the favorable concentration gradient for potassium diffusion into the urinary space [41].

Acute Interstitial Nephritis

Acute interstitial nephritis (AIN) following NSAID therapy maintains important differences from that noted with β-lactam antibiotics, which are the most frequent therapeutic agents implicated in AIN, and other culprit drugs. Acute interstitial nephritis that occurs in the setting of NSAID administration typically develops over a longer period of exposure. Treatment is often greater than one year. This contrasts development of AIN in a mean of approximately 2 weeks with β-lactam antibiotics. There is also a much lower incidence of fever, rash, and eosinophilia with NSAIDS as compared with other drugs [44]. Proteinuria is a common finding in patients with AIN from NSAIDs due to concomitant glomerular disease (minimal change disease and membranous nephropathy). On histologic evaluation, NSAID-associated AIN is similar to other forms of drug-induced AIN except that a lesser degree of interstitial inflammation, tubulitis, and eosinophilic infiltration is present. With blockade of the cyclooxygenase enzyme, shunting of arachidonic acid into the lipoxygenase pathway may underlie the development of AIN from the pro-inflammatory leukotrienes that are synthesized via this alternative pathway. The unique clinical and pathologic characteristics of AIN following treatment with NSAIDs may be explained in part by the anti-inflammatory properties of this class of drugs [45]. The similar patterns of nephrotoxicity seen with a wide range of NSAIDs suggests that injury in the kidney may relate not only to the chemical structure and immunogenicity of the agent but also to the physiologic effects of COX inhibition and possibly to the shunting of arachadonic acid metabolites into these alternative pathways that modify immune function. This has been termed the "shunting" hypothesis.

Renal Localization and Function of COX-2 Enzyme

One strategy to predict the nephrotoxic potential of selective COX-2 inhibitors is to examine the presence and importance of both COX-1 and COX-2 enzymes in the kidney. Not only is the absolute presence of the COX-2 enzyme important, but its localization in various renal compartments and its response to normal and pathologic physiologic stress are integral to understanding this issue. The next section looks into these very issues. Table 4 notes the localization of COX-2 in the kidney of various animals and humans.

Table 4. Renal Localization of Cyclooxygenase-2

Species	Vasc	Glom	MD	TAL	MIC	CD
Mouse			X			X
Rat		X	X	X	X	
Rabbit				X	X	
Dog	X		X	X	X	
Monkey	X	X				
Human	X	X	X	X	X	X

Abbreviations: Vasc, vasculature; Glom, glomerulus; MD, macula densa; TAL, thick ascending limb; MIC, medullary interstitial cells; CD, collecting duct

Animal Studies

There are several animal studies that demonstrate the presence of COX-2 enzyme in renal tissue and the importance of prostaglandins derived from COX-2 in the modulation of renal physiology. First, the COX-2 enzyme is clearly localized in discrete areas of the normal kidney. In cultured rat mesangial cells, endothelin-1 (ET-1) induced expression of COX-2 mRNA and stimulated COX-2 protein accumulation, leading to increased production of PGE_2 [46]. COX-2 has also been isolated from rat medullary thick ascending limb (MTAL) cells [12,47]. In these animals, upregulation of the COX-2 isoform and increased PGE_2 synthesis (5-fold) were noted following exposure to angiotensin II [47]. Angiotensin-II acted to increase COX-2 mRNA upregulation through stimulation of these cells to produce tumor necrosis factor. In contrast, COX-1 mRNA was not upregulated by tumor necrosis factor exposure. In this same light, angiotensin-II markedly enhanced the expression of COX-2 mRNA in cultured rat vascular smooth muscle cells, providing another example of the role of

COX-2 enzyme in the upregulation of prostaglandin synthesis to modulate renal vasoconstrictors and maintain GFR [48]. In this model, angiotensin-II increased COX-2 expression by suppressing COX-2 mRNA degradation rather than increasing gene transcription. Importantly, the COX-2 specific inhibitor NS-398 attenuated the angiotensin-II driven expression of COX-2 in these cells [48].

COX-2 has also been localized to the macula densa of the juxtaglomerular apparatus, the adjacent thick cortical ascending limb cells, and to the medullary interstitial cells at the papilla in adult rats [11,49]. Furthermore, volume contraction induced by chronic salt restriction increased COX-2 expression in the renal cortex and increased the number of COX-2 producing cells in both the macula densa and the adjacent thick ascending limb [11,49]. In this study, salt restriction did not increase COX-2 production in papillary cells nor was COX-1 detectable in cells of the macula densa. COX-2 expression in the macula densa is augmented by dietary salt restriction and renal artery constriction, two conditions in which the renin gene expression is increased [50,51]. This COX-2 localization also suggests that it has an important role in the regulation of glomerular hemodynamics through the tubuloglomerular feedback (TGF) mechanism. It is notable that administration of COX-2 inhibitors prevents TGF adaptation in the Wistar rat [52]. Absence of TGF adaptation may lead to a reduction in GFR and NaCl retention following selective COX-2 inhibitor therapy. Constitutive COX-2 expression has also been identified in rabbit medullary interstitial cells [53]. Treatment of medullary interstitial cells with COX-2 antisense downregulated COX-2 production and induced medullary cell death in vitro [53]. In a second set of experiments in rabbits, Hao and colleagues treated medullary interstitial cells with selective COX-1 inhibitors, selective COX-2 inhibitors, and traditional NSAIDs (sulindac, ibuprofen, indomethacin). All cells underwent apoptosis, however, the selective COX-2 inhibitors were 1000 times more potent than selective COX-1 inhibitors in promoting cell death.

Mouse studies localize COX- and COX-2 enzyme synthesis to the cortical collecting duct [54,55]. Immunohistochemical studies demonstrate the presence of COX-1 and COX-2 enzymes in intercalated cells of the cortical collecting duct of mice kidneys [54,55]. In contrast, neither enzyme localizes to the cortical principal cells. It appears that COX-2 is the predominant enzyme in the synthesis of prostaglandins in this nephron segment. Specifically, intercalated cells exposed to selective COX-2 inhibitors had impaired prostaglandin synthesis as compared with cells exposed to selective COX-1 inhibitors [55]. Notably, PGE_2 is an important mediator controlling salt and water reabsorption by the cortical and medullary collecting duct. Abassi and others have also shown that experimental congestive heart failure is associated with selective overexpression of COX-2 in the rat kidney medulla, a finding probably representing several important renal effects [56]. Medullary expression of COX-2 in this model maintains efficient diuresis and natriuresis despite the salt retentive state triggered by heart failure, and defends medullary blood flow in the face of decreased effective renal perfusion. Inhibition of COX-2 in the rat renal medulla also promotes sustained hypertension in rats fed a high sodium diet [57]. The effect of COX-2 inhibition on inducing hypertension was most potent with infusion of a selective inhibitor directly into the medulla as compared with intravenous administration, supporting the importance of sodium retention in the generation of hypertension. Thus the pattern of COX-2 expression and function in the kidney suggests that this isoform plays a significant role in the regulation of sodium, water and other electrolyte metabolism in both physiologic and pathophysiologic conditions.

Human Studies

Studies have also disclosed the expression of COX-2 in glomerular podocytes and arteriolar smooth muscle cells in the normal human kidney obtained from surgical nephrectomy specimens [9]. The COX-2 enzyme was identified in these renal locations using polyclonal antibodies, reverse transcription-polymerase chain reaction, and c-RNA probes. In contrast, COX-1 was expressed primarily in endothelial cells of the afferent arteriole and cells of the cortical collecting duct. COX-2 has also been detected in the macula densa of adult human kidneys. Localization of COX-2 in the macula densa was demonstrated in subjects older than 60 years of age [58] and in patients with underlying hyperreninemic states (patients with congestive heart failure) [59]. COX-2 immunoreactivity was also noted in afferent arterioles and medullary interstitial cells, with limited staining observed in the thick loops of Henle in the specimens procured from the elderly subjects [58].

These findings suggest that COX-2 derived prostaglandins contribute to the regulation of renal hemodynamics probably via production of PGI_2 (inducing arteriolar vasodilatation) as well as PGH_2, which is subsequently metabolized to thromboxane (TxA_2). However, the role of the COX-2 isoform in renal hemodynamics is probably manifest only in specific conditions that are associated with increased dependence of renal function on prostaglandins. These include decreased sodium intake, intravascular volume depletion, critical renal artery stenosis, lupus nephritis, partial renal ablation, therapy with renin-angiotensin-aldosterone system inhibitors, cirrhosis, nephrosis and congestive heart failure. Although normal regulation of renal blood flow does not depend on prostaglandins, it is possible that COX-1 has some role in normal renal hemodynamics. This function may explain the observation of a few reported cases of acute renal failure induced by NSAIDs in apparently healthy subjects [17], and the studies showing that selective COX-2 inhibitors have no effect on GFR whereas traditional NSAIDs may slightly reduce GFR in sodium-replete healthy subjects [60,61]. In contrast, the observation that selective COX-2 inhibitors reduce GFR to the same degree as non-selective NSAIDs in sodium restricted subjects and in patients with chronic stable kidney disease supports the above paradigm [62,63,64]. Thus, observations on the localization of COX-2 in the kidney, and on the increased expression of renal COX-2 under conditions known to be associated with increased renal prostaglandin dependence demonstrate the importance of constitutively expressed and upregulated COX-2 in the kidney [50,51,58,59]. Therefore, the role of COX-2 in the production of prostaglandins necessary to maintain renal hemodynamics (RBF and GFR), renin secretion and tubular function (sodium, water and potassium homeostasis) questions the earlier belief that the new class of selective COX-2 inhibitors was benign.

To summarize, it is clear that animal models demonstrate the strategic location of COX-2 expression in the kidney and intimate a key role for COX-2 enzyme in modulating renal function in patients with certain disease states. In addition, localization of COX-2 to vascular tissue and glomeruli in humans suggests a role for this isozyme in the modulation of renal hemodynamics, clearly one of the primary cyclooxygenase-mediated functions, which is interrupted by NSAIDs. Furthermore, COX-2 expression in human macula densa and medullary interstitial cells implies an integral role of this enzyme in salt and water balance. The sites of COX-2 expression suggest that selective COX-2 inhibitors may adversely affect kidney function in patients with prostaglandin-dependent disease states.

Selective COX-2 Inhibitor-Associated Nephrotoxicity

Data recently published suggest that selective COX-2 inhibitors have a renal risk profile similar to traditional NSAIDs. This is particularly true in patients at risk of adverse renal effects related to the use of NSAIDs, including patients with hypertension, cirrhosis, nephrosis and renal insufficiency. As with traditional NSAIDs, a number of clinical renal syndromes are being described with these drugs including hemodynamic ARF, edema and hypertension, and hyponatremia and hyperkalemia. Both AIN and acute papillary necrosis have also been noted with the selective COX-2 inhibitors.

Renal Blood Flow/Glomerular Filtration Rate

Hemodynamic ARF

A reduction of GFR is common with NSAID therapy, but clinically important acute renal failure occurs rarely following administration of NSAIDs. Generally, acute renal failure develops only in susceptible patients such as those with underlying volume depletion, kidney disease, congestive heart failure, diabetic nephropathy, nephrosis, cirrhosis and old age. Current evidence suggests that selective COX-2 inhibitors have a risk profile similar to traditional NSAIDs in their potential to reduce GFR in susceptible patients. The CLASS trial noted that the incidence of increased creatinine levels was in the same range observed with NSAIDs (~ 1% of patients), although at statistically significant lower values in the celecoxib arm [3]. However, it is important to note that patients with risk factors for the development of adverse renal events with NSAIDs and selective COX-2 inhibitors are rarely included in clinical studies of these agents. Indeed, different results were obtained in studies on patients that more closely resemble a "susceptible" population. These included patients with conditions associated with increased dependence on prostaglandins to preserve renal function such as a sodium-restricted diet and chronic kidney disease. The pertinent studies will be reviewed in the following sections.

Evaluation of the effects of the selective COX-2 inhibitors on kidney function in human subjects has clarified the role of the COX-2 isoform in the human kidney and provided insight into the renal effects of these drugs. As will be seen, most studies examine the effects of these drugs in patients with minimal or no risk for hemodynamic ARF. Healthy elderly patients were studied to evaluate the effect of selective COX-2 inhibition on renal hemodynamics and solute excretion [60]. After exclusion for hypertension, diabetes mellitus, or renal impairment, thirty-six patients maintained an a high sodium diet (200 mEq/day) were randomized to receive rofecoxib 50 mg/day, indomethacin 50 mg three times/day, or placebo. As compared with control, both rofecoxib and indomethacin induced a transient but significant decrease in urinary sodium excretion, which returned to baseline after approximately 72 hours of drug therapy. Urinary prostaglandins were inhibited by both rofecoxib and indomethacin (compared with placebo), whereas GFR decreased significantly in the indomethacin group only. This study demonstrates that transient sodium retention occurs with both types of NSAIDs. However, it appears that healthy elderly patients with well-preserved renal function (GFR > 80 ml/min/1.73 m^2) are at low risk to develop acute renal insufficiency with a selective COX-2 inhibitor. The study results suggested that prostaglandins produced by the COX-1 isoform regulated RBF and GFR while COX-2 prostaglandins were more important for modulation of sodium excretion.

The renal effects of celecoxib and naproxen were examined in 24 healthy elderly subjects without underlying kidney disease (GFR > 80 ml/min/1.73 m^2) who were maintained on an unrestricted diet [61]. Subjects received either five days of celecoxib 200 mg twice/day followed by an increased dose of 400 mg twice/day for another five days, or they received naproxen 500 mg twice/day for ten days. Subjects were subsequently crossed over to receive the other drug regimen. Urinary PGE_2 and 6-keto-$PGF_{1\alpha}$ were significantly decreased with celecoxib and naproxen. A small but statistically significant decrease in GFR (-7.5 ml/min/1.73 m^2) developed only in the naproxen group. Urinary sodium excretion was reduced following celecoxib (-30%) or naproxen (-38%) administration, but returned to near baseline levels by 72 hours of treatment with either drug. Thus, as in the previous study, healthy subjects who remain volume replete (ie. not sodium restricted) maintained a preserved GFR despite therapy with a selective COX-2 inhibitor. Sodium retention, however, was at least a transient problem with both selective and non-selective COX inhibitors.

Selective COX-2 and non-selective COX inhibition was examined in 40 healthy male volunteers (GFR > 100 ml/min/1.73 m^2) who were salt restricted and received a dose of diuretic [62]. To examine renal effects, subjects were entered into four groups to receive celecoxib 200 mg twice/day, celecoxib 400 mg twice/day, naproxen 500 mg twice/day or placebo for 7 days. Transient but clinically significant decreases in RBF ($\approx$ -100 ml/min) and GFR ($\approx$ -20 ml/min) were noted after 1 day of therapy only in the celecoxib 400 mg twice/day group (Figure 4). Renal Blood flow and GFR were insignificantly decreased for both celecoxib and naproxen on day 7. Urine output as well as urine sodium and potassium excretion on day 1 was significantly decreased with both doses of celecoxib and naproxen. After 7 days of therapy, urine output and urine sodium and potassium excretion were significantly depressed with both doses of celecoxib, whereas only urine potassium excretion was significantly decreased with naproxen. These data suggest that salt-depleted patients are at risk to develop a reduced GFR and impaired solute excretion when treated with a selective COX-2 inhibitor, reminiscent of traditional NSAID renal toxicity.

Multiple doses of rofecoxib and indomethacin were studied in a group of salt-restricted elderly patients to examine effects on renal function [63]. Sixty patients with stage 2-3 CKD (creatinine clearances, 30-80 ml/min/1.73 m^2), were randomized into one of 4 groups that received rofecoxib 12.5 mg/day, rofecoxib 25 mg/day, indomethacin 50 mg three times/day, or placebo for six days. Rofecoxib 12.5 mg and 25 mg doses significantly decreased glomerular filtration rate by 10.2 ml/min/1.73 m^2 and 9.6 ml/min/1.73 m^2, respectively, while indomethacin similarly decreased GFR by 7.8 ml/min (Figure 5). Neither drug produced consistent reductions in urinary sodium nor potassium excretion while indomethacin significantly increased serum potassium concentration. This study further implies that a volume depleted state from salt restriction and mild to moderate CKD creates prostaglandin-dependent renal function that requires COX-2 to synthesize compensatory renal prostaglandins.

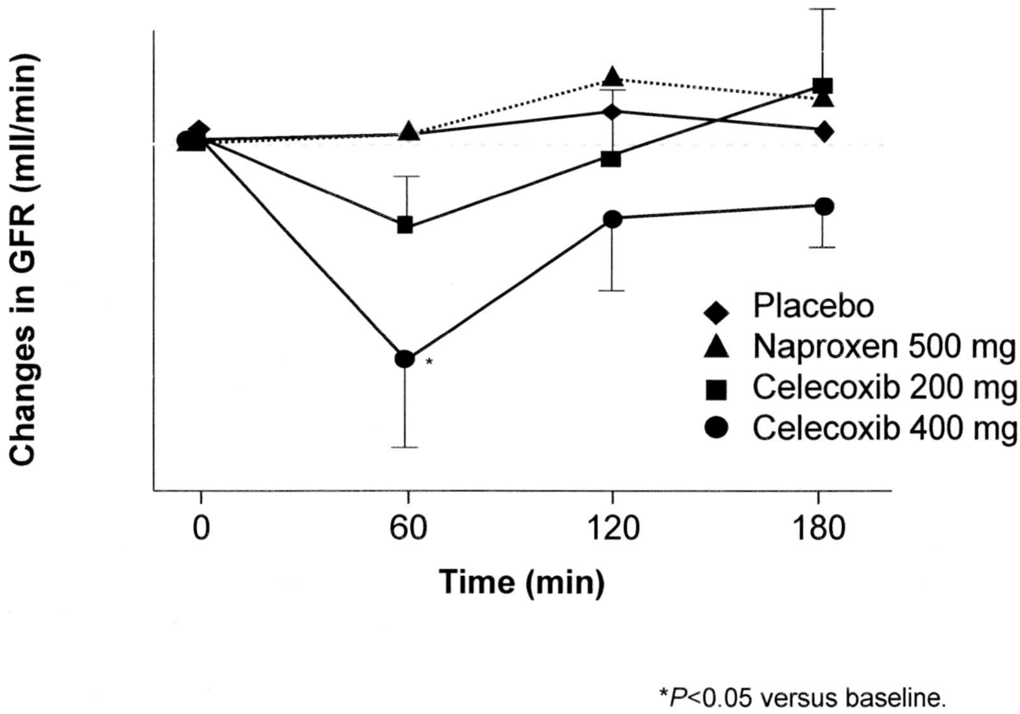

Figure 4. Effects of celecoxib 200 mg (■) and 400 mg (●), naproxen 500 mg (▲), or placebo (◆) on changes in glomerular filtration rate (GFR) over the first 3 hours in subjects on a sodium restricted diet (<50 mEq/day). Values are mean ± SE. [From ref. [62], with permission].

To summarize, in a salt restricted setting, both rofecoxib and celecoxib, reduced GFR to a similar degree as the traditional NSAIDs. Other potential states of renal stress have been studied. In patients with underlying kidney disease, celecoxib 200 mg twice/day was compared with both naproxen 500 mg twice/day and placebo for 7 days of therapy [64]. A significant reduction of GFR, similar to naproxen was noted with celecoxib. In contrast, celecoxib (400 mg, single dose) administered with irbesartan (150 mg) to healthy volunteers with slight volume depletion had no acute adverse affect on renal hemodynamics or renal salt handling [65]. It is important to recall that this was a short-term study carried out in a very limited number of healthy subjects, and therefore it cannot be used to claim renal safety for chronic therapy.

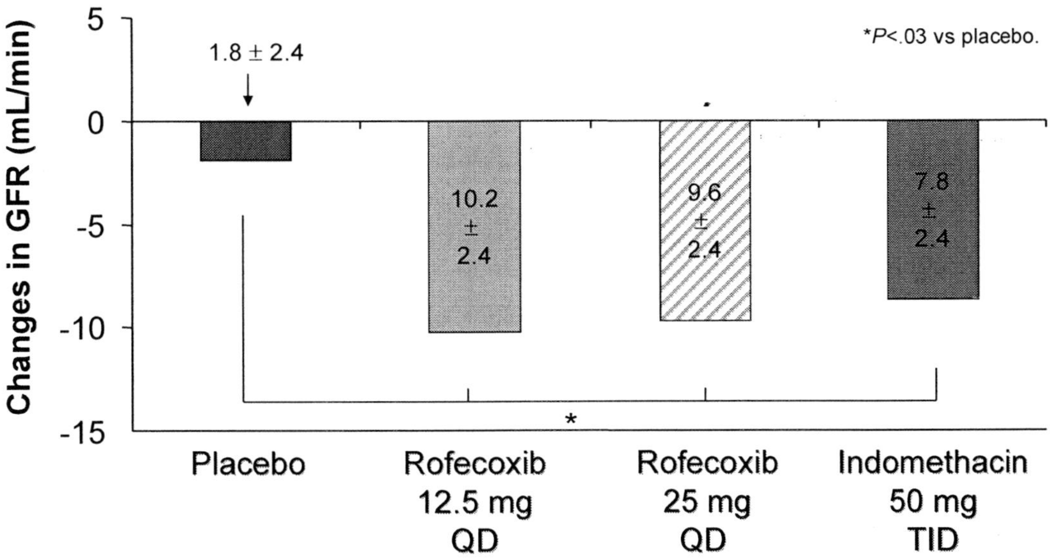

Figure 5. Effect of rofecoxib, indomethacin, or placebo on glomerular filtration rate (ml/min) in patients with mild chronic kidney disease (stages 2 and 3) on a sodium restricted diet. Measurements shown are the maximum decline in GFR (using iothalamate clearance) from baseline at day 6 of drug therapy. Bar graphs represent mean ± SE. [From ref. [63], with permission]

Selective COX-2 inhibitor therapy has also been observed to impair renal hemodynamics in several animal models. The selective COX-2 inhibitor, nimesulide significantly reduced renal blood flow and GFR in sodium-restricted dogs [66]. Another selective COX-2 inhibitor (SC-236) decreased both RBF and GFR in cirrhotic rats, although to a slightly lesser degree than ketorolac [67]. Subsequent studies suggest a lesser effect of celecoxib as compared with traditional NSAIDs on GFR in both animal and humans with compensated cirrhosis [68,69].

Clinically relevant cases of nephrotoxicity from COX-2 selective inhibitors have been published [70-76]. Three patients who developed acute renal failure and hyperkalemia following therapy with these medications (2 celecoxib, 1 rofecoxib) were the first reported by Perazella and Eras [70]. Notably, all of these patients had multiple risk factors for NSAID-induced nephrotoxicity, including factors such as underlying chronic renal failure and true or "effective" volume depletion. The acute deterioration in renal function reversed to baseline following discontinuation of COX-2 inhibitor and treatment of the associated intravascular volume disturbance. One patient required hemodialysis for severe hyperkalemia. Since this series of cases, several other reports [71-76] of renal impairment and/or electrolyte disorders have been described (Table 5). Taken together, these cases suggest that acute renal failure, hyperkalemia and sodium retention can occur with selective COX-2 inhibitor therapy in high-risk patients with prostaglandin dependent disease states.

It has been suggested that differences in renal-based adverse events between the available selective COX-2 inhibitors might reflect a peculiar difference between the agents rather than a "class"-related COX-2 pharmacologic effect. Available information, however, suggests a similar nephrotoxic potential of the selective COX-2 inhibitors represents a class effect and there are no overwhelming data to conclude in favour of a major difference in these drugs. More comparative data are necessary to demonstrate if any differences exist between the selective COX-2 inhibitors in regards to their potential to cause hemodynamic ARF. Until then, it is reasonable to conclude that the selective COX-2 inhibitors have the potential to cause acute renal failure in a manner similar to traditional NSAIDs.

Table 5. Cases of Acute Renal Failure associated with the Selective COX-2 Inhibitors

Medication Type and Dosage	Baseline Patient Characteristics	COX-2 Inhibitor Treatment: Data	Outcome After Stop COX-2 Inhibitor
Celecoxib 200 mg bid	Age-63, CKD, HTN Cr=2.8 CAD, LVH	Cr=4.9 CHF K+=5.1 Edema	Recovered within 5 days (Cr=2.9)
Celecoxib 200 mg bid	Age-68, CKD, HTN, Cr=3.5 DM, CMP	Cr=5.6 CHF K+=5.4 Edema	Recovered within 7 days (Cr=3.3)
Rofecoxib 25 mg qd	Age-73, CKD, DM Cr=2.2 CAD, PVD	Cr=9.0 Volume K+=8.5 depleted	Recovered within 8 days (Cr=2.0)
Celecoxib (n=2) Rofecoxib (n=3)	Mean Age-63 Mean GFR=60cc/min Loop diuretics (n=5) HTN (n=2), CHF (n=2)	Mean Max BUN=84 Mean Max Cr=2.8 Serum K+=5.1-6.4 Mean HCO3=19	All patients reported to recover to baseline within 2-3 weeks
Celecoxib 100 mg bi	Age-52, Cirrhosis, Cr=1.1 Gout	Cr=9.7 GI Bleed	Recovered within 3 days to baseline
Celecoxib 200 mg qd (n=3) Rofecoxib 25-50mg qd (n=2)	ACE inhibitors (n=2) Diuretics (n=3) HTN (n=3), CMP (n=4) CAD (n=3), CRF (n=5)	Mean increase Cr=2.4 Serum K+=5.6-8.5 Serum HCO3=12-18 Serum Na+=126-132 CHF (n=3)	All recovered to baseline within 2 to 8 days, 3 patients required dialysis for hyperkalemia or severe CHF
Celecoxib 400 mg qd	Age-57 Osteoarthritis Cr=1.0	Cr=3.0 HTN Edema	Recovered within 7 days to baseline
Celecoxib 200 mg qd	Age-55, Pleural effusion Cr=0.7	Cr=0.8, CHF, Edema Weight gain=4.54 kg	Recovered to baseline (+ furosemide)
Rofecoxib 25 mg qd (n=2)	Age-77, 78, DM, HTN, ACE Inhibitor (n=2) Cr=1.5, 1.9	Cr=2.8, 3.6, Edema K+=5.5 (n=1) Serum HCO3=18, 22	All 3 patients recovered within 10 to 20 days to baseline
Celecoxib 200 mg bid(n=1)	Age=19, transplant on sirolomus	ARF (Cr=?), Edema	

Abbreviations: Cr, creatinine (mg/dl); CKD, chronic kidney disease; CAD, coronary artery disease; HTN, hypertension; LVH, left ventricular hypertrophy; CMP, cardiomyopathy; DM, diabetes mellitus,; PVD, peripheral vascular disease; CHF, congestive heart failure; GFR, glomerular filtration rate; K+, potassium (mEq/L); BUN, blood urea nitrogen (mg/dl); HCO3, bicarbonate (mEq/L); ARF, acute renal failure. References[70-76]

Sodium Balance

Edema

Fluid retention is the most common NSAID-related renal effect; it has been reported to occur in approximately 5% of treated patients [28] and is due to decreased sodium excretion and mild sodium retention that occur from inhibition of renal PGE_2 synthesis. As with traditional NSAIDs, the COX-2 selective drugs can cause peripheral edema. This is not a surprising occurrence since both rofecoxib and celecoxib are capable of inducing renal sodium retention. In healthy people, during either normal or restricted sodium intake conditions, both rofecoxib and celecoxib, in separate studies, have been demonstrated to transiently reduce urinary sodium excretion rates similar to the comparator conventional NSAIDs [28,60,61,63]. In osteoarthritis studies that included approximately 6000 patients, lower extremity edema was noted in 3.6 and 3.8% of patients treated with rofecoxib at 12.5 mg and 25 mg doses, respectively [77]. These rates were similar to those observed with the comparator NSAIDs ibuprofen 800 mg three times daily (3.8%) and diclofenac 50 mg three times daily (3.4%), but higher than placebo (1.1%). In a similar fashion, celecoxib was also observed to precipitate peripheral edema formation in the large osteoarthritis trials that comprised approximately 5,200 patients [78]. The incidence of peripheral edema in patients treated with 100 mg and 200 mg twice daily of celecoxib was 1.6 and 3.0%, respectively. The edema rates were 1.3% for placebo and 2.2% for the NSAID comparator. The edema rate for celecoxib at 100 or 200 mg twice daily in data pooled from patients with osteoarthritis and rheumatoid arthritis was 2.5%, similar to the edema rate seen with naproxen (2.2%). It is probable that the slightly lower edema rates seen for both the traditional NSAIDs and celecoxib in these trials (as compared with the rofecoxib trials) reflects a different study population and/or a different edema definition.

Edema, generally in the lower extremities, is commonly reported in the selective COX-2 inhibitor clinical studies as it is during therapy with traditional NSAIDs. Edema formation with selective COX-2 inhibitors is dose-dependent and, similar to non-selective NSAIDs is associated with clinically significant weight gain in 30 to 50% of cases [79]. Although edema was a rare cause for study drop-out in the large clinical trials VIGOR and CLASS, a recent post-marketing survey noted that the development of edema led to discontinuation of the COX-2 inhibitor in 58-82% of cases [80]. Direct comparison of edema formation between rofecoxib and celecoxib has also been performed in the SUCCESS VI study [81]. Twice as many rofecoxib- compared with celecoxib-treated patients experienced edema, and a robust association emerged between the development of edema and the destabilization of hypertension control. This study and a subsequent study [82] contrasts all other studies that have demonstrated identical edema formation rates between the selective COX-2 inhibitors and traditional NSAIDs, raising questions about reliability of edema measurement in the various studies. The effect of drug half-life on edema formation (longer half-life of rofecoxib versus once daily celecoxib) also needs to be considered, since this may lead to more sodium retention over the 24-hour period. Taken together, data suggest that edema develops with both of the two approved selective COX-2 inhibitors, as seen with the traditional NSAIDs. The newer, more COX-2 selective inhibitors, such as etoricoxib do not appear to differ in respect to rofecoxib and celecoxib in terms of lower extremity edema adverse events [83]. The risk of congestive heart failure, the most serious complication of fluid retention, has been reported uncommonly in large clinical trials with selective COX-2 inhibitors, and not significantly different in respect to comparator NSAIDs.

It is of interest that rofecoxib has been noted in the rat to blunt the diuretic-induced increase in urinary prostaglandin excretion, and to attenuate dose-dependently diuresis and natriuresis, as well as the stimulation of the renin-angiotensin system induced by furosemide and thiazides [84]. This likely explains the edema formation and diuretic resistance seen in humans treated with these drugs.

Hypertension

Based on blood pressure data generated from traditional NSAIDs, one might also expect that the COX-2 selective drugs would also induce or exacerbate hypertension in predisposed patients (treated and borderline hypertensive patients). As noted, a number of mechanisms have been proposed to explain the increased blood pressure associated with NSAID treatment. Inhibition of renal prostaglandin synthesis causes sodium and water retention, secondarily expanding plasma volume. Inhibition of prostacyclin synthesis by NSAIDs may increase peripheral resistance by blunting the potent vasodilator effect of prostacyclin. Negating the counter-regulatory role of vasodilator prostaglandins may unfavourably derange the balance achieved with reflex-mediated pressor mechanisms induced by initiation of anti-hypertensive therapy [85]. Finally, loss of the inhibitory action of prostaglandins on the renal synthesis of endothelin-1 may lead to both salt and water retention as well as increased peripheral vascular resistance [86].

The relative contributions of the COX-1 and COX-2 isoforms in the production of vasodilatory prostaglandins, and possibly of endothelin-1 are not currently known. Thus, the potential differences of the selective COX-2 inhibitors as compared with traditional NSAIDs in the ability to induce hypertension cannot be predicted in the absence of direct comparisons. Current data suggest that selective COX-2 inhibitors have a blood pressure raising profile similar to traditional NSAIDs. The effect of these drugs to reduce prostaglandin production and renal sodium excretion in patients as described in the previous studies [60-63] suggests that elevation of blood pressure could occur in "salt-sensitive" patients. Although the large osteoarthritis trials that studied rofecoxib and celecoxib demonstrated only small increments in blood pressure with both of these drugs, the populations examined in these trials were relatively healthy and possessed minimal risk for the development of hypertension. As such, the absence of severe hypertension in the selective COX-2 trials is not an unexpected finding, since the normotensive patients in the studies that evaluated the hypertensive effects of traditional NSAIDs also did not develop significant elevations in blood pressure [36-38].

To support the possibility of a blood pressure-raising effect of the selective COX-2 inhibitors, a few studies in experimental animals provide insight into the pressor effect of these drugs. Hocherl and coworkers confirmed that the COX-2 isoform may be implicated in these hypertensive mechanisms [87]. They demonstrated that rofecoxib increased systolic blood pressure in rats through inhibition of prostacyclin synthesis, and that this alteration can be prevented by salt deprivation (supporting the notion that hypertension can occur in salt sensitive groups). This latter finding confirms previous observations that hypertension is exacerbated by selective COX-2 inhibitors therapy in rats with salt-dependent hypertension [88]. Celecoxib reduced prostacyclin formation, induced weight gain and raised blood pressure (as compared with vehicle) in both normotensive and hypertensive rats [89]. Selective inhibition of COX-2 in rat renal medulla also causes hypertension in rats fed a high sodium diet [57]. Interestingly, these observations have their clinical counterpart in a study conducted in humans [81]. Hypertension and edema developed concurrently during selective COX-2 inhibitor therapy (celecoxib and rofecoxib), thus suggesting that appropriate diuretic therapy to reduce sodium retention may be an important component in re-establishing blood pressure control.

Clinically, the data on the hypertensive effects of COX-2 inhibitors are abundant but heterogenous. It does appear that treatment with rofecoxib (12.5, 25, 50 mg once/day) causes a dose-related increase in the incidence of hypertension [90]. At therapeutic doses, the incidence of hypertension is similar to those observed with comparator NSAIDs. Furthermore, in clinical trials with celecoxib, hypertension occurred in the same range observed with conventional NSAIDs (~ 2% of patients), although the incidence of hypertension was statistically significantly lower than in the the conventional NSAID group [3]. These results need to be analyzed carefully because the doses of selective COX-2 inhibitors and comparator NSAIDs utilized in the studies were not equivalent, the use of ACE inhibitors was unbalanced between arms, and hypertension was reported by investigators rather than confirmed by objective measures. Differences in the pharmacokinetics of selective COX-2 inhibitors and traditional NSAIDs were not taken into account in reference to the time when blood pressure was measured. Additionally, there was no direct comparison between the available selective COX-2 inhibitors.

Subsequent studies were performed to address some of these residual questions on the hypertensive properties of various COX-2 inihibitors. The SUCCESS VI Study, a randomized, double-blind trial in hypertensive, osteoarthritic patients older than 65 treated with either celecoxib (200 mg/day) or rofecoxib (25 mg/day) demonstrated a small, but statistically significant increase in systolic hypertension with rofecoxib as compared with celecoxib [81]. However, a few caveats from this study should be noted. First, the two arms differed in terms of numbers of patients on ACE inhibitor therapy (more frequent in the celecoxib group). It is unclear how the imbalance in ACE inhibitor use might influence the results (negatively or positively) and therefore makes the results difficult to interpret. Second, the doses of drugs employed may not have been equivalent in regards to efficacy as suggested in some studies [91]. Finally, blood pressure measurements were aimed to target trough effect, which favoured the drug with the shorter half-life (celecoxib). Measurement of blood pressure throughout the 24-hour period would have provided more accurate information about drug-associated hypertensive effect. A similar 6-week study of the blood pressure effects of celecoxib (200 mg/day) and rofecoxib (25 mg/day) was undertaken in osteoarthritic patients, the majority of which were hypertensive [92]. The major difference between this study and the previously described study was that blood pressure was measured at peak (within hours of drug administration). The development of hypertension was not different between the drug groups. In a double-blind, placebo controlled study on 67 healthy elders maintained on a 200 mEq/day sodium diet (documented sodium balance with 24 hour urine collections), equipotent doses of rofecoxib, celecoxib and naproxen were examined to assess the effect on renal sodium excretion and blood pressure [93]. Sodium balance was achieved and documented with daily 24-hour urinary sodium measurements for 8 to 13 days prior to entry into the study. All treatment arms experienced an increase in systolic blood pressure (rofecoxib, 3.4 mmHg ± 2.0 mmHg; celecoxib, 4.3 mmHg ± 2.0 mmHg; naproxen, 3.1 mmHg ± 2.0 mmHg) as compared with placebo (-1.4 mmHg ± 2.0 mmHg). No significant difference on renal sodium excretion between agents was observed, although sodium retention was increased with all three medications as compared with the placebo group. It is important to note that these were not hypertensive patients on blood pressure lowering medications. It is possible that a different effect may have occurred in hypertensive patients.

Investigators have sought to examine the effects of COX-2 inhibitors on diurnal blood pressure variations. In a study of hypertensive osteoarthritis patients with controlled blood pressure, subjects received either 25 mg rofecoxib once daily or nabumetone (a non-selective NSAID) 2000 mg once daily for 1 week of treatment and 1000 mg for the following 3 weeks [94]. Twenty-four hour arterial blood pressure monitoring was performed. Rofecoxib treatment did not change arterial blood pressure during daytime, however, there was a distinct increase in night-time systolic and diastolic blood pressure leading to a disappearance of the physiological diurnal variation. Nabumetone, on the other hand, caused a moderate increase of day and night blood pressure, without changes in biological diurnal variation.

Another clinically pertinent question is whether COX-2 inhibitors interfere with the efficiacy of antihypertensive agents. White and colleagues studied 91 patients with controlled hypertension on linsinopril (10 to 40 mg/day) and randomized them to placebo or celecoxib (200 mg bid) and monitored them with 24-hour ambulatory blood pressure recordings over 4 weeks [95]. Celecoxib had no significant effect on the mean changes of the 24-hour systolic and diastolic blood pressures during therapy with the ACE inhibitor. Similarly, a recent review of this issue in data from rofecoxib phase IIb/III osteoarthritis database containing over 5000 patients noted that there was no change in blood pressure control when rofecoxib therapy was commenced in patients on ACE inhibitors [79]. Furthermore, none of the recorded classes of antihypertensive agents (ACE inhibitors, beta-blockers, diuretics, calcium channel blockers) posed an increased risk of having a hypertension-related adverse event with rofecoxib therapy.

While most of the studies reviewed thus far reveal that selective COX-2 inhibitors increase blood pressure to only a small degree in some patients, an obvious difference between the various COX-2 inhibitors has not yet been appreciated. An fair amount of more recent data, however, suggest there are some differences in the hypertensive properties of various COX-2 inhibitors, with rofecoxib possessing greater hypertensive potency. For example, a large study comprising 404 diabetic patients with controlled hypertension and osteoarthritis, examined the effects of celecoxib (200 mg daily), rofecoxib (25 mg daily) or naproxen (500 mg twice daily) on 24-hour ambulatory blood pressure [96]. Baseline antihypertensive therapy was similar among all treatment groups. Patients treated with rofecoxib for 6 weeks had higher systolic blood pressures (approximately 4 mm Hg), than patients treated with celecoxib and traditional NSAIDs. After 12 weeks, the differences remained between rofecoxib and celecoxib, but not between rofecoxib and naproxen, as this latter group manifested similar increases in systolic blood pressure at this time period. Rofecoxib also increased the proportion of patients (30%) with controlled hypertension (24-hour systolic blood pressure <135 mm Hg) who developed ambulatory hypertension by week 6 to a greater extent than celecoxib (16%) or naproxen (19%). Unlike the findings of a previous study [94], diurnal variation of blood pressure was not affected by any of the agents.

Three other reports similarly suggest that rofecoxib induces greater elevations in BP than celecoxib. A case-control study by Solomon and colleagues, involving 17,844 patients of 65 years of age or greater, found that rofecoxib users had an increased relative risk of developing new onset hypertension compared with those taking celecoxib (odds ratio [OR] 1.6), non-specific NSAIDs (OR 1.4) or no NSAID (OR 1.6) [97]. These risks were similarly elevated for doses of rofecoxib $\leq$ 25 mg daily or > 25 mg daily. In contrast, even those patients taking higher doses of celecoxib (> 200 mg daily) did not have an increased risk of hypertension.

Another retrospective analysis examined changes in blood pressure in 121 Native Americans patients who switched selective COX-2 inhibitor therapy from celecoxib to rofecoxib [98]. Systolic blood pressure was 2.9 mm Hg higher and mean diastolic blood pressure was 1.5 mm Hg higher on rofecoxib compared with celecoxib. These differences were even greater in hypertensive patients (4.8 and 2.0 mm Hg, respectively). Twelve of the 121 patients experienced a systolic blood pressure rise of > 20 mm Hg after the switch. Unfortunately, no analysis was performed of a contrary pharmacologic switch (rofecoxib to celecoxib).

Finally, a retrospective analysis of spontaneous adverse events in the US FDA database revealed approximately a 4-fold greater frequency of hospitalization for acute blood pressure elevation with rofecoxib use compared with celecoxib use [99]. This occurred despite a higher prevalence of chronic hypertension in the celecoxib group (88 vs. 67%). The median time to hospitalization after initiation of use was 10 days, and mean time was approximately 30 days. Most of the blood pressure events occurred on 25 mg daily or less of rofecoxib, while only 4 of the 26 patients were taking greater than 25 mg.

Perhaps the most convincing data that there indeed differences amongst the selective COX-2 inhibitors in regards to their hypertension-inducing properties are garnered from the largest randomized, controlled trial directly comparing celecoxib and rofecoxib in 1,095 elderly, osteoarthritic patients with treated and controlled hypertension [82]. After 6 weeks of therapy, more patients in the rofecoxib group compared with the celecoxib group had a higher incidence of clinically significant systolic blood pressure elevations (change > 20 mm Hg plus absolute value > 140 mm Hg) at any time point (14.9% versus 6.9%, $p<0.01$). The rofecoxib-treated patients experienced a mean increase in SBP of approximately 3 mm Hg, while mean SBP in the celecoxib group did not change. As in the SUCCESS VI study [81] approximately twice as many rofecoxib- compared with celecoxib-treated patients experienced edema (7.7% vs 4.7%, $p= 0.045$). Interestingly, the rofecoxib-induced BP differences were only statistically significant in those patients treated with ACE inhibitors and beta-blockers alone or in combination with a diuretic. In comparison, patients treated at baseline with calcium channel blockers or diuretics alone did not experience significant blood pressure changes. Presuming that the increases in blood pressure are volume dependent (likely, given the sodium retentive properties of rofecoxib and the higher propensity to edema formation in the rofecoxib group in this study), then it would intuitively follow that ACE inhibitors and beta-blocking agents would be less effective antihypertensive agents in this setting [100]. In contrast, calcium channel antagonists, and of course, diuretics, are excellent antihypertensive agents in the setting of volume expansion.

Finally, a recent meta-analysis has attempted to assess the pooled effect of selective COX-2 inhibitors on blood pressure. Nineteen randomized controlled trials consisting of a total of 45,451 patients were analyzed. Selective COX-2 inhibitors, as a whole, caused a weighted mean difference point estimate increase in systolic and diastolic blood pressure compared with placebo (3.85/1.06 mm Hg) and non-selective NSAIDs (2.83/1.34) [101]. Selective COX-2 inhibitors, as a general class again, resulted in a non-significant trend towards increases in de novo hypertension versus both placebo and non-selective NSAIDs.

When investigating the hypertensive propensity for the specific selective COX-2 inhibitors, rofecoxib resulted in elevations in systolic blood pressure compared with celecoxib and non-selective NSAIDs (Table 6). Celecoxib induced only minimal increases in systolic and diastolic blood pressure when compared with placebo, but no increase when compared with non-selective NSAIDs (Table 7).

Table 6. Effect of Rofecoxib on BP or HTN in comparison with other NSAIDs or other Selective COX-2 Inhibitors

Study	Comparison	Number of Pts	Type of Study	Difference in BP or HTN
81	Rof vs. Cel	810	RC	+
82	Rof vs. Cel	1092	RC	+
92	Rof vs. Cel	N/A	RC	-
93	Rof vs. Cel	34	RC	-
93	Rof vs. NSAID	34	RC	-
94	Rof vs. Name	N/A	RC	-
96	Rof vs. Cel	274	RC	+
96	Rof vs. Nap	268	RC	+
97	Rof vs. Cel	1264	CC	+
97	Rof vs. NSAID	1255	CC	+
98	Rof vs. Cel	121	Retrospective	+
99	Rof vs. Cel	N/A	Retrospective*	+
116	Rof vs. Nap	439	RC	+
117	Rof vs. Nap	5557	RC	-

Abbreviations: BP, blood pressure; HTN, hypertension; Rof, rofecoxib; Nap, naproxen; NSAID, nonsteroidal anti-inflammatory drug; Name, namebutone; RC, randomized, controlled trial; CC, case-control study.

*Analysis of FDA database examining cases of hypertensive urgencies induced by selective COX-2 inhibitors

Table 7. Effect of Celecoxib on BP or HTN in comparison with other NSAIDs or Selective COX-2 Inhibitors

Study	Comparison	Number of Patients	Type of Study	Difference in BP or HTN
3	Cel vs. NSAID	655	RC	-*
96	Cel vs. Nap	266	RC	-
97	Cel vs. NSAID	1747	CC	-
118	Cel vs. Diclof	655	RC	-
119	Cel vs. Nap	918	RC	-

Abbreviations: BP, blood pressure; HTN, hypertension; Cel, celecoxib; Nap, naproxen; NSAID, nonsteroidal anti-inflammatory drug; diclof, dicofenac; RC, randomized, controlled trial; CC, case-control study

* BP statistically significantly lower in celecoxib group

In conclusion, hypertension appears to be a dose-related class effect of selective COX-2 inhibitors, similar to conventional NSAIDs. At this point in time, one can conservatively conclude that while both of these drugs cause little hypertension in the general population, both are capable of significantly elevating blood pressure in patients with underlying hypertension. Animal studies and initial human studies have suggested a relative equivalence among different selective COX-2 inhibitors in regard to their hypertensive effects. However, the preponderance of evidence seems to now indicate that rofecoxib possesses greater hypertensive potency than other selective COX-2 inhibitors (Table 6). The reason for this apparent difference is not well understood. One potential hypothesis is that rofecoxib results in reductions in aldosterone metabolism, as has been suggested by some authors, however, in Wistar-Kyoto rats and spontaneously hypertensive rats treated with rofecoxib, plasma aldosterone concentrations were unaffected [102]. A second hypothesis for the difference in the hypertensive properties of rofecoxib and celecoxib is that celecoxib, through inhibition of carbonic anhydrase, results in a modest natriuresis that is enough to compensate for the alterations in renal blood flow and prostaglandin-dependent renal sodium handling. However, clinically, acetazolamide, the prototypical carbonic anhydrase inhibitor, is not an effective hypertensive agent, simply because of the lack of any significant diuretic action of the agent.

Thus, hypertensive patients treated with selective COX-2 inhibitors, and in particular rofecoxib, as with NSAIDs, should be carefully monitored in the initial phase of treatment for loss of blood pressure control. If hypertension worsens, the doses of anti-hypertensive agents should be accordingly modified. Further, it should be clearly recognized that changes in blood pressure are small if expressed as group averages, but they can underestimate individual changes [104]. Nevertheless, the importance of relatively small variations in blood pressure can be great due to its relevant public health implications. In many large clinical trials, sustained increases in systolic pressure of only 3 mmHg explained a 10 to 20% increase in congestive heart failure [105], a 15 to 20% increase in stroke risk (49), and a 12% increase in angina risk [106]. These findings have meaningful clinical implications for the maintenance of adequate blood pressure control, since a small but persistent loss of adequate blood pressure control can lead to an increase in adverse cardiovascular events.

Water and Potassium Balance

Hyponatremia and Hyperkalemia

The effect of the selective COX-2 inhibitors on water and potassium metabolism has not been specifically investigated in the large clinical trials that preceded their introduction on the market. Hyponatremia may occurs from water retention induced by the selective COX-2 [73]. Four out of five patients developed hyponatremia (serum Na^+ concentrations 126 mEq/L-132 mEq/L) following therapy with these drugs. In addition, selective COX-2 inhibitors decrease urinary potassium excretion in healthy subjects and patients with other risk factors for hyperkalemia [62,63]. Not surprisingly, several cases were reported that raise concern about the risk of hyponatremia, severe hyperkalemia and type-4 renal tubular acidosis in particular clinical settings with the selective COX-inhibitors [70,73]. In nine out of 14 cases where serum potassium concentration was measured, hyperkalemia (serum K^+

concentration 5.1 mEq/L-8.5 mEq/l) occurred following therapy with a selective COX-2 inhibitor [73]. In the cases where hyperkalemia developed, contemporaneous use of ACE inhibitors, angiotensin receptor blockers, spironolactone, potassium supplements, as well as concomitant diabetes mellitus with hyporeninemic hypoaldosteronism, and renal failure were present. It is interesting that the hyperkalemic effects of the selective COX-2 inhibitors are indistinguishable from traditional NSAIDs.

AIN from Selective COX-2 Inhibitors

As noted previously, traditional NSAIDs are a well-known cause of AIN. Recently, several cases of AIN following treatment with the selective COX-2 inhibitors, rofecoxib and celecoxib, were reported [106-114]. At least 9 cases of well-documented AIN from selective COX-2 inhibitors have been described (celecoxib, n=6, rofecoxib, n=3). The details are noted in Table 8. There is no obvious pattern to the clinical presentation as one case of AIN developed within 3 days, four cases occurred after 3-4 weeks of therapy, two developed at 6 to 7 months, and the two others developed after a year or greater of consumption. Eosinophilia was present in only 2/7 cases, while all cases had some level of proteinuria. The urine sediment was active in 8/9 cases with pyuria and hematuria the predominant cellular elements. Peak serum creatinine concentration following drug treatment ranged between 1.6 mg/dl and 13.6 mg/dl. Hemodialysis was required in 3/9 patients, 6 patients received corticosteroids, and all recovered renal function with serum creatinine concentrations ranging from 0.9 to 1.4 mg/dl. One of the cases of celecoxib-associated AIN also had concurrent minimal change disease, while two cases had membranous glomerulonephritis on renal biopsy, findings that have also been described with traditional NSAIDs [110,111]. One case of minimal change disease associated with acute tubular necrosis (without AIN) was noted to be a complication of celecoxib therapy [115].

Table 8. Cases of Acute Interstitial Nephritis associated with the Selective COX-2 Inhibitors

Drug	Dose	Peak SCr	Treatment	Final SCr
Celecoxib	400 mg/day	1.6 mg/dl	Steroids	0.9 mg/dl
Celecoxib	200 mg/day	4.5 mg/dl	Steroids	1.2 mg/dl
Celecoxib	200 mg/day	2.1 mg/dl	Steroids	1.1 mg/dl
Celecoxib	400 mg/day	11.8 mg/dl	Hemodialysis	1.1 mg/dl
Celecoxib	400 mg/day	5.9 mg/dl	Steroids	1.2 mg/dl
Rofecoxib	25 mg/day	8.7 mg/dl	Hemodialysis Steroids	1.4 mg/dl
Rofecoxib	25 mg/day	13.6 mg/dl	Hemodialysis	1.3 mg/dl
Rofecoxib	25 mg/day	2.5 mg/day	Steroids	Baseline

Abbreviations: SCr, serum creatinine concentration.
References [99-105]

Conclusion

Based on data presented in this chapter, selective COX-2 inhibitors should be considered to have equivalent nephrotoxicity as traditional NSAIDs. Therefore, patients considered at high risk for adverse renal events, such as those treated with diuretics and ACE inhibitors or angiotensin receptor blockers, volume depleted patients, the elderly, and patients with congestive heart failure, diabetic nephropathy, lupus nephritis, nephrosis, acute and chronic kidney disease and cirrhosis should be treated cautiously with selective COX-2 inhibitors. Treatment with these drugs should prompt careful monitoring for edema, hypertension, hyperkalemia, hyponatremia and acute renal failure. Finally, since selective COX-2 inhibitors have better gastrointestinal tolerance, patients may be more likely to consume doses greater than prescribed for longer periods of time, increasing risk for adverse renal events. Since the hypertensive and renal effects of selective COX-2 inhibitors are dose-dependent, patients should be alerted to strictly adhere to the prescribed regimen and contact their physician if edema, hypertension or other problems develop. As with traditional NSAIDs, both AIN and glomerular disease (membranous glomerulonephritis and minimal change disease) may complicate therapy with the selective COX-2 inhibitors.

References

[1] Cryer B, Feldman M. Cyclooxygenase-1 and Cyclooxygenase-2 selectivity of widely used nonsteroidal anti-inflammatory drugs. *Am J Med* 1998;104:413-421.

[2] Crofford LJ. COX-1 and COX-2 Tissue expression: Implications and predictions. *J Rheumatol* 1997;(suppl 49) 24:15-9.

[3] Silverstein FE, Faich G, Goldstein JL, et al. Gastrointestinal toxicity with celecoxib vs nonsteroidal anti-inflammatory drugs for osteoarthritis and rheumatoid arthritis. The CLASS study: a randomised controlled trial. *JAMA* 2000;284: 1247-1255.

[4] Bombardier C, Laine L, Reicin A, et al. Comparison of upper gastrointestinal toxicity of rofecoxib and naproxen in patients with rheumatoid arthritis. *N Engl J Med* 2000; 343:1520-1528.

[5] Clive DM, Stoff JS: Renal syndromes associated with nonsteroidal anti-inflammatory drugs. *N Engl J Med* 1984; 310: 563-672.

[6] Schlondorf D. Renal complications of nonsteroidal anti-inflammatory drugs. Kidney Int 1993;44:643-653.

[7] Smith WL, DeWitt DL. Biochemistry and prostaglandin endoperoxide H synthase-1 and synthase-2 and their differential susceptibility to nonsteroidal anti-inflammatory drugs. *Sem Nephrol* 1995; 15 (3):179-194.

[8] Morham SG, Langenback R, Loftin CD. Prostaglandin synthase 2 gene disruption causes severe renal pathology in the mouse. *Cell* 1995;83:473-482.

[9] Komhoff M, Gróne H-J, Klein T, Seyberth HW, Núsing RM. Localization of cyclooxygenase-1 and –2 in adult and fetal human kidney: implication for renal function. *Am J Physiol* 1997;272: F460-468.

[10] Hao CM, Komhoff M, Guan Y, Redha R, Breyer MD. Selective targeting of cyclooxygenase-2 reveals its role in renal medullary interstitial survival. *Am J Physiol* 1999;277(Renal Physiol. 46):F352-F359.

[11] Harris RC, McKanna JA, Akai Y, Jacobson HR, Dubois RN, Breyer MD: Cyclooxygenase-2 is associated with the macula densa of rat kidney and increases with salt restriction. *J Clin Invest* 1994;94: 2504-2510.

[12] Ferreri NR, Escalante BA, Zhao Y, An S, McGiff JC. Angiotensin II induces TNF products by the thick ascending limb: functional implications. *Am J Physiol* 1998;274:F148-F155.

[13] Niwa T, Maeda K, Shibata M. Urinary prostaglandins and thromboxane in patients with chronic glomerulonephritis. *Nephron* 1987;46:281-287.

[14] Palmer BF, Henrich WL. Clinical acute renal failure with nonsteroidal anti-inflammatory drugs. *Sem Nephrol* 1995;15 (3):214-227.

[15] Smith, WL. Prostanoid biosynthesis and mechanisms of action. *Am J Physiol* 1982;263:F181-187.

[16] Nath, K.A., Chmielewski DH, Hostetter TH. Regulatory role of prostanoids in glomerular microcirculation of remnant nephrons. *Am. J. Physiol.* 1987;252 (Renal Fluid Electrolyte Physiol. 21): F829-F837.

[17] Perazella MA, Buller GK: NSAID nephrotoxicity revisited: parenteral ketorolac-induced acute renal failure. *South Med J* 1993; 86:1421-1424.

[18] Kimberly RP, Gill JR, Bowden RE, Keiser HR, Plotz PH. Elevated urinary prostaglandins and the effects of aspirin on renal function in lupus erythematosus. *Ann Intern Med* 1978;89:336-341.

[19] Eras J, Perazella MA: NSAIDs and the kidney revisited: Are selective cyclooxygenase-2 inhibitors safe? *Am J Med Sci* 2001; 321: 181-190.

[20] Eriksson LO, Sturfelt G, Thysell H, Wollheim FA. Effects of sulindac and naproxen on prostaglandin excretion in patients with impaired renal function and rheumatoid arthritis. *Am J Med* 1990;89: 313-321.

[21] Cook E, Wallin JD, Thakur VD, et. al. Comparative effects of nabumetone, sulindac, and ibuprofen on renal function. *J. Rheumatol* 1997;24:1137-44.

[22] Ciabattoni G, Cinotti GA, Pierucci A, et al. Effects of sulindac and ibuprofen in patients with chronic glomerular disease. *N Engl J Med* 1984;310:279-283.

[23] Murray MD, Brater DC, Tierney WM, Hui SL, McDonald CJ. Ibuprofen-associated renal impairment in a large general internal medicine practice. *Am J Med Sci* 1990;299 (4):222-229.

[24] Bouvy ML, Heerdink ER, Hoes AW, Leufkens HG. Effects of NSAIDs on the incidence of hospitalizations for renal dysfunction in users of ACE inhibitors. *Drug Safety* 2003;26 (13): 983-989.

[25] Perez-Gutthann SP, Garcia-Rodriguez LA, Raiford DS, Duque Oliart A, Romeu JR. Nonsteroidal anti-inflammatory drugs and the risk of hospitalization for acute renal failure. *Arch Intern Med* 1996;156 (21):2433-2439.

[26] Huerta C, Castellsague J, Varas-Lorenzo C, Rodriguea LAG. Nonsteroidal anti-inflammatory drugs and risk of ARF in the general population. *Am J Kidney Dis* 2005;45 (2) 531-539.

[27] Griffin MR, Yared A, Ray WA. Nonsteroidal anti-inflammatory drugs and acute renal failure in elderly persons. *Am J Epidemiol* 2000;151:488-496.

[28] Whelton A. Nephrotoxicity of nonsteroidal anti-inflammatory drugs: physiologic foundations and clinical implications. *Am J Med* 1999;106 (5B): 13S-24S.

[29] Heerdink ER, Leufkens HG, Herings RMC, et al. NSAIDs associated with increased risk of congestive heart failure in elderly patients taking diuretics. *Arch Intern Med* 1998;158:1108-1112.

[30] Page J, Henry D. Consumption of NSAIDs and the development of congestive heart failure in elderly patients. *Arch Intern Med* 2000;160:777-784.

[31] Schooley RT, Wagley PF, Lietman P. *JAMA* 1977;237:1716.

[32] Nies AS, Gal J, Fadul S, et al. Indomethacin-furosemide interaction: the importance of renal blood flow. *J Pharmacol Exp Thr* 1983;226:27-31.

[33] Greven J, Farjam A. Effect of inhibitors of prostaglandin synthesis on the furosemide action in the loop of Henle. *Pflugers Arch* 1988;41:579-585

[34] Levenson DJ, Simmons CE, Brenner BM. Arachidonic acid metabolism, prostaglandins and the kidney. *Am J Med* 1982;72:354-362.

[35] Gurwitz JH, Avron J, Bonh RL, Glynn RJ, Monane M, Mogun H. Initiation of antihypertensive treatment during nonsteroidal anti-inflammatory drug therapy. *JAMA* 1994;272:781-786.

[36] Johnson AG, Nguyen TV, Day RO. Do nonsteroidal anti-inflammatory drugs affect blood pressure? A metaanalysis. *Ann Intern Me*d 1994;121:289-300.

[37] Pope JE, Anderson JJ, Felson DT. A meta-analysis of the effects of nonsteroidal anti-inflammatory drugs on blood pressure. *Arch Intern Med* 1993;153:477-484.

[38] Houston MC. Nonsteroidal anti-inflammatory drugs and antihypertensives. *Am J Med* 1991;90:42-47.

[39] Kim SW, Kim JW, Choi KC, et al. Indomethacin enhances shuttling of aquaporin-2 despite decreased abundance in rat kidney. *J Am Soc Nephrol* 2004;15:2998-3005.

[40] Whelton A, Hamilton CW. Nonsteroidal anti-inflammatory drugs: Effects on kidney function. *J Clin Pharmacol* 1991;31:588-598.

[41] Perazella MA. Drug-induced hyperkalemia: old culprits and new offenders. *Am J Med* 2000;109:307-314.

[42] Tan SY, Shapiro R, Franco R, Stockard H, Mulro PJ. Indomethacin-induced prostaglandin inhibition with hyperkalemia. A reversible cause of hyporeninemic hypoaldosteronism. *Ann Intern Med* 1979;90:783-785.

[43] Galler M, Folkert VW, SchlondorffD. Revesible acute renal insufficiency and hyperkalemia following indomethacin therapy. *JAMA* 1981;246:154-155.

[44] Pirani CL, Valeri A, D'Agati V, Appel GB. Renal toxicity of nonsteroidal anti-inflammatory drugs. *Contr Nephrol* 1987;55:159-175.

[45] Border WA, Lehman DH, Egan JD, Sass HJ, Glode JE, Wilson CB. Antitubular basement-membrane antibodies in methicillin-associated interstitial nephritis. *N Engl J Med* 1974;291:381-384.

[46] Kester M, Coroneos E, Thomas P, Dunn MJ. Endothelin stimulates prostaglandin endoperoxide synthase-2 mRNA expression and protein synthesis through tyrosine kinase signaling pathway in rat cells. *J Biol Chem* 1994;269:22574-22580.

[47] Ferreri NR, An S-J, McGiff JC. Cyclooxygenase-2 expression and function in the medullary thick asending limb. *Am J Physiol* 1999;277: F360-368.

[48] Ohnaka K, Numaguchi K, Yamakawa T, Inagami T. Induction of cyclooxygenase-2 by angiotensin II in cultured rat vascular smooth muscle cells. *Hypertension* 1999;35:68-75.

[49] Harris RC, Wang JL, Cheng HF, Zhang MZ, McKanna JA. Prostaglandins in macula densa function. *Kidney Int* 1998;67:S49-52.

[50] Yang T, Singh I, Pham H, Sun D, Smart A, Schnermann JB, Briggs JP. Regulation of cyclooxygenase expression in the kidney by dietary salt intake. *Am J Physiol* 1998;274:F481-489.

[51] Hartner A, Goppelt-Struebe M, Hilgers KF. Coordinate expression of cyclooxygenase-2 and rennin in the rat kidney in renovascular hypertension. *Hypertension* 1998;31: 201-205.

[52] Deng A, Wead LM, Blantz RC. Temporal adaptation of Tubuloglomerular feedback: Effects of COX-2. *Kidney Int* 2004;66:2348-2353.

[53] Hao CM, Yull F, Blackwell T, et al. Dehydration activates an NF-κB-driven, COX2-dependent survival mechanism in renal medullary interstitial cells. *J Clin Invest* 2000;106:973-982.

[54] Ferguson S, Hébert RL, Laneuville O. NS-398 upregulates constitutive cyclooxygenase-2 expression in the M-1 cortical collecting duct cell line. J Am Soc Nephrol 1999;10: 2261-2271.

[55] Harding P, Sigmon DH, Alfle ME, et al. Cyclooxygenase-2 mediates increased renin content induced by low-sodium diet. *Hypertension* 1997;29:297-302.

[56] Abassi Z, Brodsky S, Gealekman O, Rubinstein I, Hoffman A, Winaver J. Intrarenal expression and distribution of cyclooxygenase isoforms in rats with experimental heart failure. *Am J Physiol Renal Physiol* 2001;280: F43-F53.

[57] Zewde T, Mattson DL. Inhibition of cyclooxygenase-2 in the rat renal medulla leads to sodium-sensitive hypertension. *Hypertension* 2004;44:424-428.

[58] Nantel F, Meadows E, Denis D, Connolly B, Metters KM, Giaid A. Immunolocalization of cyclooxigenase-2 in the macula densa of human elderly. *FEBS letters* 1999;457:475-477.

[59] Komhoff M, Jeck NDM, Seyberth HW, et al. Cyclooxygenase-2 expression is associated with the renal macula densa of patients with Bartter-like syndrome. *Kidney Int* 2000; 58:2410-2424.

[60] Catella-Lawson F, McAdam B, Morrison BW, et al. Effects of specific inhibition of cyclooxygenase-2 on sodium balance, hemodynamics, and vasoactive eicosanoids. *J Pharmacol Exp Ther* 1999;289: 735-741.

[61] Whelton A. Nephrotoxicity of nonsteroidal anti-inflammatory drugs: physiologic foundations and clinical implications. *Am J Med* 1999;106 (5B): 13S-24S.

[62] Rossat J, Maillard M, Nussberger J, Brunner HR, Burnier M. Renal effects of selective cyclooxygenase-2 inhibition in normotensive salt-depleted subjects. *Clin Pharmacol Ther* 1999;66: 76-84.

[63] Swan SK, Rudy DW, Lasseter KC, et al. Effect of cyclooxygenase-2 inhibition on renal function in elderly persons receiving a low-salt diet. A randomized, controlled trial. *Ann Intern Med* 2000;133: 1-9.

[64] FDA Arthritis Advisory Committee. Celebrex: Briefing Document: Renal Effects, 1998. Available at: http://www.fda.gov/cder/foi/adcomm/98/celebrex.htm

[65] Kistler T, Ambuhl PM. Renal safety of combined cyclooxygenase 2 (COX-2) inhibitor and angiotensin II receptor blocker administration in mild volume depletion. *Swiss Med Wkly* 2001;131: 193-198.

[66] Llinás MT, López R, Rodríguez F, Roig F, Salazar FJ. Role of COX-2-derived metabolites in regulation of the renal hemodynamic response to norepinephrine. *Am J Physiol Renal Physiol* 2001;281: F975-F982.

[67] Bosch-Marce M, Claria J, Titos E, et al. Selective inhibition of cyclooxygenase 2 spares renal function and prostaglandin synthesis in cirrhotic rats with ascites. *Gastroenterology* 1999;116:1167-1175.

[68] Guevara M, Abecasis R, Terg R. Effect of celecoxib on renal function in cirrhotic patients with ascites. A pilot study. *Scand J Gastroenterol* 2004;39:385-386.

[69] Claria J, Kent JD, Lopez-Parra M, et al. Effects of celecoxib and naproxen on renal function in nonazotemic patients with cirrhosis and ascites. *Hepatology* 2005;41:579-587.

[70] Perazella MA, Eras J. Are selective COX-2 inhibitors nephrotoxic? *Am J Kidney Dis* 2000;35:937-940.

[71] Braden GL, O'Shea M, Mulhern J, Germain MJ. COX-2 inhibitor acute renal failure: Association with hyperkalemia and type IV renal tubular acidosis. *Nephrol Dial Transplant* 2004; 19:1149-1153.

[72] Stafford C, Bestoso JT. Celecoxib-induced acute renal failure. *J Am Soc Nephrol* (abstract) 2000;11:134A.

[73] Perazella MA, Tray K. Selective COX-2 inhibitors: a pattern of nephrotoxicity similar to traditional nonsteroidal anti-inflammatory drugs. *Am J Med* 2001;111: 64-67.

[74] Graham MG: Acute renal failure related to high-dose celecoxib. *Ann Intern Med* 2001;135:69-70.

[75] Pfister AK, Crisalli RJ, Carter WH. Cyclooxygenase-2 inhibition and renal function. *Ann Intern Med* 2001;134:1077.

[76] Gadalean F, Barreto G, Epstein M. Acute renal failure induced by COX-2 specific inhibitors. *J Am Soc Nephrol* 2001;12:779A.

[77] Daniels B, Seidenberg B. Cardiovascular safety profile of rofecoxib in controlled clinical trials. *Arthritis Rheum* 1999;42 (suppl):143.

[78] Whelton A, Maurath CJ, Verburg KM, Geis GS. Renal safety and tolerability of celecoxib, a novel cyclooxygenase-2 inhibitor. *Am J Ther* 2000;7:159-175.

[79] Gertz BJ, Krupa D, Bolognese JA, Sperling RS, Reicin A. A comparison of adverse renovascular experiences among osteoartritis patients treated with rofecoxib and comparator non-selective non-steroidal anti-inflammatory agents. *Curr Med Res Opin* 2002;18:82-91.

[80] Osterhaus JT, Burke TA, May C, Wentworth C, Whelton A, Bristol S. Physician-reported management of edema and destabilized blood pressure in cyclooxygenase-2-

specific inhibitor users with osteoarthritis and treated hypertension. *Clin Ther* 2002;24:969-989.

[81] Whelton A, Fort JG, Puma JA, Normandin D, Bello AE, Verburg KM. Cyclooxygenase-2-specific inhibitors and cardiorenal function: a randomized, controlled trial of celecoxib and rofecoxib in older hypertensive osteoarthritis patients. *Am J Therapeut* 2001;8:85-95.

[82] Whelton A, White WB, Bello AE, Puma JA, Fort JG. Effects of celecoxib and rofecoxib on blood pressure and edema in patients ≥ 65 years of age with systemic hypertension and osteoarthritis. *Am J Cardiol* 2002;90:959-963.

[83] Collantes E, Curtis SP, Wing Lee K, et al. A multinational randomized, controlled,clinical trial of etoricoxib in the treatment of rheumatoid arthritis. *BMC Family Practice* 2002;3: 1-10.

[84] Kammerl MC, Nusing RM, Richthammer W, Kramer BK, Kurtz A. Inhibition of COX-2 counteracts the effects of diuretics in rats. *Kidney Int* 2001;60:1684-1691.

[85] De Leeuw PW. Nonsteroidal anti-inflammatory drugs and hypertension. The risks in perspective. *Drugs* 1996;51:179-187.

[86] Johnson AG. NSAIDs and blood pressure. Clinical importance for older patients. *Drugs Aging* 1998;12: 17-27.

[87] Johnson AG, Nguyen TV, Owe-Young R, Williamson DJ, Day RO. Potential mechanisms by which nonsteroidal anti-inflammatory drugs elevate blood pressure: the role of endothelin-1. *J Hum Hypertens* 1996;10: 257-261.

[88] Hocherl K, Endemann D, Kammerl MC, Grobecker HF, Kurtz A. Cyclo-oxygenase-2 inhibition increases blood pressure in rats. *Br J Pharmacol* 2002;136: 1117-1126.

[89] Muscara MN, Vergnolle N, Lovren F, Triggle CR, Elliott SN, Asfaha S, Wallace JL. Selective cyclooxygenase-2 inhibition with celecoxib elevates blood pressure and promotes leukocyte adherence. *Br J Pharmacol* 2000 ;129: 1423-1430.

[90] Vioxx® [package insert]. Whitehouse Station, NJ : Merck and Co., Inc., March 2000 (Cited by Whelton 2001)

[91] FDA Arthritis Advisory Committee. Cardiovascular safety review of rofecoxib. Available at: http://www.fda.gov/ohrms/ac/01/briefing/3677b2_06_cardio.pdf.2001

[92] Geba GP, Polis AB, Dixon ME, et al. Comparative blood pressure effects of rofecoxib, celecoxib and placebo in patients with osteoarthritis (OA): A randomized controlled trial. *Proceedings from XVI EULAR Congress* (2001)

[93] Schwartz JI, Vandormael K, Malice MP, et al. Comparison of rofecoxib, celecoxib, and naproxen on renal function in elderly subjects receiving a normal-salt diet. *Clin Pharmacol Ther* 2002;72:50-61.

[94] Reitblat T, Zamir D, Estis L, Priluk R, Drogenikov T, Viskoper JR. The different patterns of blood pressure elevation by rofecoxib and nabumetone: *J Hum Hypertens* 2002;16: 431-434.

[95] White WB, Kent J, Taylor A, Verburg KM, Lefkowith JB, Whelton A. Effects of celecoxib on ambulatory blood pressure in hypertensive patients on ACE inhibitors. *Hypertension* 2002;39:929-934.

[96] Sowers JR, White WB, Pitt B, et al. The effects of cyclooxygenase-2 inhibitors and nonsteroidal anti-inflammatory therapy on 24-hour blood pressure in patients with

hypertension, osteoarthritis, and type 2 diabetes mellitus. *Arch Intern Med* 2005;165:161-168.

[97] Solomon DH, Schneeweiss S, Levin R, Avron J. Relationship between cox-2 specific inhibitors and hypertension. *Hypertension* 2004;44:140-145.

[98] Fredy J, Diggins DA, Morrill GB. Blood pressure in Native Americans switched from celecoxib to rofecoxib. *Ann Pharmacother* 2005;39:797-802.

[99] Brinker A, Goldkind L, Bonnel R, Beitz J. Spontaneous reports of hypertension leading to hospitalizations in association with rofecoxib, celecoxib, nabumetone, and oxaprozin. *Drugs Aging* 2004;21:479-484.

[100] Weir MR. The role of combination antihypertensive therapy in the prevention and treatment of chronic kidney disease. *Am J Hypertension* 2005; 18:100S-105S.

[101] Aw TJ, Haas SJ, Liew D, Krum H. Meta-analysis of cyclooxygenase-2 inhibitors and their effects on blood pressure. *Arch Intern Med* 2005;165:490-496.

[102] Hocherl K, Endemann D, Kammerl MC, Grobecker HF, Kurtz A. Cyclo-oxygenase-2 inhibition increases blood pressure in rats. *Br J Pharm* 2002;135:1117-1126.

[103] Fitzgerald GA, Patrono C. The coxibs, selective inhibitors of cyclooxygenase-2. *N Engl J Med* 2001;345:433-442.

[104] Graves JW, Hunder IA. Worsening of hypertension by cyclo-oxygenase-2 inhibitors. *J Clin Hypertens* 2000;2:396-398.

[105] ALLHAT Collaborative Research Group: Major cardiovascular events in hypertensive patients randomized to doxazosin vs chlortalidone: the antihypertensive and lipid-lowering tratment to prevent heart attack trial (ALLHAT). *JAMA* 2000;283:1967-1975.

[106] Collins R, Peto R, MacMahon S, et al. Blood pressure, stroke, and coronary heart disease. Part 2: short-term reductions in blood pressure: overview of randomised drug trials in their epidemiological context. *Lancet* 1990;335:827-838.

[107] Hypertension Detection and Follow-up Program Cooperative Group: Effect of stepped care treatment on the incidence of myocardial infarction and angina pectoris: 5-year findings of the Hypertension Detection and Follow-up Program. *Hypertension* 1984;6:1198-1206.

[108] Rocha JL, Fernandez-Alonso J. Acute tubulointerstitial nephritis associated with the selective COX-2 enzyme inhibitor, rofecoxib. *Lancet* 2001;357:1946-1947.

[109] Alper AB, Meleg-Smith S, Krane NK. Nephrotic syndrome and interstitial nephritis associated with celecoxib. *Am J Kidney Dis* 2002;40:1086-1090.

[110] Henao J, Hisamuddin I, Nzerue CM, Vasadani G, Hewan-Lowe K. Celecoxib-induced acute interstitial nephritis. *Am J Kidney Dis* 2002;39:1313-1317.

[111] Markowitz GS, Falkowitz DC, Isom R, et al. Membranous glomerulopathy and acute interstitial nephritis following treatment with celecoxib. *Clin Nephrol* 2003;59:137-142.

[112] Brewster UC, Perazella MA. Acute tubulointerstitial nephritis associated with celecoxib. *Nephrol Dial Transplant* 2004;19:1017-1018.

[113] Chow KM, Szeto CC, Li P, Lai FM. Acute interstitial nephritis and COX-2 inhibition. *Hosp Med* 2003;64:429.

[114] Esteve JB, Launay-Vachar V, Brocheriou I, Grimaldi A, Izzedine H. COX-2 inhibitors and acute interstitial nephritis: case report and review of the literature. *Clin Nephrol* 2005;63:385-389.

[115] Almansori M, Kovithavongs T, Quarri MU. Cyclooxygenase-2 inhibitor-associated minimal change disease. *Clin Nephrol* 2005;63:381-384.

[116] Hawkey CJ, Laine L, Simon T, Quan H, Shingo S, Evans J. Incidence of gastroduodenal ulcers in patients with rheumatoid arthritis after 12 weeks of rofecoxib, naproxen, or placebo: a multicentre, randomized, double blind study. *Gut* 2003;52:820-826.

[117] Lisse JR, Perlman M, Johansson G, et al. Gastrointestinal tolerability and effectiveness of rofecoxib versus naproxen in the treatment of osteoarthritis: a randomized, controlled trial. *Ann Intern Med* 2003;139:539-546.

[118] Emery P, Zeidler H, Kvien TK, et al. Celecoxib versus diclofenac in long-term management of rheumatoid arthritis: randomized double-blind comparison. *Lancet* 1999;354:2106-2111.

[119] Simon LS, Weaver AL, Graham DY, et al. Anti-inflammatory and upper gastrointestinal effects of celecoxib in rheumatoid arthritis: a randomized controlled trial. *JAMA* 1999;282:1921-1928.

In: Drug Toxicity: New Research
Editor: Cam E. Vellotis, pp.223-261
ISBN 978-1-60456-320-7

Chapter 7

Ethanol Induced Adaptive Changes in Structure and Function of NMDA Receptors

József Nagy,* Sándor Kolok, András Boros and Péter Dezső
Gedeon Richter Ltd., Pharmacological and Drug Safety Research
Laboratory of Molecular and Cellular Biology, Budapest, Hungary

Abstract

Ethanol is a small molecule acting on several neurotransmitter systems in the brain. Accumulating evidences suggest that the primary excitatory – i.e. the glutamatergic – neurotransmitter system is a particularly important site of ethanol's action. Several studies showed that ethanol is a potent and selective inhibitor of the N-methyl-D-aspartate (NMDA) receptors and prolonged ethanol exposition leads to a compensatory "up-regulation" of these receptors resulting in enhanced NMDA receptor mediated functions after removal of ethanol. These alterations are supposed to contribute to the development of ethanol tolerance, dependence as well as the acute and delayed signs of ethanol withdrawal. Recently, alterations in subunit composition of NMDA receptors were reported after long-term ethanol exposure. mRNA and/or protein levels of NR2A and NR2B types of subunits were found elevated both by *in vivo* and *in vitro* experiments. In primary cultures of rat hippocampal or cortical neurons, especially the NR2B subunit expression and levels of certain NR1 splice variants were increased after 3 days of intermittent ethanol treatment. According to the high calcium permeability, the increased agonist sensitivity and the relatively slow closing kinetics of NMDA ion channels composed of NR1 and NR2B subunits, these changes may underlie the enhanced NMDA receptor activation observed after long-term ethanol exposure. Consequently, novel type of NMDA receptor antagonists - the NR2B subunit selective agents potently inhibited the neurotoxic effect of ethanol withdrawal seen in primary cultures of rat cortical neurons pre-treated with ethanol. Consistent with these

* Fax: 36-1-2605000; e-mail: jozsef.nagy@richter.hu

observations, enhanced NR2B type of NMDA receptor subunit expression is likely involved in development of alcohol dependence and withdrawal symptoms, therefore this subunit may serve as a possible drug target in pharmacological interventions against alcoholism.

Introduction

Alcohol use disorders represent a substantial public health problem all over the world. The World Health Organization (WHO) estimated 2 billion alcohol users in 2000, compared with 1.3 billion smokers and 185 million users of other psychoactive drugs. According to the data released by WHO in 2003, the global prevalence of alcohol use disorders was 1.7%, and these disorders accounted for 1.4% of the total world disease burden. Data released by The National Institute on Alcohol Abuse and Alcoholism (NIAAA) in August 2004 showed that whereas in 1991–1992 the total prevalence of 12-month alcohol abuse and dependence – according to the "Diagnostic and Statistical Manual of Mental Disorders, Fourth Edition" (DSM-IV) – was 7.41% in the USA representing 13.8 million adult Americans, this prevalence rose to 8.46% representing 17.6 million Americans in 2001–2002. As it was published by the editorial board of an international general medical journal, The Lancet, in March 2004, alcohol use is the fourth largest cause of disability in men and the tenth largest in women in developed regions of the world. Given the harmful effects of alcohol use disorder on the afflicted individuals and society as a whole, alcohol use disorders continue to represent a substantial public health problem (Grant 2004).

Investigation of the mechanisms underlying the actions of ethanol in the central nervous system (CNS) has been ongoing for more than a century. Early research on acute alcohol actions focused on the physical properties of alcohols and related anesthetics and established the widely appreciated Meyer-Overton relation that describes the direct relationship between the hydrophobicity of an alcohol and its potency for producing intoxication (Meyer 1901; Overton 1896). According to this "lipid theory" of alcohols' action, ethanol is thought to produce its behavior effects by actions on the membrane lipids bringing about changes in the function of the membrane proteins. Consistent with this hypothesis, the intoxicating potency of aliphatic n-alcohols with up to five carbon atoms is correlated with both their lipid solubility and their membrane lipid disordering potency. However, the potency of aliphatic n-alcohols for producing intoxication reaches a maximum at six to eight carbon atoms and then decreases (Peoples and Weight 1995; Godden 2001; Akinshola 2001). The molecular bases of this "cut-off" effect cannot be explained by the "lipid theory", since both lipid solubility and membrane lipid disordering potency increase exponentially with the increase in the carbon chain length. The hypothesis of ethanol's non-specific membrane effects has also been challenged by data demonstrating definite subunit compositions and certain amino-acid residues of sensitive receptors critical for allosteric modulation by ethanol (Allgaier 2002; Mihic 1997; Kumari and Ticku 2000; Ueno 2000).

Effect of Ethanol on Neurotransmission

Although, the exact mechanism by which ethanol exerts its effect is still a matter of debate, studies over the last decade showed that ethanol affecting several neurotransmitter systems differentially modifies neurotransmission processes in the CNS. Besides altering the release of neurotransmitters like dopamine (DA) – resulting in increased DA levels in the "central reward" pathway –, ethanol alters the function of a number of neurotransmitter receptors (e.g.: γ-amino butyric acid A ($GABA_A$), glycine, glutamate, norepinephrine, DA, serotonin, acetylcholine) as well as transporters (adenosine, norepinephrine, DA, serotonin). Especially the ligand-gated ion channels including the brain's major amino acid neurotransmitter systems – the inhibitory GABA and the excitatory glutamate – were shown highly sensitive to the acute effect of ethanol at relevant (<100 mM) concentrations (Lovinger 1990, Li 1994, Franks and Lieb 1994). In the past years, there has been increasing evidence that acute ethanol facilitates GABAergic transmission by enhancing chloride conductance through the $GABA_A$ receptors, and inhibits glutamatergic function by decreasing cationic conductance especially through the N-methyl-D-aspartate (NMDA) activated subclass of glutamate receptors. Conversely, the development of tolerance and dependence associated with chronic ethanol consumption leads to reduced GABAergic and increased glutamatergic functions.

Structure and Function of NMDA Receptors

NMDA receptors (NMDARs) belong to the family of ionotropic glutamate receptors. These receptors are highly expressed in the CNS. The involvement of these receptors in diverse processes like excitatory synaptic transmission, synaptic plasticity, and excitotoxicity rests upon their unique features. Their special characteristics are the high permeability to Ca^{2+} ions, the relatively slow activation / deactivation kinetics and their voltage-sensitive blockage by extracellular Mg^{2+} ions. The Mg^{2+} block results in a unique mechanism of channel activation. Glutamate, the native agonist of the NMDARs, can open the ion-channel only if the plasma membrane became depolarized and the Mg^{2+} blockage was displaced. Thus, NMDARs act as coincidence perceptive elements, which become active only when electrical and chemical signals are present concurrently.

Besides glutamate, NMDARs are sensitive to several other endogenous modulators. For full receptor activation, the co-agonist glycine (Meguro et al., 1992) or D-serine (Mothet 2000) must also bind to the receptor. Endogenous polyamines, spermine and spermidine also facilitate (Lerma 1992; Rock and Macdonald 1992), whereas extracellular Zn^{2+} ions (Christine and Choi 1990) and protons (Tang 1990; Traynelis and Cull-Candy 1990) suppress NMDAR activation. In addition, NMDARs interact with various intracellular scaffolding, anchoring, and signaling molecules associated with the postsynaptic density (Figure 1). The sensitivity of NMDARs to different ligands, its permeation, and block by divalent ions, kinetic properties, and interaction with intracellular proteins highly depend on their subunit composition (Danysz and Parsons 1998; Husi and Grant 2001).

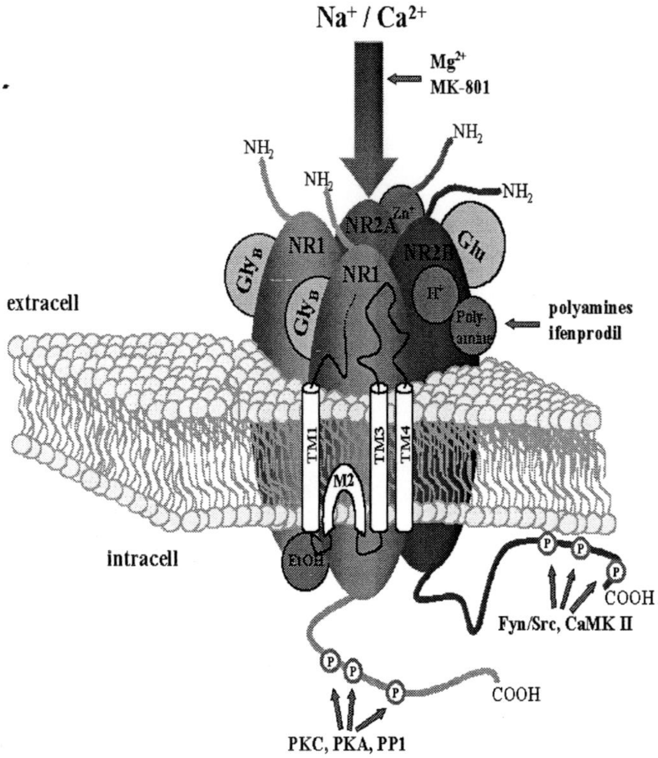

Figure 1. Schematic model of the NMDA receptor showing the heteromeric assemblies of four subunits in NMDA receptors. Each subunit has four hydrophobic regions, although only three form membrane-spanning domains (TM1, TM3, and TM4). M2 makes a hairpin bend within the membrane and forms the channel pore. Functional NMDA receptor complexes are formed by combinations of NR1 and NR2 subunits, which contain the glycine and glutamate recognition sites, respectively. Supposed binding sites of agonists, some antagonists, and other modulators are shown.
From: József Nagy (2004) NR2B type of NMDA receptor subunits: a possible target in treatment for alcohol dependence. *Current Drug Targets – CNS & Neurological Disorders 3,* 169-179.

NMDARs, like other ion-channel receptors, are multimeric transmembrane proteins, made up of different types of subunits. Several distinct NMDAR subunits have been identified in neurons (Figure 2). The ubiquitously expressed NR1 subunit occurs as eight distinct isoforms because of three independent sites (N1, C1 and C2 cassettes) of alternative splicing. Families of four distinct NR2 (A, B, C and D) and two NR3 (A, B) subunits are also identified (Moriyoshi 1991; Hollmann 1999; Das 1998). Although, the precise subunit composition and stoichiometry of native NMDARs are difficult to determine and largely unknown (Premkumar and Auerbach 1997; Laube 1998), it is believed that NMDARs exist as

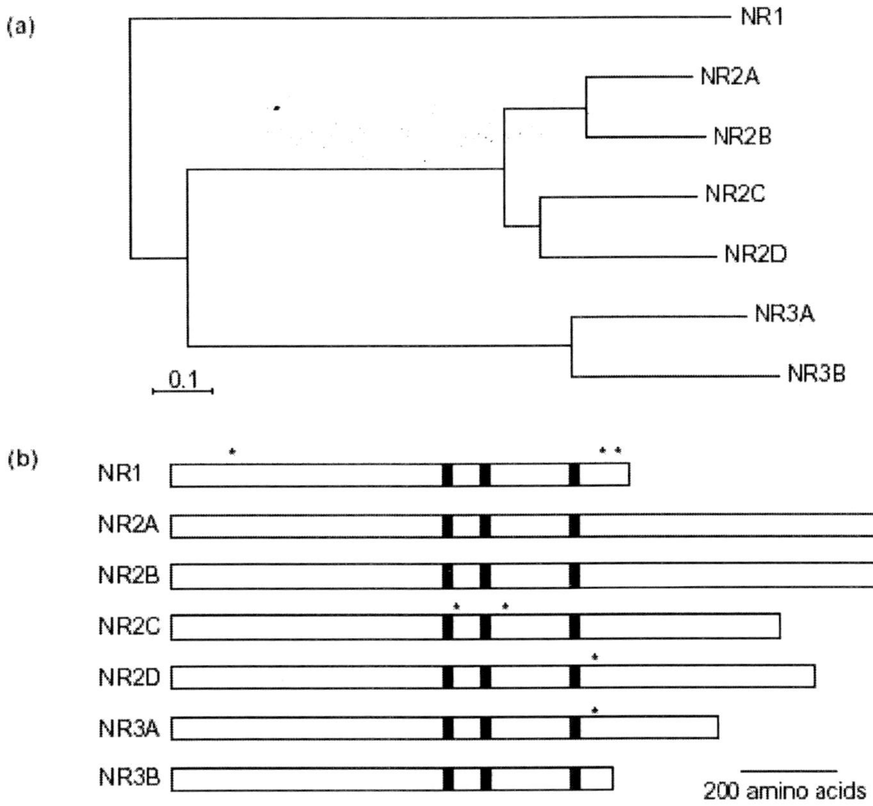

Figure 2. NMDAR subunit diversity. (a) Dendrogram of complete amino-acid sequences for rat NMDAR subunits (except NR3B; human). Sequences were aligned using ClustalX and the tree was generated with NJPlot (http://pbil.univ-lyon1.fr/software/njplot.html) ClustalX (ftp://ftp-igbmc.u-strasbg.fr/pub/ClustalX). (b) Representation of NMDAR subunit polypeptides. Black boxes indicate transmembrane domains, and grey boxes show the transmembrane TM2 re-entrant loop. Asterisks denote regions at which alternative splicing takes place. This is best characterized for the NR1 subunit, which has three regions of alternative splicing: the amino-terminal N1 cassette (exon 5); and the carboxy-terminal C1 (exon 21) and C2 (exon 22) cassettes. Splicing at these sites can generate eight distinct isoforms of NR1 subunit (NR1-1a, -1b, -2a, -2b, -3a, -3b, -4a and -4b). Splicing of the NR2C subunit leads to truncated polypeptides ending after TM1 or TM3. The NR2D subunit can be spliced in the carboxyl terminus, producing a 33-amino-acid insert. Likewise, NR3A splicing leads to a 20-aminoacid insert in the carboxy-terminal domain. NR2B, NR2C and NR2D also have splice sites in their 5′-untranslated regions but no splice variants have been reported for NR2A.
From: Stuart Cull-Candy, Stephen Brickley and Mark Farrant (2001) NMDA receptor subunits: diversity, development and disease. *Current Opinion in Neurobiology 11,* 327–335.

tetrameric complexes consisting of at least one NR1 and one NR2 subunits (Moriyoshi 1991; Monyer 1992, 1994). The subunits are most probably arranged as dimer of dimers with an NR1-NR1-NR2-NR2 orientation in the channel (Schorge 2003). Each subunit has four hydrophobic regions, although only three of them form membrane-spanning domains (TM1, TM3, and TM4). The fourth one (M2) makes a hairpin bend within the membrane and participate in the formation of the ion-channel pore (Danysz and Parsons 1998).

Two important composition dependent properties of the NMDARs include their single-channel conductance (Brimecombe 1997) and their block by extracellular Mg^{2+} ions. Diheteromeric NMDARs composed of NR1/NR2A or NR1/NR2B subunits generate 'high-conductance' channel openings with a high sensitivity to Mg^{2+} blockade. On the contrary, receptors containing NR2C or NR2D subunits give rise to 'low-conductance' channels with a lower sensitivity to extracellular Mg^{2+} ions. The NR3 subunits are thought to be regulatory in nature since they do not form functional channels alone but co-assemble with NR1/NR2 complexes (Das 1998). NMDARs containing NR3 subunits form 'low-conductance' channels; insertion of an NR3 subunit into NR1/NR2A complexes show a roughly fivefold reduction in relative Ca^{2+} permeability compared to those composed of merely NR1/NR2A subunits (Perez-Otano 2001).

One of the NR2 subunits, the NR2B type appears to be specifically important in respect of several functional properties of the NMDAR. It participates in regulation of the Mg^{2+} block, since replacement of Trp607 of this subunit to Asp or Ala greatly attenuates while substitution of this amino acid side chain for Leu completely abolishes the Mg^{2+} block. According to these observations, Williams et al. (1998) proposed a model in which the M2 loop of the NR2B subunit containing the Trp607 is part of the binding site for Mg^{2+} ions. The presence of an NR2B subunit in the receptor complex affects the binding of the co-agonist glycine as well. Whereas the binding site for glycine is thought to be located on the NR1 subunit (Danysz and Parsons 1998), a high-affinity site for CGP61594, a glycine site antagonist, was shown exclusively displayed by NR1/NR2B receptors as compared with receptors containing other types of NR2 subunits (Honer 1998). One of the unique characteristics of the NR2B subunit is that it binds polyamines. Polyamines appear to facilitate NMDAR function, probably by reducing the inhibitory impact of protons (Gallagher 1997). The NR2B subunit is a highly relevant candidate for mediating the modulatory effects of polyamines, such as spermine and spermidine. In addition, similarly to polyamines, ifenprodil (Avenet 1996), the prototype of the recently discovered NR2B subunit selective NMDAR antagonists (SSNAs) and related compounds – e.g. eliprodil, CP-101,606, Ro25-6981, RG-1103 (Avenet 1997; Williams 1993, 1995; Kashiwagi 1996; Gallagher 1996; Borza 2003) – selectively antagonize NMDA responses in those receptors that contain NR2B subunit.

Ethanol is a Potent Inhibitor of NMDA Receptors

Glutamatergic system is considered an important factor in the mediation of the addictive effect of alcohol (Di Chiara 1998). Among glutamate receptors, AMPA and especially NMDA type of receptors represent the highest affinity targets for ethanol in the CNS (Lovinger 1989; Hoffman 1990; Grant 1995). Biochemical, electrophysiological and behavioral evidences show that ethanol is a potent and selective inhibitor of these receptors (Dildy 1989; Hoffman 1989; Lovinger 1989; Lovinger 1993; Costa 2000) (Table 1A).

Table 1A. Effect of Acute Ethanol Treatment on NMDA Ion Channels

Effects	Ethanol conc.	Preparation	References
Inhibition of NMDA-evoked currents	2.5 – 100 mM	Hippocampal neurons, sensory neurons, Recombinant NR1, ε1/ζ1 and ε2/ζ1, as well as NR1/NR2A, NR1/NR2B and NR1/NR2A/NR2B subunits expressed in Xenopus oocytes	Lovinger 1989, White 1990, Koltchine 1993, Masood 1994, Mirshahi and Woodward 1995
Inhibition of NMDA-mediated signal transmission	1 – 50 mM	rat hippocampal slice preparation	Lovinger 1990
Inhibition of NMDA-induced cytoplasmic Ca^{2+}-increase	10 – 100 mM	Newborn rat neurons, Cerebellar granule cells	Dildy and Leslie 1989, Hoffman 1989a
Inhibition of NMDA- induced cGMP production	10 – 50 mM	Cerebellar granule cells	Hoffman 1989a, 1989b
Inhibition of NMDA excitotoxicity	100 mM	Rat cortical culture	Lustig 1992
Increase the possibility of open state of NMDA channels	1.74 – 174 mM	Rat hippocampal culture	Lima-Landman and Albuquerque 1989

Several studies involving recombinant receptors have demonstrated that receptors containing different types of NR2 subunits have differential sensitivity to the inhibitory effect of ethanol (Popp 1998; Smothers 2001). The ability of ethanol to depress NMDA evoked currents paralleled with the neuroprotective action of ifenprodil in rat cultured cortical neurons (Lovinger 1995). Similar results were obtained when NMDA-induced release of (^{3}H)-norepinephrine was measured in slices from rat cerebral cortex (Fink and Göthert 1996). Since ifenprodil is known as an NR2B subunit selective NMDAR antagonist (Williams 1993), it was assumed that ethanol acts on the NR2B subunit. Indeed, studies performed on recombinant NMDARs showed that heteromers containing either NR2A or NR2B subunits are preferentially sensitive to ethanol inhibition vs. heteromers containing NR2C or NR2D subunits (Kuner 1993; Masood 1994; Buller 1995; Chu 1995; Mirshahi 1995; Wirkner 1999). Moreover, NMDARs with NR1/NR2B subunit combination were more susceptible to the effect of ethanol compared to those composed of NR1/NR2A subunits (Blevins 1995, 1997; Anders 1999; Smothers 2001).

Earlier it was thought that ethanol binds to a hydrophobic pocket distinct from other modulatory binding sites of the NMDAR (Peoples and Weight 1995; Peoples 1997). Recently it was suggested that this pocket is associated with the third transmembrane domain (TM3) of the NR1 subunit. While mutation of Phe639 to Ala in this region of the NR1 subunit expressed in either oocytes or HEK-293 cells significantly decreased the inhibitory effect of ethanol, the substitution of this residue for Trp resulted in receptors that were slightly more sensitive to ethanol inhibition than the wild-type receptors. These observations suggest that the 639 position of the NR1 subunit is an important determinant of ethanol sensitivity (Ronald 2001; Allgaier 2002).

Action of ethanol on NMDARs may also be mediated by changes in the phosphorylation status of the receptor subunits. According to Alvestad et al. (2003) tyrosine phosphorylation of NR2A and NR2B subunits was significantly reduced following *in situ* exposure of hippocampal slices to 100 mM ethanol. Specifically, phosphorylation of Tyr1472 of the NR2B subunit was reduced by 23.5 percent. Addition of a phosphotyrosine phosphatase inhibitor – bpV(phen) – in the recording medium prior to and during ethanol exposure significantly reduced the inhibitory effect of ethanol on NMDAR mediated excitatory postsynaptic potentials (Alvestad 2003; Ferrani-Kile 2003). These data suggest a possible mechanism by which ethanol may inhibit the NMDAR via activation of a tyrosine phosphatase and phosphatase-mediated dephosphorylation of NMDAR subunits may play a role in mediating the inhibitory effect of ethanol.

Effect of Chronic Ethanol Treatment on NMDA Receptors

Changes in NMDAR Functions

Data from studies on neuroadaptation following chronic ethanol exposure indicate a significant role of NMDARs in expression of alcohol withdrawal syndrome as well as in associated neuronal damage (Table 1B). Initial *in vivo* studies showed that seizures evoked by withdrawal of ethanol in alcohol dependent animals were attenuated by NMDAR antagonists and exacerbated by administration of NMDA at doses that are not convulsant in control animals. According to these data, it has been hypothesized that an enhancement of NMDAR mediated neurotransmission following the removal of ethanol blockade mediates ethanol withdrawal seizures (Grant 1990; Gonzalez 2001).

Indeed, several papers reported that chronic ethanol exposure leads to a selective enhancement of NMDAR function in cultured hippocampal and cortical neurons (Hoffman 1996; Smothers 1997; Chandler 1999; Nagy 2001; Floyd 2003). For instance, whereas in hippocampal (Whittington 1995; Thomas 1998) and cortical (Ibbotson 1997) slices prepared from ethanol-naive animals, synaptic potentials were rather AMPA-mediated, in slices from mice chronically treated with ethanol the electrical stimulation evoked synaptic potentials involved a large extent of NMDA-mediated components. In addition, when ethanol was superfused for one hour, in naïve slices a transient depression of NMDA-induced depolarization developed, which vanished at the end of the superfusion period and washout of ethanol caused a withdrawal-type increase in NMDA responses. Similarly, while the amount of non-viable cells in hippocampal brain slice explants was significantly reduced in presence of ethanol, cytotoxic effect of NMDA was significantly higher in ethanol-exposed samples after 24h withdrawal. These data also suggest that acute administration of ethanol has a minor neuroprotective effect but following long-term ethanol exposure and withdrawal neurons became more sensitive to NMDA (Thomas 2000; Harris 2003). Correspondingly, when cultures of rat cortical cells were treated with ethanol the morphology of neurons was not altered, whereas obvious signs of neuronal damage and increased release of lactate dehydrogenase (LDH) were observed after 24 hours of withdrawal (Figure 3A) (Nagy 2001). Interestingly, neurotoxic effect of ethanol withdrawal was observed only in those cultures which were pre-treated with ethanol repeatedly, once daily at least for three consecutive days (Figure 3B) (Nagy 2002). This kind of daily ethanol treatment produced an *in vitro* neuronal model of alcohol-dependence similar to that of Hu and Ticku (1997) who used chronic but intermittent ethanol treatment (CIE, 12h ethanol : 12h withdrawal) providing a feasible model for studying the mechanism underlying the CIE-induced kindling-like phenomenon observed in humans (Ballenger 1978; Becker 1993). This *in vitro* test system, when ethanol treatment is interrupted and the cycle of treatment and withdrawal is repeated several times, may be a useful model for studying the development of ethanol dependence and withdrawal symptoms observed in alcoholics who consume alcohol intermittently for an extended period.

Table 1B. Effect of chronic ethanol treatment on NMDA ion channels

	Effects	Duration of treatment	Ethanol conc.	Preparation	References
in vitro experiments	Enhancement of NMDA-induced cytoplasmic Ca^{2+}-increase	2 – 4 days	20 – 100 mM	Rat cortical culture, Cerebellar granule cells	Blevins 1995 Iorio 1992
	Enhancement of NMDA excitotoxicity	3 – 4 days	100 mM	Rat cortical culture, Cerebellar granule cells	Chandler 1993a, Iorio 1993 Nagy and Laszlo 2002
	Enhancement of NMDA-induced NO production	4 days	100 mM	Rat cortical culture	Chandler 1997
	Increase of NR2B mRNA levels	5 days	50 mM	Rat cortical culture	Hu 1996
	Increase of NR2B protein levels	3 days, intermittent	100 mM	Rat cortical culture Rat hippocampal culture	Nagy 2003
	Enhancement of inhibitory potential of NR2B subunit selective NMDA receptor antagonists	3 days, intermittent	100 mM	Rat cortical culture	Nagy 2003
in vivo experiments	Increase of MK-801 binding	7 days	7% ethanol in liquid diet	hippocampus, cortex, striatum of C57BL mice	Grant 1990, Gulya 1991
	Increase of NR1 immuno-labeling	12 weeks	5% ethanol in liquid diet	Rat hippocampus	Trevisan 1994
	Increase of NR2A and NR2B mRNA levels	5 days	20% ethanol intragastrically	Rat brain	Follesa and Ticku 1995
	Increase of ornithine decarboxylase enzyme activity	5 days	>2 mg/ml blood alcohol level	Rat hippocampus	Davidson 1998
	Enhancement of glutamate release	4 days + 12h withdrawal	1 – 3 g/kg	Rat nucleus accumbens and hippocampus	Dahchour 1996, 1999, 2000

After such kind of ethanol treatment, NMDA responses and sensitivity of NMDARs for ethanol were enhanced in primary cultures of rat cortical neurons (Figure 4) (Nagy 2002). Furthermore, the neurotoxic effect of withdrawal could be reduced by re-addition of ethanol or administration of NMDAR antagonists (Figure 5). On the other hand, the effect of the $GABA_A$ receptor agonist muscimol was insignificant. These observations support the conception that NMDARs may play a role in the development of *in vitro* ethanol dependence and in alcohol-withdrawal evoked neurotoxicity.

A. Control

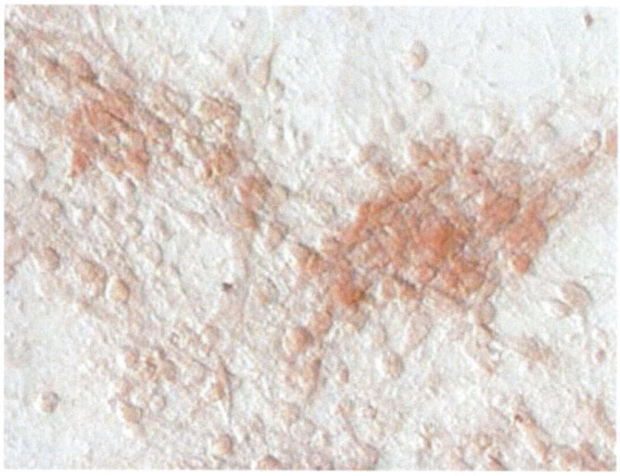

B. Pre-treated with 50 mM ethanol for 3 days and withdrawn for 24h

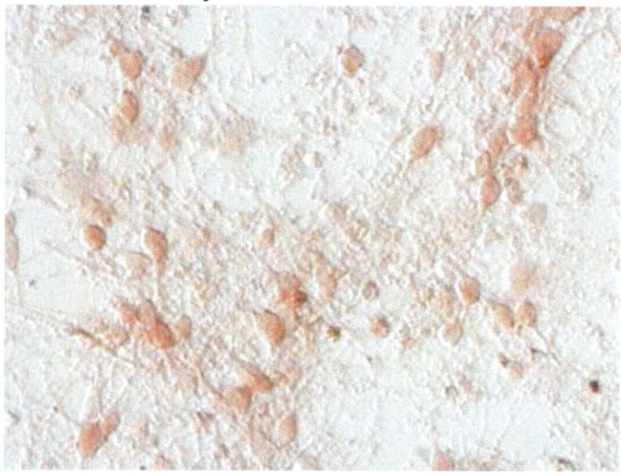

C. Pre-treated with 50 mM ethanol for 3 days and treated with 50 mM ethanol for 24h

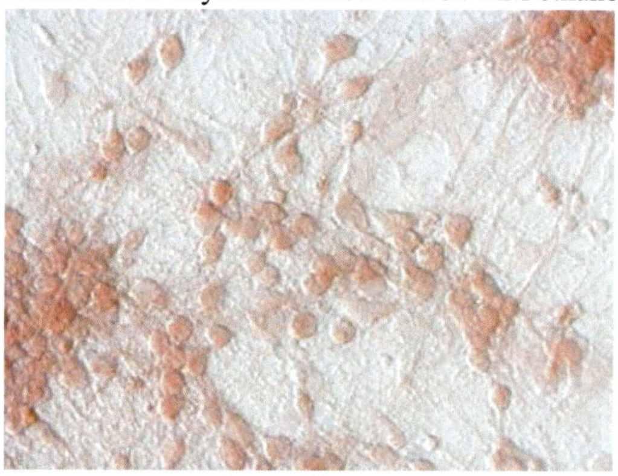

Figure 3A. In vitro model of ethanol dependence and withdrawal
Differential interference photomicrographs of control primary cultures of rat cortical neurons (A) and cultures previously adapted to 50 mM alcohol for 3 days (B, C). 24 hours before fixation cultures were exposed to control medium (A, B), or medium containing 50 mM ethanol (C). Red coloured neurons are immuno-labelled with anti-neurofilament antibody. Note the extensive granulation and disintegration of neuritic processes and cell bodies in culture under alcohol-withdrawal (B) and its protection by ethanol (C). (magnification: 200x)
From: Nagy J., Müller F., László L. (2001) Cytotoxic effect of alcohol-withdrawal on primary cultures of cortical neurons. *Drug Alcohol Depend. 61,* 155–162.

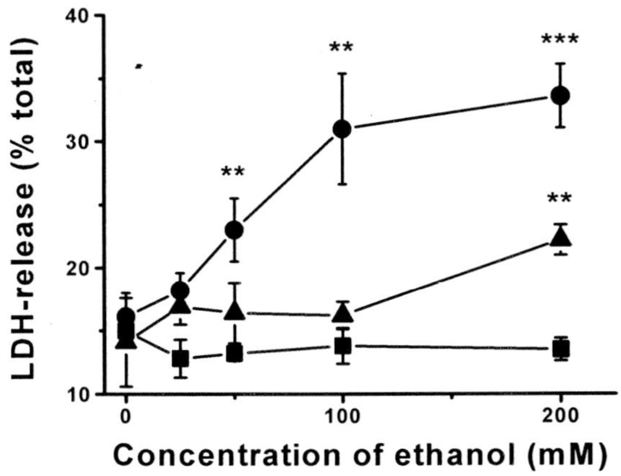

Figure 3B. Toxic effect of 24-hour ethanol-withdrawal and its inhibition by re-addition of ethanol in ethanol pre-treated primary cortical cultures.

LDH activity of the culture medium expressed as percentage of total activity was measured in cultures pre-treated with different concentrations of ethanol once for 24 (squares) or 72 (triangles) hours as well as daily for 3 successive days (circles).

(*: p<0.05, **: p<0.01, ***: p<0.001 as compared to the respective control not treated with ethanol)

From: Nagy J., László L. (2002) Increased sensitivity to NMDA is involved in alcohol-withdrawal induced cytotoxicity observed in primary cultures of cortical neurons chronically pre-treated with ethanol. *Neurochem. Int. 40,* 585–591.

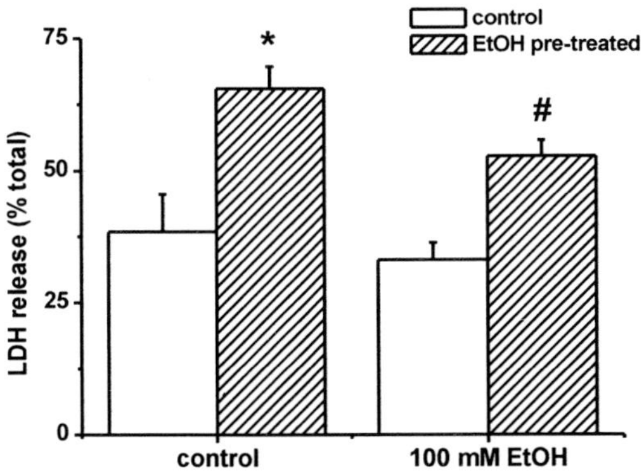

Figure 4A. Altered excitotoxic effect of NMDA after ethanol pre-treatment. Effect of acute and chronic ethanol treatment on NMDA induced cytotoxicity. Control cortical cultures (open columns) and cortical cultures pre-treated with 100mM ethanol repeatedly, once daily for 3 days (dashed columns) were exposed to 300 μM NMDA for 15 min in presence or absence of 100 mM ethanol. LDH-release, expressed as percentage of total LDH content, was measured 24h after NMDA wash out.

(*, P < 0.01 compared to NMDA induced LDH-release in control cultures; #, P < 0.01 compared to LDH-release in absence of ethanol).

From: József Nagy (2004) Renaissance of NMDA receptor antagonists: Do they have a role in the pharmacotherapy for alcoholism? *IDrugs: The Investigational Drugs Journal 7(4),* 339-350.

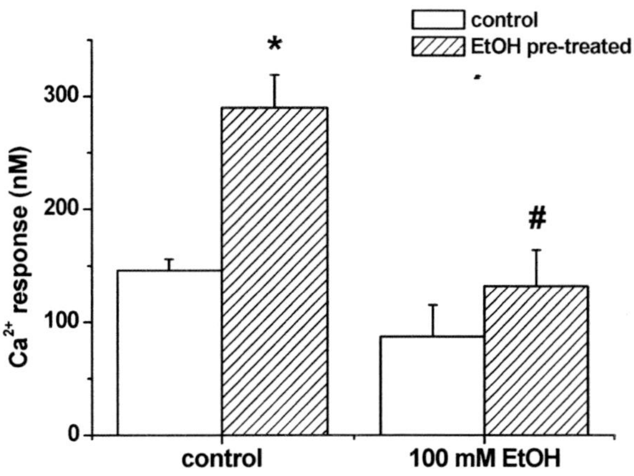

Figure 4B. Altered NMDA evoked calcium signals after ethanol pre-treatment.
Effect of chronic ethanol pre-treatment on NMDA induced changes in cytosolic calcium ion concentration. Control cortical cultures (open columns) and cortical cultures pre-treated with 100mM ethanol repeatedly, once daily for 3 days (dashed columns) were exposed to 10 μM NMDA in presence or absence of 100 mM ethanol. (*, $P < 0.01$ compared to NMDA induced elevation of [Ca2+]i in control cultures; #, $P < 0.05$ compared to elevation of [Ca2+]i in absence of ethanol).
From: József Nagy (2004) Renaissance of NMDA receptor antagonists: Do they have a role in the pharmacotherapy for alcoholism? *IDrugs: The Investigational Drugs Journal 7(4),* 339-350.

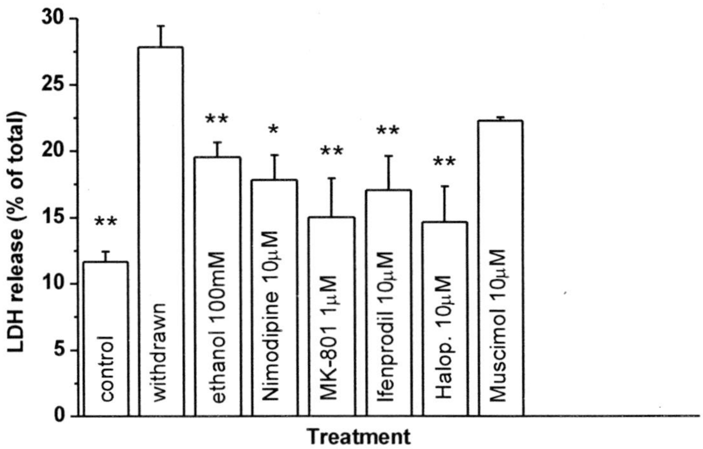

Figure 5. Inhibition of alcohol-withdrawal induced cytotoxicity by re-addition of ethanol and by treatment with different drugs. Columns represent LDH-release after 24 hours of the indicated treatment in primary cultures of rat cortical neurons pre-treated with 100 mM ethanol daily for 3 successive days. Control column shows LDH-release in cultures not adapted to ethanol.
(*: $p<0.05$, **: $p<0.01$ compared to the alcohol-adapted and withdrawn group)
From: József Nagy (2004) NR2B type of NMDA receptor subunits: a possible target in treatment for alcohol dependence. *Current Drug Targets – CNS & Neurological Disorders 3,* 169-179.

Changes in Structure of NMDARs

According to earlier reports, it was hypothesized that chronic ethanol treatment leads to an increase in the number of NMDARs leading to facilitated receptor function (Wirkner 1999). However, up-regulation of NMDAR expression has not been found in all studies after chronic ethanol exposition (Rudolph 1997; Ferreira 2001). According to the recently emerging view, the increased NMDAR function is presumably due to a differential up-regulation of the various NMDAR subunits. This conception is supported by several papers presenting evidence for altered NMDAR subunit composition after chronic ethanol treatment.

Notwithstanding, there is a disagreement in respect of the expression of the different NR1 splice variant forms and NR2 subunits. On the one hand, some authors reported no changes in subunit expression at all (Cebere 1999) and others found changes solely in the expression of the NR2A subunit due to long-term ethanol exposure (Darstein 2000). On the other hand, there are papers concluding that besides several other types of subunits and certain NR1 splice variants the expression of the NR2B subunit is increased. Lots of *in vitro* studies showed increased NR2B subunit mRNA levels, with no change in NR1 and/or NR2A subunit transcription in cultured cortical neurons following chronic ethanol administration (Morrow 1994; Hu 1996; Hardy 1999). On the contrary, the levels of NR2B as well as NR2A and NR1 subunit proteins were found increased in the cortex and hippocampus of rats or mice (Trevisan 1994; Follesa 1996a, 1996b; Kalluri 1998; Narita 2000; Henniger 2003). Furthermore, in cultured cerebellar granule cells, the 'developmental switch' of NR2B subunit for NR2A was found delayed resulting in higher NR2B and lower NR2A subunit levels (Snell 2001).

Similarly to these later observations, in primary cultures of rat cortical neurons treated with ethanol for three consecutive days, whereas the efficiency of the non-subunit selective NMDAR antagonists was not changed, the maximal inhibitory effect of ethanol as well as the NR2B subunit selective NMDAR antagonists tested was significantly increased (Figure 6, Table 2). Accordingly, whereas the immuno-labelling of the NR2A, NR2C, and NR2D subunits was not changed, increased NR2B immuno-labelling was observed in ethanol pre-treated compared to control cultures of rat cortical as well as hippocampal neurons. In addition, the expression of the C1 and C2' cassette containing splice variant forms of the NR1 subunit was also increased in these cultures (Figure 7) (Nagy 2003). Considering that i) the deactivation time of NMDARs composed of NR1/NR2B subunits is longer than those built up of NR1/NR2A subunits (Monyer 1992), ii) the deactivation rate is four times faster for receptors composed of NR1 subunit containing the N1 cassette than those lacking this cassette (Rumbaugh 2000; Cull-Candy 2001), and iii) NMDARs assembled of NR1 splice variants containing C1 and/or C2 cassettes may form functionally more active ion channels (Rameau 2000), the increased expression of the C1 and C2' cassette containing splice variant forms of the NR1 and/or the NR2B subunits may underlie the enhanced NMDAR function and subsequently the increased sensitivity of neurons to excitotoxic insults seen after ethanol withdrawal.

Table 2. Maximal Inhibition and Calculated IC_{50} Values of NMDAR Antagonists

Compound	Control		Ethanol pre-treated	
	I_{max} (%)	IC_{50}	I_{max} (%)	IC_{50}
MK-801	89 ± 4	104 ± 18 nM	92 ± 5	126 ± 18 nM
5,7-DCK	82 ± 2	23 ± 2 μM	85 ± 6	20 ± 4 μM
ethanol	34 ± 1	242 ± 6 mM	56 ± 6 *	177 ± 14 mM *
t-ifenprodil	63 ± 2	210 ± 29 nM	74 ± 6 *	167 ± 40 nM
CP-101606	48 ± 4	18 ± 3 nM	69 ± 6 *	18 ± 6 nM
CI-1041	51 ± 6	17 ± 5 nM	83 ± 9 **	12 ± 3 nM

Note: Maximal inhibition value (I_{max}) shows the mean ± S.E. of inhibition produced by the given antagonist at the maximal concentration used. IC_{50} data indicate the mean ± S.E. of the calculated IC_{50} values of individual measurements using Microcal™ Origin® 6.0 data analysis software.

From: Nagy, J., Kolok, S., Dezső, P., Boros, A., Szombathelyi, Z. (2003) Differential alterations in the expression of NMDA receptor subunits following chronic ethanol treatment in primary cultures of rat cortical and hippocampal neurons. ***Neurochem. Int. 42(1),*** 35-43.

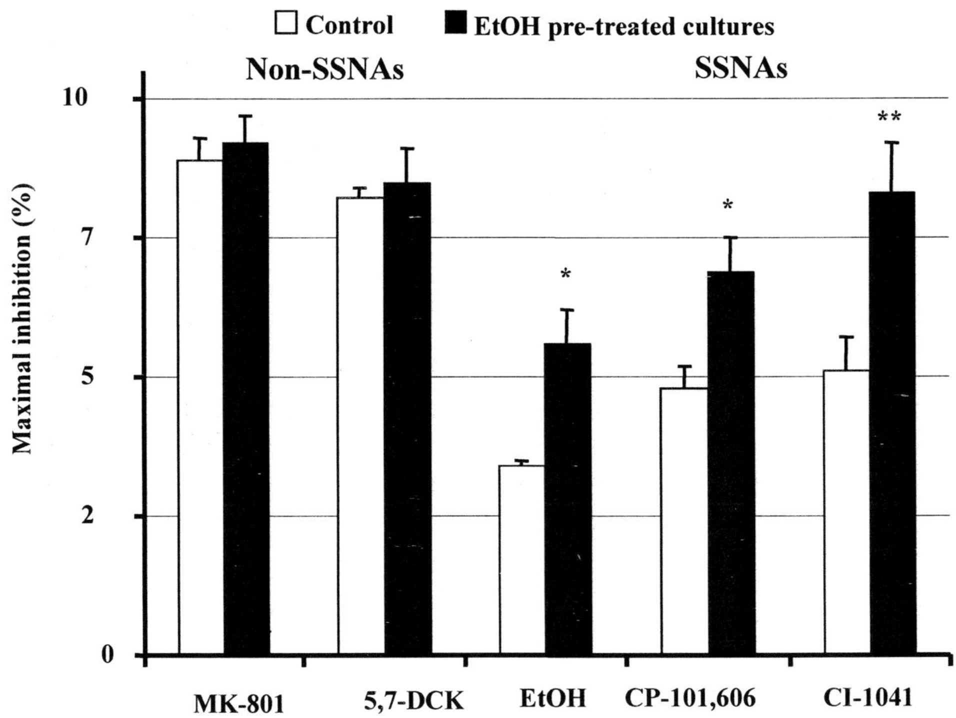

Figure 6. Effect of chronic ethanol pre-treatment on the inhibitory potential of different NMDA receptor antagonists

Maximal inhibitory effect of different NMDAR antagonists on NMDA induced cytosolic calcium elevation in control (white columns) and 100 mM ethanol pre-treated (black columns) primary rat cortical cultures. (*, $P < 0.05$; **, $P < 0.01$ compared to the adequate NMDA induced calcium increase in control cultures).

From: Nagy, J., Kolok, S., Dezső, P., Boros, A. (2003) Szombathelyi, Z. Differential alterations in the expression of NMDA receptor subunits following chronic ethanol treatment in primary cultures of rat cortical and hippocampal neurons. *Neurochem. Int., 42(1),* 35-43.

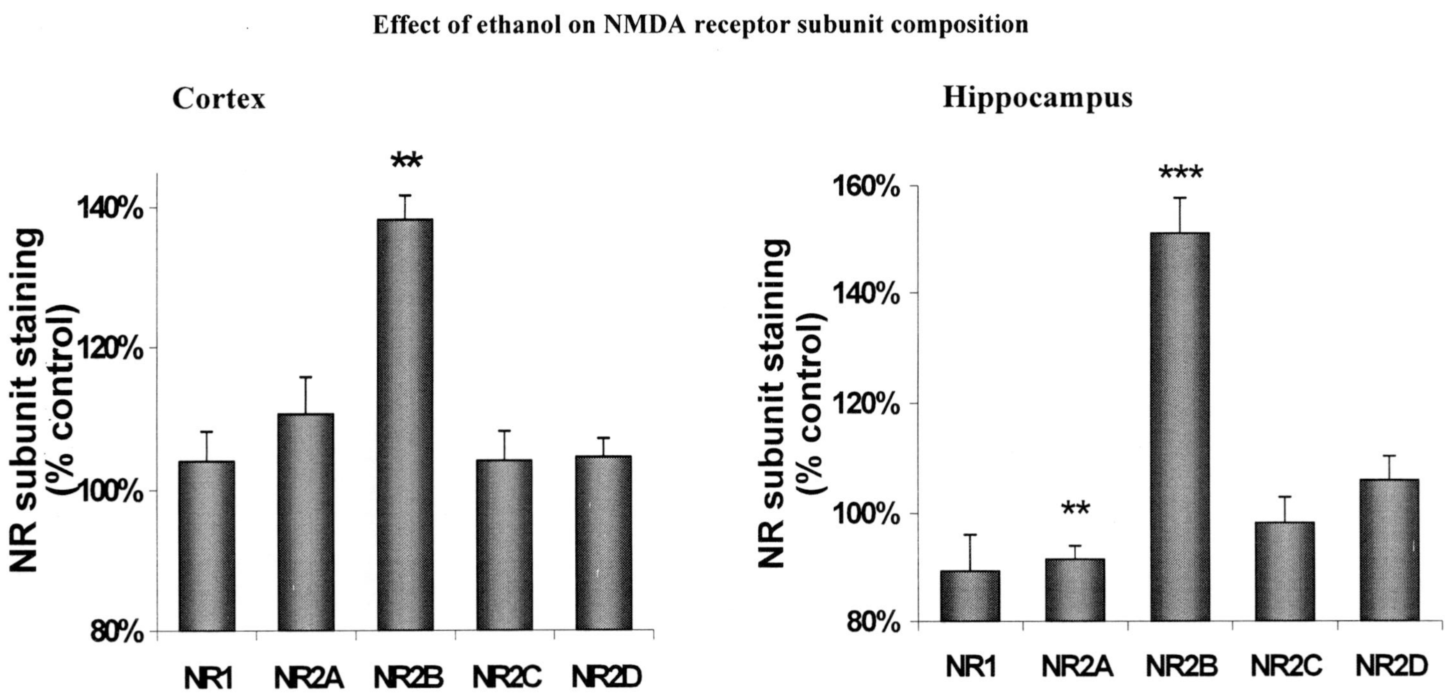

Figure 7. Effect of chronic ethanol pre-treatment on the expression of NMDA receptor subunits and NR1 splice cassettes

Expression of NMDA receptor subunit proteins was estimated by a flow-cytometry based immuno-cytochemical method in primary cultures of rat cortical and hippocampal neurones. Background related fluorescence values measured in 100 mM ethanol pre-treated cultures are expressed as percentage of those obtained in control cultures. (Continued on next page.)

(*, $P < 0.05$; **, $P < 0.01$; ***, $P < 0.001$ compared to control).

From: Nagy, J., Kolok, S., Dezső, P., Boros, A. (2003) Szombathelyi, Z. Differential alterations in the expression of NMDA receptor subunits following chronic ethanol treatment in primary cultures of rat cortical and hippocampal neurons. *Neurochem. Int., 42(1),* 35-43.

Effect of ethanol on the expression of NR1 splice cassettes

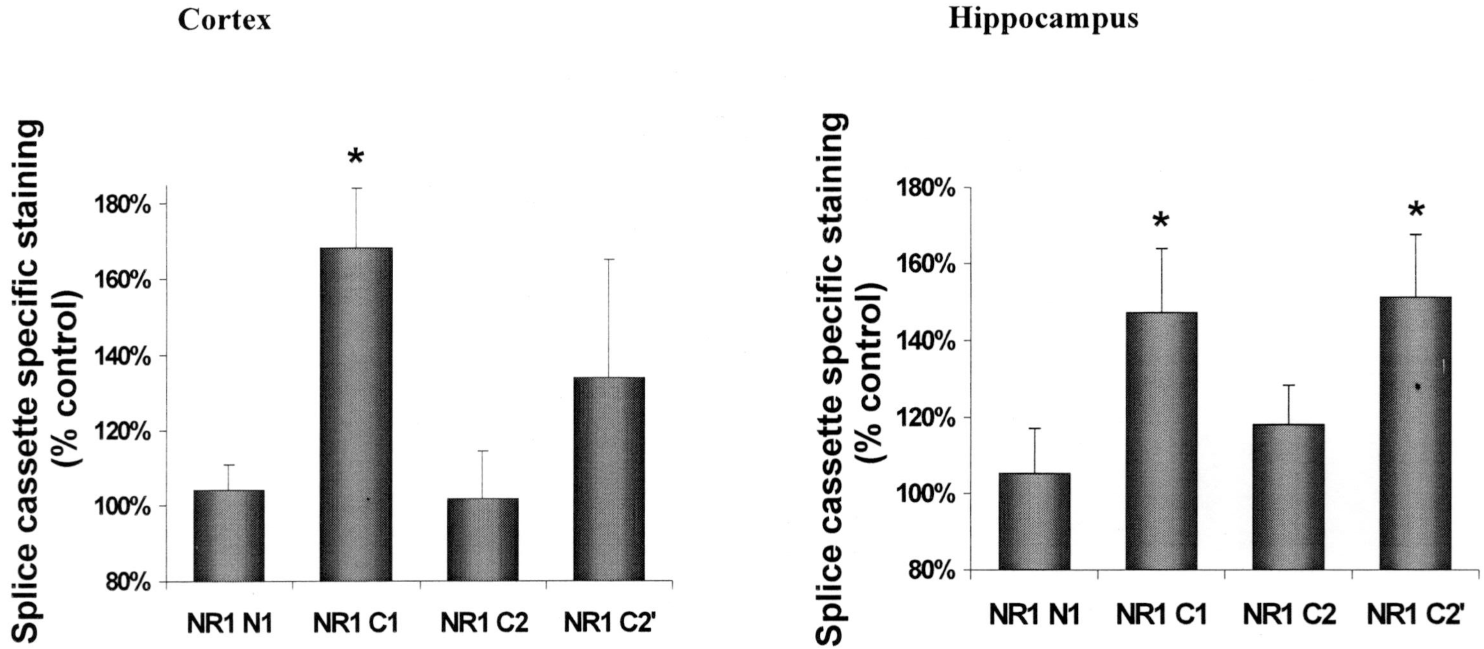

Figure 7. Effect of chronic ethanol pre-treatment on the expression of NMDA receptor subunits and NR1 splice cassettes

Expression of NMDA receptor subunit proteins was estimated by a flow-cytometry based immuno-cytochemical method in primary cultures of rat cortical and hippocampal neurones. Background related fluorescence values measured in 100 mM ethanol pre-treated cultures are expressed as percentage of those obtained in control cultures.

(*, $P < 0.05$; **, $P < 0.01$; ***, $P < 0.001$ compared to control).

From: Nagy, J., Kolok, S., Dezső, P., Boros, A. (2003) Szombathelyi, Z. Differential alterations in the expression of NMDA receptor subunits following chronic ethanol treatment in primary cultures of rat cortical and hippocampal neurons. *Neurochem. Int., 42(1),* 35-43.

According to Carpenter-Hyland et al. (2004), the co-localization of NR1 clusters with the presynaptic marker protein synapsin was increased in rat hippocampal neurons exposed to 50 mM ethanol for 4 days. This was accompanied by significant increases in the size and density of these synapsin-associated clusters with no change observed in non synapsin-associated NR1 clusters. Similar effects were observed with NR2B clustering after chronic ethanol exposure. The increase in synaptic NMDA receptor clustering was prevented by addition of a protein kinase A inhibitor or by co-exposure to a low concentration of NMDA and was reversed when ethanol was removed from the cultures. On the contrary, no changes were observed in the synaptic content, cluster size, or density of AMPA receptors after ethanol exposure. Electrophysiological measurements on ethanol-treated neurons revealed a similar enhancement in synaptic NMDA currents with no change in AMPA-mediated events.

It is known that Src family of protein tyrosine kinases, specifically Src and Fyn, up-regulates NMDAR function (Salter and Kalia 2004) thereby reducing the sensitivity of NMDARs to ethanol. Previously it was shown that both c-Src and Fyn kinases potentiate the NMDA-activated currents in *in vitro* recombinant systems (Chen and Leonard 1996; Kohr and Seeburg 1996; Anders 1999; Salter and Kalia 2004) as well as in spinal neurons (Wang and Salter 1994). Furthermore, phosphorylation status of NR1 and NR2B subunits was found increased in consequence of ethanol exposure (Miyakawa 1997). Concerning the NR1 subunit, truncation ($NR1_{858stop}$) (Anders 2000) or phosphorylation of Ser897 of this subunit (Maldve 2002) decreased the ability of ethanol to inhibit NMDA receptor function. In addition, the reduced sensitivity of NMDARs to ethanol was linked up with the dopamine receptor-1 activation via dopamine and cAMP-regulated phosphoprotein-32 kD (DARPP-32) phosphorylation (Maldve 2002). According to Yaka et al. (2003a, 2003b), the scaffolding protein RACK1 that binds Fyn kinase to the NR2B subunit dissociates from the complex due to ethanol exposure, consequently facilitating Fyn-mediated phosphorylation of the NR2B subunit leading to enhanced channel activity counteracting the inhibitory actions of ethanol. In addition, transgenic mice over-expressing the Fyn tyrosine kinase and withdrawn from alcohol failed to show any increase of anxiety-like behavior or reduction of exploratory activity like it was observed in case of their wild-type littermates (Stork 2002). This apparent lack of alcohol withdrawal-induced behavioral effects was associated with increased Fyn kinase activity and tyrosine phosphorylation of several proteins including the NR2B subunit.

Taken together, the changes in subunit expression, phosphorylation states and synaptic clustering of NMDAR subunits due to ethanol exposure may lead to the enhancement of NMDA responses. These changes may also explain the occurrence of acute ethanol tolerance leading to reinforcement of ethanol consumption and may underlie the development of ethanol dependence.

Consequences of Increased NMDAR Function

Presumably, in consequence of the increased function of NMDARs, enhanced release of glutamate was observed after chronic ethanol exposure both in *in vitro* as well as *in vivo* experiments. Besides several other factors (e.g. adaptive changes in GABA receptors and calcium channels), the NMDARs are major contributors to the increased glutamate release during alcohol withdrawal since in the brain of ethanol-dependent rats, the extracellular concentration of glutamate shows a transient, NMDAR mediated increase after cessation of ethanol intake and these changes are time-locked to the behavioral signs of ethanol withdrawal (Rossetti 1995; Fadda 1998). This enhanced glutamate release may contribute to the further shift towards the excitatory dominance in the CNS after ethanol withdrawal. Furthermore, the up-regulation of the NMDARs can enhance the activity of the noradrenergic system (Engberg and Hajos 1992a, 1992b) as well, that may account for the vegetative instability seen in serious states of alcohol withdrawal, especially in delirium tremens (Tsai 1995, 1998).

Recently, it has been hypothesized that the same neuronal system including the mesolimbic dopaminergic pathway mediates the reinforcement for alcohol and other addictive drugs like opiates or cocaine (Koob 1992; Nestler 1993). Indeed, ethanol has been reported to stimulate dopamine (DA) release in the nucleus accumbens (Imperato 1986) and electrophysiological studies have demonstrated a concomitant ethanol-induced increase in the activity of ventral tegmental dopaminergic neurons (Brodie 1990, 1999). On the other hand, systemic administration of NMDAR antagonists increases burst firing of dopaminergic neurons (Zhang 1992) and can stimulate release of DA from dopaminergic terminal areas suggesting that glutamate – acting through NMDARs – exerts a tonic inhibitory action on DA release in the nucleus accumbens (Hoffman 1996; Kretschmer 1999). According to the model of Fadda and Rossetti (1998), blockade of the NMDARs by acute ethanol treatment disinhibits dopaminergic neurons via GABAergic interneurons possessing NMDARs. Withdrawal of alcohol, similarly to withdrawal of opiates or cocaine, has been found associated with decreased DA release in the limbic forebrain areas (Rossetti 1992) due to decreased firing rate of dopaminergic neurons (Diana 1993). Thus, reduced dopaminergic functions seen after ethanol withdrawal may arise as a consequence of enhanced NMDA responses induced by chronic ethanol exposure.

All the above-discussed findings suggest the possibility that increased NMDA mediated neurotransmission may constitute the basis of both the motor signs (e.g. tremor, seizures etc.) and the affective or emotional disturbances (e.g. craving, dysphoria) associated with alcohol withdrawal. Bearing in mind that besides the glutamatergic system other transmitter mechanisms are also involved in the adaptive changes induced by chronic ethanol treatment and that *in vitro* experiments allow only limited conclusions to deduce for a whole organism, it is clear that alterations in NMDAR function play a critical role in these processes leading to the development of alcohol dependence and withdrawal symptoms. According to this view of the pathomechanism of alcohol withdrawal syndrome (AWS), the NMDAR may be a possible target and NMDAR antagonists may be useful agents for the treatment of both the physical and the psychical signs of alcohol withdrawal.

NMDAR Antagonists in Pharmacotherapy for Alcohol Withdrawal

In the early 90s, it was already hypothesized that NMDAR antagonists can block alcohol withdrawal induced seizures in ethanol dependent animals. Since then, extensive literature on animal experimental and preliminary clinical data suggest that NMDAR antagonists are promising candidates for the treatment of AWS, inasmuch as these compounds may attenuate not only the physical but also the affective and motivational components of AWS.

Competitive NMDA Receptor Antagonists

So far, mostly the classic competitive and channel blocking NMDAR antagonists were tested and proved to be useful in *in vitro* or animal models of alcoholism. Early experiments showed that competitive NMDA receptor antagonists acting at the glutamate site (e.g. CGP 39551, D-CPP-ene) decreased handling-induced hyperactivity after withdrawal from chronic ethanol treatment in mice (Liljequist 1991; Lamblin 1993; Ripley 1995). These compounds increased the threshold for population spikes in hippocampal slices from the same animals. NMDA antagonists acting within the ion channel (e.g. ketamine, MK-801 and ADCI) were also shown to suppress withdrawal-induced seizures effectively in both rats and mice (Fidecka 1989; Morrisett 1990; Grant 1996). Unfortunately, preclinical studies indicated that most of these compounds produce psychotomimetic or sedative effects, ataxia, muscle relaxation, neuronal damages (e.g. in the cingulate cortex) as well as motor and learning impairment.

These serious side effects impeded their introduction to the human therapy (Koek 1990; Murata 1993; Carter 1994; Parsons 1998; Yenari 1998; Breese 2002). However, due to immense therapeutic promise of NMDA antagonists in acute and/or chronic neurodegenerative and psychiatric disorders efforts have been made to develop compounds lacking these side effects. More encouraging approaches were performed with low affinity channel blockers like memantine or with NMDA antagonists acting on the glycine binding site (L-701,324) having more tolerable side effect profiles.

Channel Blockers

Novel channel blockers like memantine (1-amino-3,5-dimethyl-adamantane) and its analogue neramexane (MRZ 2/579, 1-amino-1,3,3,5,5-pentamethyl-cyclohexane hydrochloride) have improved side effect profile probably due to their moderate potency and rapid, strongly voltage-dependent blocking kinetics (Parsons 1999). These compounds greatly inhibited alcohol consumption without affecting water or food intake during relapse in a rat craving model (Hölter 1996, 2000; Shelton 1997; Piasecki 1998). In addition, neramexane as well as memantine effectively suppressed ethanol withdrawal induced seizures in alcohol dependent rats (Bienkowski 2001).

Glycine Site Antagonists

There are several observations that glycine and D-cycloserine can reverse the inhibitory effects of and rapid tolerance to ethanol (Rabe 1990; Woodward 1990; Buller 1995; Khanna 1995; Moraes-Ferreira 1997). Glycine-B site antagonists also attenuated the expression of withdrawal symptoms. A member of this type of NMDA receptor antagonists, L-701,324 (7-chloro-4-hydroxy-3-3-phenoxyphenyl-2-1H–quinolone) produced a dose-dependent inhibition of audiogenic seizures associated with alcohol withdrawal (Kotlinska and Liljequist 1996) and potently blocked the acquisition of ethanol-induced conditioned place preference (Biala and Kotlinska 1999).

Preliminary problems with glycine site antagonists included poor systemic availability has now been overcome with agents like GV196771A ((E)-4,6-Dichloro-3-(2-oxo-1-phenylpyrrolidin-3-ylidenemethyl)-1H-indole-2-carboxylic acid sodium salt) or SM-31900 (3(S)-(2- (4- (Amino methyl) -2- (1(R)-carboxyethoxy)phenylamino) -2- oxoethyl) -7- chloro -1,3,4,5- tetrahydrobenzo(c,d)indole -2- carboxylic acid hydrochloride) which are not only of very high affinity, but also have improved pharmacokinetic and physicochemical properties, such as good brain permeation and solubility (Jansen and Dannhardt 2003). Although these compounds were not tested in animal models related to alcoholism, the facts that SM-31900 has a potent anticonvulsant activity (Katayama 2001), GV196771A can inhibit the development of morphine tolerance (Quartaroli 2001) and both compounds are devoid of behavioral side effects (hyperactivity, motor dysfunction) make these compounds promising candidates also in the treatment of alcoholism.

Acamprosate

The American Food and Drug Administration (FDA) recently granted the approval of a novel anti-alcohol medication Campral (acamprosate calcium) to maintain abstinence in patients with alcohol dependence. In Europe, more than 4 million people have been treated with this agent since 1989 when it became commercially available in France. According to several human studies, acamprosate has a consistent effect on prolonging abstinence and reducing the rate of relapse, in conjunction with an equally consistent absence of effect on self-reported craving, suggesting that it can be used as a relapse-prevention medication.

In previous animal studies, it was observed that acamprosate dose-dependently reduced alcohol consumption with no effects on food and water intake. It could also lessen the increase in extracellular glutamate level and hypermotility during ethanol withdrawal (Dahchour 1998; Dahchour and De Witte 1999; Rammes 2001). The ability of acamprosate to reduce the glutamate level in microdialysates from nucleus accumbens during ethanol withdrawal was an important finding for the therapeutic use of this agent.

The exact mechanism of action of acamprosate, originally developed as a GABA analogue, was intensively investigated in the past years. According to several studies, acamprosate had no direct effect on NMDA responses in primary neuronal cultures (Popp and Lovinger 2000; Mayer 2002a; Nagy 2004). In spite of these findings, acamprosate effectively reduced the ethanol-withdrawal evoked neuronal cell death in ethanol pre-treated organotypic hippocampal (Mayer 2002b) or primary cortical cultures from the rat (Figure 8) (al-Qatari 2001; Nagy 2004). On the other hand, acamprosate was reported by several other authors to have an inhibitory effect on the native or recombinant NMDA-receptors (Spanagel 1997b; Allgaier 2000; Rammes 2001). alQatari et al. (1998) argued that acamprosate may have an excitatory or inhibitory effect on NMDA receptors depending upon the experimental conditions indicating that acamprosate, at least partly, acts as a 'partial agonist' at the NMDA receptor (alQatari 1998). In addition, acamprosate was shown to bind to a spermidine-sensitive site on the NMDAR and to modulate the function of NMDARs (Naassila 1998). Based on these observations a glutamatergic hypothesis for the action of acamprosate and a causal relationship between NMDA antagonism and the anticraving properties of acamprosate has been suggested (Lhuintre 1985, 1990; Spanagel and Zieglgansberger 1997a; Holter 1997; Heyser 1998; Dahchour 1998; Bolo 1998).

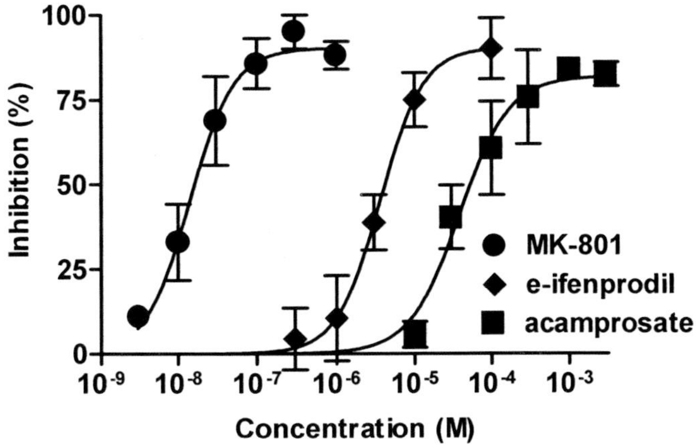

Figure 8. Inhibitory effect of different compounds on ethanol-withdrawal-induced neurotoxicity Neuronal cell death caused by 24-hour ethanol-withdrawal in primary cultures of rat cortical neurones pre-treated with 100 mM ethanol for 3 consecutive days was quantified by measuring LDH-release. Different concentrations of MK-801, erythro-ifenprodil and acamprosate were present during the withdrawal period. Each point represents the percentage of inhibition (mean ± S.E. (error bars)). *From:* Nagy, J., Horváth, C., Farkas, S., Kolok, S., Szombathelyi, Z. (2004a) NR2B subunit selective NMDA antagonists inhibit neurotoxic effect of alcohol-withdrawal in primary cultures of rat cortical neurons. *Neurochem. Int., 44(1),* 17-23.

NR2B Subunit Selective Antagonists

In recent years, a novel type of NMDAR antagonists, the NR2B subunit selective ones have emerged and received considerable attention. This type of compounds showed potency in models of neurodegeneration (Kew 1998), Parkinson disease (Nash 1999, 2000; Wright 2000; Steece-Collier 2000), and hyperalgesia (Boyce 1999; Carter 2000; Fillhard 2000; Chizh 2001). It was also realized that this type of compounds lacks the serious side effects of the classic NMDAR antagonists' (Nikam and Meltzer 2002). Although, like other un-competitive NMDAR antagonists they may have some adverse effect on learning and memory, it was proved that they have a wider separation between doses that are effective in seizure or stroke models and those that disrupt learning and memory. The limited information on the novel NR2B SSNAs such as CP-101,606 (traxoprodil) (Chenard 1995; Kemp and McKernan 2002), Ro25-6981 (Fischer 1997), Co-101244 (Zhou 1999), CI-1041 (Chizh 2002) and RG-1103 (Borza 2003) (Figure 9, Table 3) also suggests that these drugs are better tolerated and are largely devoid of adverse CNS effects at antinociceptive doses, at least with respect to psychotomimetic, ataxic and sedative effects (Taniguchi 1997; Boyce 1999; Carter 2000; Fillhard 2000; Murray 2000; Chizh 2001).

Table 3. Selectivity of Novel NR2B Subunit Selective NMDA Antagonists

Compound	Inhibition of NMDA evoked Ca^{2+} responses (IC_{50} values)		Selectivity (NR2B vs. 2A)
	NR1/NR2A	NR1/NR2B	
CP-101,606	> 30 μM	30.0 ± 3.6 nM	> 1000
Ro-25-6981	> 10 μM	57 ± 10 nM	> 175
Co-101244	> 30 μM	4.8 ± 0.7 nM	> 6250
CI-1041	> 50 μM	8.4 ± 1.4 nM	> 5950
RG-13579	> 30 μM	19.9 ± 4.5 nM	> 1600
RG-1103	> 30 μM	2.1 ± 0.4 nM	> 13600

Compounds were tested for their inhibitory activity on 100 μM NMDA induced calcium elevation in HEK 293 cells stably expressing recombinant NMDA receptor (Nagy 2003b). IC_{50} values were determined and degrees of selectivity were evaluated as the ratio of IC_{50} values obtained in cells expressing NR1/NR2A and NR1/NR2B receptors.

From: József Nagy, Csilla Horváth, Sándor Farkas, Sándor Kolok, Zsolt Szombathelyi (2004) NR2B subunit selective NMDA antagonists inhibit neurotoxic effect of alcohol-withdrawal in primary cultures of rat cortical neurons. *Neurochemistry International 44(1),* 17-23.

The initial chemical leads of NR2B SSNAs – ifenprodil and eliprodil – were found effective in animal models of alcohol dependence. According to Malinowska et al. (1999), ifenprodil potently reduced the severity of withdrawal-induced seizures. Oral administration of increasing doses of eliprodil produced a dose-dependent and almost complete inhibition of ethanol withdrawal produced audiogenic seizures in alcohol dependent Sprague-Dawley rats (Kotlinska and Liljequist 1996). This effect of eliprodil was achieved at doses that by themselves did not alter the basal locomotor activity of untreated control animals. Similar results were observed in alcohol dependent male C57BL/6J mice (Narita 2000). The expression of spontaneous ethanol withdrawal signs (piloerection, jerk, tremor) occurring 6 – 12 hours after the discontinuation of ethanol treatment was suppressed by ifenprodil and was accompanied by a marked up-regulation of the NR2B subunit in the limbic forebrain of ethanol treated mice. According to Kotlinska and Liljequist (1997), eliprodil effectively reversed the reduction in extracellular DA level during ethanol withdrawal but only partially and dose-independently substituted ethanol indicating that it has no discriminative stimulus properties similar to those produced by ethanol.

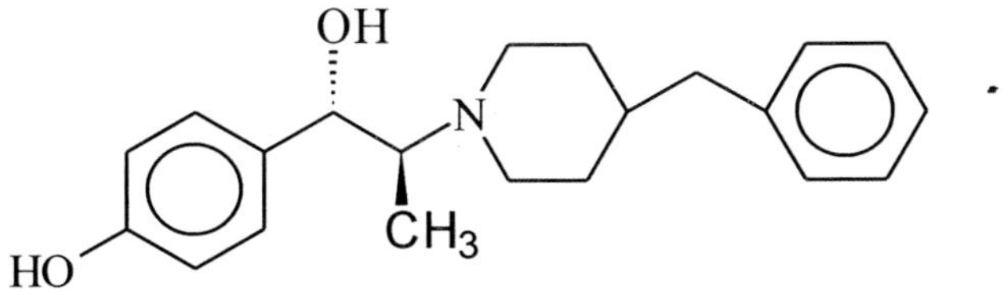

ifenprodil

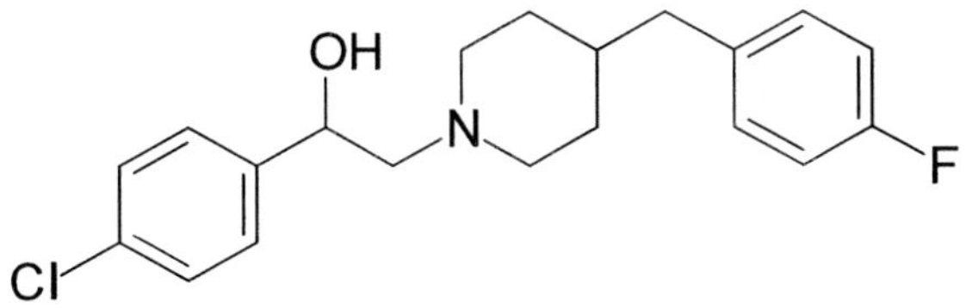

eliprodil

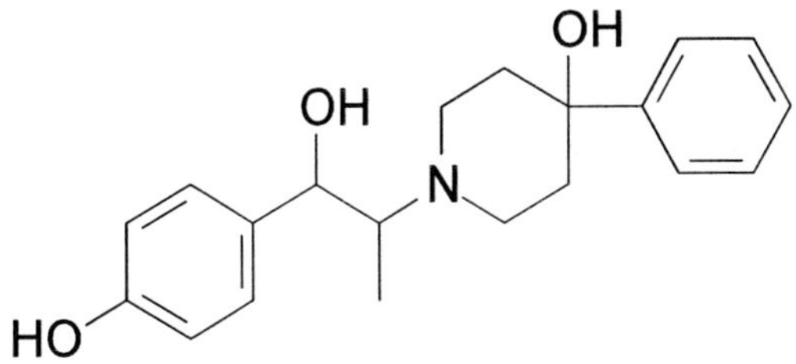

CP-101,606

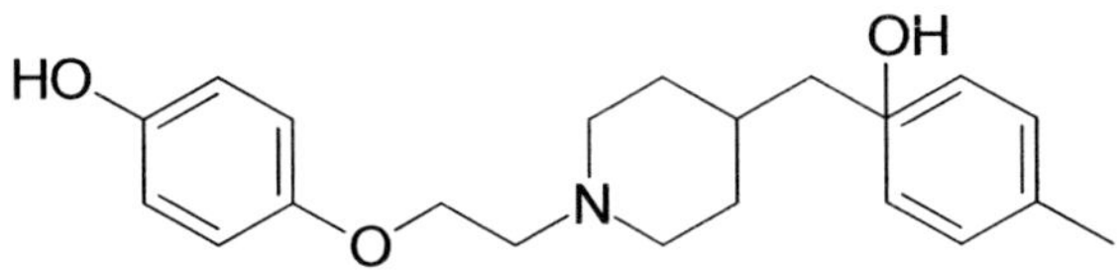

Co-101244

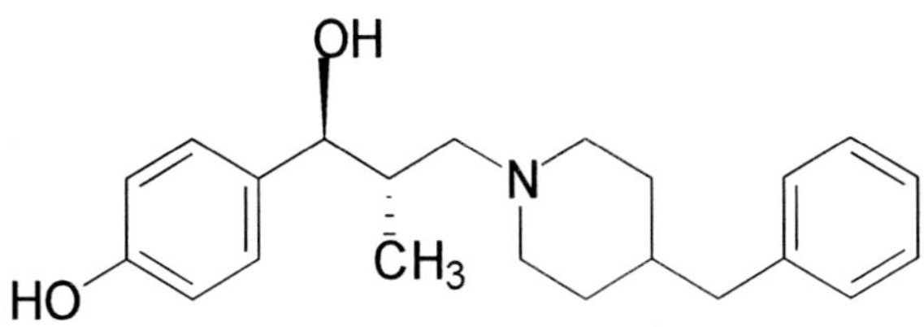

Ro-25-6981

Figure 9. NR2B subunit selective NMDAR antagonists. (Continued on mext page.)

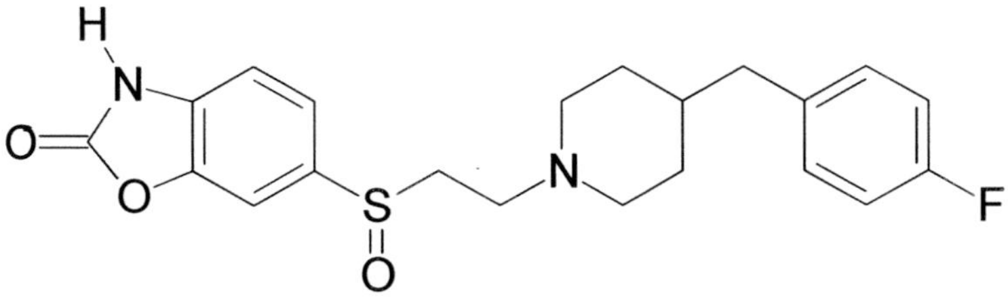

CI-1041

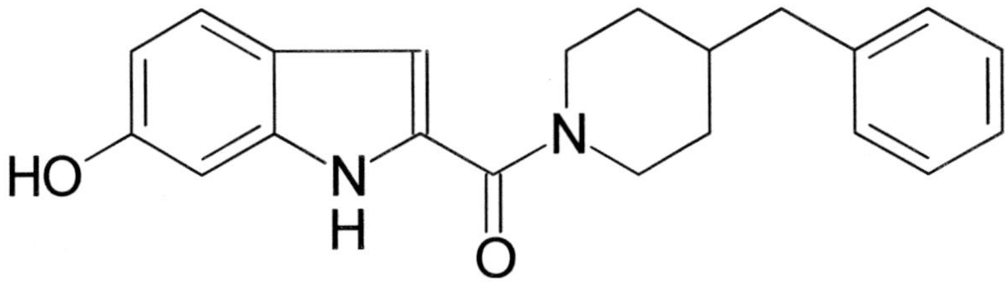

RGH-13579

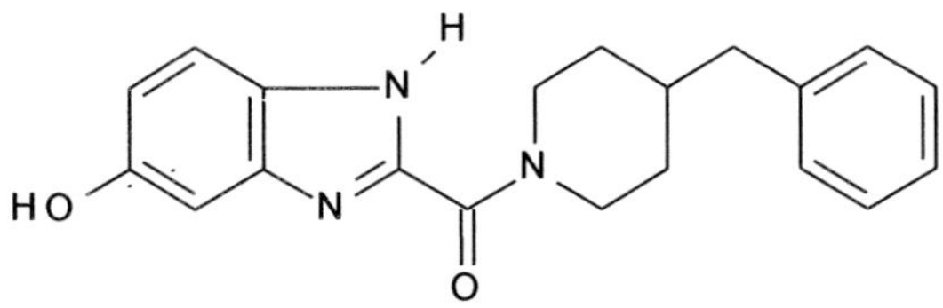

RGH-1103

Figure 9. NR2B subunit selective NMDAR antagonists

In primary cultures of cortical neurons from rats pretreated with ethanol intermittently for 3 days, some of the novel indole-2-carboxamide derivative NR2B SSNAs (RGH-13579 and RGH-1103 (Borza 2003)) as well as CP-101,606, Co-101244 and CI-1041 potently and dose-dependently reduced the withdrawal-evoked LDH release (Figure 10). One of the novel compounds (RGH-1103) was as effective as MK-801, the most potent but not subunit selective, channel blocker NMDAR antagonist. The inhibitory potencies of the NR2B SSNAs for withdrawal-induced toxicity was in good linear relation with their effectiveness for inhibition of NMDA induced cytosolic calcium elevation (Table 4) (Nagy 2004a).

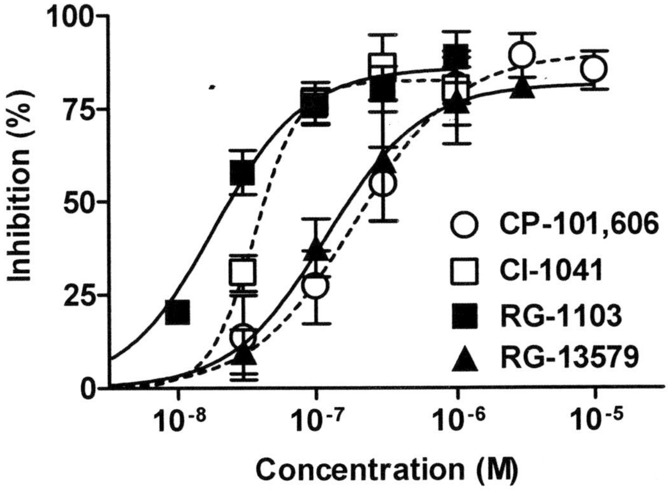

Figure 10. Inhibitory effect of NR2B SSNAs on ethanol-withdrawal-induced neurotoxicity Neuronal cell death caused by 24-hour ethanol-withdrawal in primary cultures of rat cortical neurones pre-treated with 100 mM ethanol for 3 consecutive days was quantified by measuring LDH-release. Different concentrations of some known (open symbols, dashed lines) and novel (filled symbols, straight lines) NR2B SSNAs were present during the withdrawal period. Each point represents the percentage of inhibition (mean ± S.E. (error bars)).

From: Nagy, J., Horváth, C., Farkas, S., Kolok, S., Szombathelyi, Z. (2004) NR2B subunit selective NMDA antagonists inhibit neurotoxic effect of alcohol-withdrawal in primary cultures of rat cortical neurons. *Neurochem. Int., 44(1),* 17-23.

Table 4. Inhibitory Effect of NMDA Antagonists on Cytosolic Calcium Rises and Ethanol Withdrawal Induced Neurotoxicity

Compound	NMDA evoked Ca^{2+} elevation		withdrawal induced toxicity	
	I_{max} (%)	IC_{50} (μM)	I_{max} (%)	IC_{50} (μM)
MK-801	100 ± 5	0.037 ± 0.002	90 ± 5	0.020 ± 0.004
CP-101,606	58 ± 2	0.041 ± 0.005	89 ± 9	0.201 ± 0.061
Co-101244	67 ± 2	0.024 ± 0.003	101 ± 5	0.206 ± 0.045
CI-1041	70 ± 3	0:007 ± 0.001	82 ± 6	0.037 ± 0.008
RGH-13579	77 ± 3	0.018 ± 0.004	81 ± 18	0.137 ± 0.067
RGH-1103	74 ± 2	0.002 ± 0.0004	87 ± 6	0.019 ± 0.005
Acamprosate	−1.2 ± 2.9	> 300	82 ± 8	40 ± 13

Compounds were tested for their inhibitory effect on cytosolic calcium elevation evoked by 40 μM NMDA and on ethanol-withdrawal produced neurotoxicity in primary cultures of rat cortical neurons.

From: József Nagy, Csilla Horváth, Sándor Farkas, Sándor Kolok, Zsolt Szombathelyi (2004) NR2B subunit selective NMDA antagonists inhibit neurotoxic effect of alcohol-withdrawal in primary cultures of rat cortical neurons. *Neurochemistry International 44(1),* 17-23.

Summary

According to the recently emerged glutamatergic theory of the pathomechanism of alcohol withdrawal syndrome, increased NMDA receptor function plays a central role in the development of alcohol dependence and manifestation of the withdrawal symptoms. Furthermore, at least partly, an increase in the expression of the NR2B subunit underlies the alcohol-induced alterations (Nagy 2004b, 2004c). Since NMDA receptor antagonists can reduce hyperactivity, seizures, and neuronal cell loss associated with alcohol withdrawal, novel NMDA receptor antagonists, especially NR2B subunit selective ones, may be effective in the treatment of the physical symptoms of withdrawal. Since NMDAR antagonists can also restore the reduced DA brain levels associated with ethanol withdrawal and thereby can reduce psychical symptoms of alcohol dependence, novel type of NMDAR antagonists could be promising agents to prevent relapse and maintain abstinence as well.

In the last decade, great achievements have been made in research for novel, subunit selective NMDA antagonists. Several such agents potent in animal models of a number of CNS diseases and showing improved side-effect profile have been identified and characterized. Although, only few of them have been examined and found effective in animal models of alcoholism, their *in vitro* and – according to the available preliminary data – *in vivo* efficiency is encouraging. To answer the question whether these agents will be useful in the pharmacotherapy for alcohol dependence is a major challenge for the forthcoming years.

References

Akinshola, B.E. (2001) Straight-chain alcohols exhibit a cutoff in potency for the inhibition of recombinant glutamate receptor subunits. *Br. J. Pharmacol., 133(5),* 651-658.

Allgaier, C., Franke, H., Sobottka, H., Scheibler, P. (2000) Acamprosate inhibits Ca2+ influx mediated by NMDA receptors and voltage-sensitive Ca2+ channels in cultured rat mesencephalic neurones. *Naunyn Schmiedebergs Arch. Pharmacol., 362(4-5),* 440-443.

Allgaier, C. (2002) Ethanol sensitivity of NMDA receptors. *Neurochem. Int.,41(6),* 377-382.

Alvestad, R.M., Grosshans, D.R., Coultrap, S.J., Nakazawa, T., Yamamoto, T., Browning, M.D. (2003) Tyrosine dephosphorylation and ethanol inhibition of N-Methyl-D-aspartate receptor function. *J. Biol. Chem., 278(13),* 11020-11025.

Anders, D.L., Blevins, T., Sutton, G., Chandler, L.J., Woodward, J.J. (1999) Effects of c-Src tyrosine kinase on ethanol sensitivity of recombinant NMDA receptors expressed in HEK 293 cells. *Alcohol Clin. Exp. Res., 23(2),* 357-362.

Anders, D.L., Blevins, T., Smothers, C.T., Woodward, J.J. (2000) Reduced ethanol inhibition of N-methyl-D-aspartate receptors by deletion of the NR1 C0 domain or overexpression of alpha-actinin-2 proteins. *J. Biol. Chem., 275(20),* 5019-5024.

Avenet, P., Leonardon, J., Besnard, F., Graham, D., Frost, J., Depoortere, H., Langer, S.Z., Scatton, B. (1996) Antagonist properties of the stereoisomers of ifenprodil at NR1A/NR2A and NR1A/NR2B subtypes of the NMDA receptor expressed in Xenopus oocytes. *Eur. J. Pharmacol., 296(2),* 209-213.

Avenet, P., Leonardon, J., Besnard, F., Graham, D., Depoortere, H., Scatton, B. (1997) Antagonist properties of eliprodil and other NMDA receptor antagonists at rat NR1A/NR2A and NR1A/NR2B receptors expressed in Xenopus oocytes. *Neurosci. Lett., 223(2),* 133-136.

Ballenger, J.C. & Post, R.M. (1978) Kindling as a model for alcohol withdrawal syndromes. *Br. J. Psychiatry., 133,* 1-14.

Becker, H.C. & Hale, R.L. (1993) Repeated episodes of ethanol withdrawal potentiate the severity of subsequent withdrawal seizures: an animal model of alcohol withdrawal "kindling". *Alcohol Clin. Exp. Res., 17(1),* 94-98.

Biala, G. & Kotlinska, J. (1999) Blockade of the acquisition of ethanol-induced conditioned place preference by N-methyl-D-aspartate receptor antagonists. *Alcohol Alcohol., 34(2),* 175-182.

Bienkowski, P., Krzascik, P., Koros, E., Kostowski, W., Scinska, A., Danysz, W. (2001) Effects of a novel uncompetitive NMDA receptor antagonist, MRZ 2/579 on ethanol self-administration and ethanol withdrawal seizures in the rat. *Eur. J. Pharmacol., 413(1),* 81-89.

Blevins, T., Mirshahi, T., Woodward, J., (1995) Increased agonist and antagonist sensitivity of N-methyl-D-aspartate stimulated calcium flux in cultured neurons following chronic ethanol exposure. *Neurosci. Lett., 200,* 214-218.

Blevins, T., Mirshahi, T., Chandler, L.J., Woodward, J.J. (1997) Effects of acute and chronic ethanol exposure on heteromeric N-methyl-D-aspartate receptors expressed in HEK 293 cells. *J. Neurochem., 69(6),* 2345-2354.

Borza, I., Kolok, S., Gere, A., Agai-Csongor, E., Agai, B., Tarkanyi, G., Horvath, C., Barta-Szalai, G., Bozo, E., Kiss, C., Bielik, A., Nagy, J., Farkas, S., Domany, G. (2003) Indole-2-carboxamides as novel NR2B selective NMDA receptor antagonists. *Bioorganic & Medicinal Chemistry Letters, 13,* 3859–3861.

Boyce, S., Wyatt, A., Webb, J.K., O'Donnell, R., Mason, G., Rigby, M., Sirinathsinghji, D., Hill, R.G., Rupniak, N.M. (1999) Selective NMDA NR2B antagonists induce antinociception without motor dysfunction: correlation with restricted localisation of NR2B subunit in dorsal horn. *Neuropharmacology, 38(5),* 611-623.

Breese, G.R., Knapp, D.J., Moy, S.S. (2002) Integrative role for serotonergic and glutamatergic receptor mechanisms in the action of NMDA antagonists: potential relationships to antipsychotic drug actions on NMDA antagonist responsiveness. *Neurosci. Biobehav. Rev., 26(4),* 441-455.

Brimecombe, J.C., Boeckman, F.A. and Aizenman E. (1997) Functional consequences of NR2 subunit composition in single recombinant N-methyl-D-aspartate receptors. *Proc. Natl. Acad. Sci. USA, 94,* 11019-11024.

Brodie, M.S., Shefner, S.A., Dunwiddie, T.V. (1990) Ethanol increases the firing rate of dopamine neurons of the rat ventral tegmental area in vitro. *Brain Res., 508(1),* 65-69.

Brodie, M.S., Pesold, C., Appel, S.B. (1999) Ethanol directly excites dopaminergic ventral tegmental area reward neurons. *Alcohol Clin. Exp. Res., 23(11),* 1848-1852.

Buller, A.L., Larson, H.C., Morrisett, R.A., Monaghan, D.T., (1995) Glycine modulates ethanol inhibition of heteromeric N-methyl-D-aspartate receptors expressed in Xenopus oocytes. *Mol. Pharmacol., 48(4),* 717-723.

Carpenter-Hyland E.P., Woodward J.J., Chandler L.J. (2004) Chronic Ethanol Induces Synaptic But Not Extrasynaptic Targeting of NMDA Receptors. *J. Neurosci., 24(36),* 7859 –7868.

Carter, A.J., (1994) Many agents that antagonize the NMDA receptor-channel complex in vivo also cause disturbances of motor coordination. *J. Pharmacol. Exp. Ther., 269(2),* 573-580.

Carter, R.B., Wilent, W., Huber, M., Xu, Z., Vanover, K.E., Woodward R.M. (2000) Anti-allodynic and anti-hyperalgesic effects of the nr2b subunit-selective nmda antagonist ci-1041 in rat models of inflammation and neuropathy *Soc. Neurosci. Abstr., 26,* 617.3.

Cebere, A., Cebers, G., Liljequist, S. (1999) Enhancement of NMDA-induced functional responses without concomitant NMDA receptor changes following chronic ethanol exposure in cerebellar granule cells. *Naunyn Schmiedebergs Arch. Pharmacol., 360(6),* 623-632.

Chandler, L.J., Norwood, D., Sutton, G. (1999) Chronic ethanol upregulates NMDA and AMPA, but not kainate receptor subunit proteins in rat primary cortical cultures. *Alcohol Clin. Exp. Res., 23(2),* 363-370.

Chen, C, Leonard, J.P. (1996) Protein tyrosine kinase-mediated potentiation of currents from cloned NMDA receptors. *J. Neurochem., 67(1),* 194-200.

Chenard, B.L., Bordner, J., Butler, T.W., Chambers, L.K., Collins, M.A., De Costa, D.L., Ducat, M.F., Dumont, M.L., Fox, C.B., Mena, E.E., et al. (1995) (1S,2S)-1-(4-hydroxyphenyl)-2-(4-hydroxy-4-phenylpiperidino)-1-propanol: a potent new neuroprotectant which blocks N-methyl-D-aspartate responses. *J. Med. Chem., 38(16),* 3138-3145.

Chizh, B.A., Headley, P.M., Tzschentke, T.M. (2001) NMDA receptor antagonists as analgesics: focus on the NR2B subtype. *Trends Pharmacol. Sci., 22(12),* 636-642.

Chizh, B.A., (2002) Novel approaches to targeting glutamate receptors for the treatment of chronic pain: Review article *Amino Acids, 23,* 169-176.

Christine, C.W., Choi, D.W. (1990) Effect of zinc on NMDA receptor-mediated channel currents in cortical neurons. *J. Neurosci., 10(1),* 108-116.

Chu, B., Anantharam, V., Treistman, S.N. (1995) Ethanol inhibition of recombinant heteromeric NMDA channels in the presence and absence of modulators. *J. Neurochem., 65(1),* 140-148.

Costa, E.T., Savage, D.D., Valenzuela, C.F. (2000) Acute effects of ethanol on kainate receptors in cultured hippocampal neurons. *Alcohol Clin. Exp. Res., 24(5),* 706-715.

Cull-Candy, S., Brickley, S., Farrant, M. (2001) NMDA receptor subunits: diversity, development and disease. *Current Opinion in Neurobiology, 11,* 327–335.

Dahchour, A., De Witte, P., Bolo, N., Nedelec, J.F., Muzet, M., Durbin, P., Macher, J.P. (1998) Central effects of acamprosate: part 1. Acamprosate blocks the glutamate increase in the nucleus accumbens microdialysate in ethanol withdrawn rats. *Psychiatry Res., 82(2),* 107-114.

Dahchour, A. & De Witte, P. (1999) Effect of repeated ethanol withdrawal on glutamate microdialysate in the hippocampus. *Alcohol Clin. Exp. Res., 23(10),* 1698-1703.

Dahchour, A. & De Witte, P. (2000) Ethanol and amino acids in the central nervous system: assessment of the pharmacological actions of acamprosate. *Pro. Neurobiol., 60(4),* 343-362.

Danysz, W. & Parsons, C.G. (1998) Glycine and N-methyl-D-aspartate receptors: physiological significance and possible therapeutic applications. *Pharmacological Reviews, 50(4),* 597-664.

Darstein, M.B., Landwehrmeyer, G.B., Feuerstein, T.J. (2000) Changes in NMDA receptor subunit gene expression in the rat brain following withdrawal from forced long-term ethanol intake. *Naunyn Schmiedebergs Arch. Pharmacol., 361(2),* 206-213.

Das, S., Sasaki, Y F., Rothe, T., Premkumar, L S., Takasu, M., Crandall, J E., Dikkes, P., Conner, D A., Rayudu, P V., Cheung, W., Chen, H S., Lipton, S A., Nakanishi, N. (1998) Increased NMDA current and spine density in mice lacking the NMDA receptor subunit NR3A. *Nature, 393(6683),* 377-381.

Davies, M. (2003) The role of GABAA receptors in mediating the effects of alcohol in the central nervous system. *J. Psychiatry Neurosci., 28(4),* 263-274.

Di Chiara, G., Tanda G., Cadoni, C., Aquas E., Bassareo, V., Carboni, E. (1998) Homologies and differences in the action of drugs of abuse and a conventional reinforcer (food) on dopamine transmission: an interpretative framework of the mechanism of drug dependenc *Adv. Pharmacol., 42,* 983-987.

Diana, M., Pistis, M., Carboni, S., Gessa, G L., Rossetti, Z L. (1993) Profound decrement of mesolimbic dopaminergic neuronal activity during ethanol withdrawal syndrome in rats: electrophysiological and biochemical evidence. *Proc. Natl. Acad. Sci. USA, 90(17),* 7966-7969.

Dildy, J.E. & Leslie, S.W. (1989) Ethanol inhibits NMDA-induced increases in free intracellular Ca2+ in dissociated brain cells. *Brain Res., 499,* 383-387.

Editorial (2004) Time for coordinated action on alcohol. *The Lancet, 363,* 9414.

Engberg, G. & Hajos, M. (1992) Ethanol attenuates the response of locus coeruleus neurons to excitatory amino acid agonists in vivo. *Naunyn Schmiedebergs Arch. Pharmacol., 345(2),* 222-226

Engberg, G. & Hajos, M. (1992b) Alcohol withdrawal reaction as a result of adaptive changes of excitatory amino acid receptors. *Naunyn Schmiedebergs Arch. Pharmacol., 346(4),* 437-441.

Fadda, F. & Rossetti, Z.L. (1998) Chronic ethanol consumption: from neuroadaptation to neurodegeneration. *Prog. Neurobiol., 56(4),* 385-431.

Ferrani-Kile, K., Randall, P.K., Leslie, S.W. (2003) Acute ethanol affects phosphorylation state of the NMDA receptor complex: implication of tyrosine phosphatases and protein kinase A. *Brain Res. Mol. Brain Res., 115(1),* 78-86.

Ferreira, V.M., Frausto, S., Browning, M.D., Savage, D.D., Morato, G.S., Valenzuela, C.F. (2001) Ionotropic glutamate receptor subunit expression in the rat hippocampus: lack of an effect of a long-term ethanol exposure paradigm. *Alcohol Clin. Exp. Res., 25(10),* 1536-1541.

Fidecka, S., Langwinski, R. (1989) Interaction between ketamine and ethanol in rats and mice. *Pol. J. Pharmacol. Pharm., 41(1),* 23-32.

Fillhard, J.A., Kinsora J.J., Meltzer L.T. (2000) The effects of ci-1041 in two tests of analgesia: acetic acid-induced writing test and formalin foot pad test. Soc. *Neurosci. Abstr., 26,* 617.4.

Fink, K. & Göthert, M. (1996) Both ethanol and ifenprodil inhibit NMDA-evoked release of various neurotransmitters at different, yet proportional potency: potential relation to NMDA receptor subunit composition. *Naunyn Schmiedebergs Arch. Pharmacol., 354(3),* 312-319.

Fischer, G., Mutel, V., Trube, G., Malherbe, P., Kew, J.N., Mohacsi, E., Heitz, M.P., Kemp, J.A. (1997) Ro 25-6981, a highly potent and selective blocker of N-methyl-D-aspartate receptors containing the NR2B subunit. Characterization in vitro. *J. Pharmacol. Exp. Ther., 283(3),* 1285-1292.

Floyd, D.W., Jung, K.Y., McCool, B.A. (2003) Chronic ethanol ingestion facilitates N-methyl-D-aspartate receptor function and expression in rat lateral/basolateral amygdala neurons. *J. Pharmacol. Exp. Ther., 307(3),* 1020-1029.

Follesa, P. & Ticku, M.K. (1996a) NMDA receptor upregulation: molecular studies in cultured mouse cortical neurons after chronic antagonist exposure. *J. Neurosci., 16,* 2172-2178.

Follesa, P. & Ticku, M.K. (1996b) Chronic ethanol-mediated up-regulation of the N-methyl-D-aspartate receptor polypeptide subunits in mouse cortical neurons in culture. *J. Biol. Chem., 271(23),* 13297-13299.

Franks, N.P. & Lieb, W.R. (1994) Molecular and cellular mechanisms of general anaesthesia. *Nature, 367(6464),* 607-614.

Gallagher, M.J., Huang, H., Pritchett, D.B., Lynch, D.R. (1996) Interactions between ifenprodil and the NR2B subunit of the N-methyl-D-aspartate receptor. *J. Biol. Chem., 271(16),* 9603- 9611

Gallagher, M J, Huang, H, Grant, E R, Lynch, D R. (1997) The NR2B-specific interactions of polyamines and protons with the N-methyl-D-aspartate receptor. *J. Biol. Chem., 272(40),* 24971-24979.

Godden, E.L., Harris, R.A., Dunwiddie, T.V. (2001). Correlation between molecular volume and effects of n-alcohols on human neuronal nicotinic acetylcholine receptors expressed in Xenopus oocytes. *J. Pharmacol. Exp. Ther., 296(3),* 716-722.

Gonzalez, L.P., Veatch, L.M., Ticku, M.K., Becker, H.C. (2001) Alcohol withdrawal kindling: mechanisms and implications for treatment. *Alcohol Clin. Exp. Res., 25,* 197S-201S.

Grant, K.A., Valverius, P., Hudspith, M., Tabakoff, B. (1990) Ethanol withdrawal seizures and the NMDA receptor complex. *Eur. J. Pharmacol., 176,* 289-296.

Grant, K.A., Lovinger, D.M. (1995) Cellular and behavioral neurobiology of alcohol: receptor-mediated neuronal processes. *Clin. Neurosci., 3(3),* 155-164.

Grant, K.A., Colombo, G., Grant, J., Rogawski, M.A. (1996) Dizocilpine-like discriminative stimulus effects of low-affinity uncompetitive NMDA antagonists. *Neuropharmacology, 35(12),* 1709-1719.

Grant, B.F., Dawson, D.A., Stinson, F.S., Chou, S.P., Dufour, M.C., Pickering, R.P. (2004). The 12-month prevalence and trends in DSM-IV alcohol abuse and dependence: United States, 1991–1992 and 2001–2002. *Drug and Alcohol Dependence, 74,* 223–234.

Hardy, P.A., Chen, W., Wilce, P.A., (1999) Chronic ethanol exposure and withdrawal influence NMDA receptor subunit and splice variant mRNA expression in the rat cerebral cortex. *Brain Res., 819(1-2),* 33-39.

Harris, B.R., Gibson, D.A., Prendergast, M.A., Blanchard, J.A., Holley, R.C., Hart, S.R., Scotland, R.L., Foster, T.C., Pedigo, N.W., Littleton, J.M. (2003) The neurotoxicity induced by ethanol withdrawal in mature organotypic hippocampal slices might involve cross-talk between metabotropic glutamate type 5 receptors and N-methyl-D-aspartate receptors. *Alcohol Clin. Exp. Res., 27(11),* 1724-1735.

Henniger, M.S., Wotjak, C.T., Holter, S.M. (2003) Long-term voluntary ethanol drinking increases expression of NMDA receptor 2B subunits in rat frontal cortex. *Eur. J. Pharmacol., 470(1-2),* 33-36.

Heyser, C.J., Schulteis, G., Durbin, P., Koob, G.F. (1998) Chronic acamprosate eliminates the alcohol deprivation effect while having limited effects on baseline responding for ethanol in rats. *Neuropsychopharmacology, 18(2),* 125-133.

Hoffman, P.L., Rabe, C.S., Moses, F., Tabakoff, B. (1989) N-methyl-D-aspartate receptors and ethanol: inhibition of calcium flux and cyclic GMP production. *J. Neurochem., 52,* 61937-61940.

Hoffman, P.L., Rabe, C.S., Grant, K.A., Valverius, P., Hudspith, M., Tabakoff, B. (1990) Ethanol and the NMDA receptor *Alcohol., 7(3),* 229-231.

Hoffman, P.L. & Tabakoff, B. (1996) Alcohol dependence: a commentary on mechanisms. *Alcohol Alcohol., 31(4),* 333-340.

Hollmann, M. Structure of ionotropic glutamate receptors. In Ionotropic Glutamate Receptors in the CNS. Edited by Jonas, P., Monyer, H., Berlin: Springer, 1999, 1-98.

Hölter, S.M., Danysz, W., Spanagel, R. (1996) Evidence for alcohol anti-craving properties of memantine. *Eur. J. Pharmacol., 314,* R1–R2.

Hölter, SM., Landgraf, R., Zieglgansberger, W., Spanagel, R. (1997) Time course of acamprosate action on operant ethanol self-administration after ethanol deprivation. *Alcohol Clin. Exp. Res., 21(5),* 862-868.

Hölter, S.M., Danysz, W., Spanagel, R. (2000) Novel Uncompetitive N-Methyl-D-Aspartate (NMDA)-Receptor Antagonist MRZ 2/579 Suppresses Ethanol Intake in Long-Term Ethanol-Experienced Rats and Generalizes to Ethanol Cue in Drug Discrimination Procedure. *J. Pharmacol. Exp. Ther., 292,* 545–552.

Honer, M., Benke, D., Laube, B., Kuhse, J., Heckendorn, R., Allgeier, H., Angst, C., Monyer, H., Seeburg, P H., Betz, H., Mohler, H. (1998) Differentiation of glycine antagonist sites of N-methyl-D-aspartate receptor subtypes. Preferential interaction of CGP 61594 with NR1/2B receptors. *J. Biol. Chem., 273(18),* 11158-11163.

Hu, X.J., Follesa, P., Ticku, M.K. (1996) Chronic ethanol treatment produces a selective upregulation of the NMDA receptor subunit gene expression in mammalian cultured cortical neurons. *Brain Res. Mol. Brain Res., 36,* 211-218.

Hu, X.J. & Ticku, M.K. (1997) Functional characterization of a kindling-like model of ethanol withdrawal in cortical cultured neurons after chronic intermittent ethanol exposure. *Brain Res., 767(2),* 228-234.

Husi, H. & Grant, S.G. (2001) Isolation of 2000-kDa complexes of N-methyl-D-aspartate receptor and postsynaptic density 95 from mouse brain. *J. Neurochem., 77(1),* 281-291.

Ibbotson, T., Field, M.J., Boden, P.R. (1997) Effect of chronic ethanol treatment in vivo on excitability in mouse cortical neurones in vitro. *Br. J. Pharmacol., 122(5),* 956-962.

Imperato, A. & Di Chiara, G. (1986) Preferential stimulation of dopamine release in the nucleus accumbens of freely moving rats by ethanol. *J. Pharmacol. Exp. Ther., 239(1),* 219-228.

Jansen, M., Dannhardt, G. (2003) Antagonists and agonists at the glycine site of the NMDA receptor for therapeutic interventions. *European Journal of Medicinal Chemistry, 38,* 661-670.

Kalluri, H.S., Mehta, A.K., Ticku, M.K. (1998) Up-regulation of NMDA receptor subunits in rat brain following chronic ethanol treatment. *Brain Res. Mol. Brain Res., 58(1-2),* 221-224.

Kashiwagi, K., Fukuchi, J., Chao, J., Igarashi, K., Williams, K. (1996) An aspartate residue in the extracellular loop of the N-methyl-D-aspartate receptor controls sensitivity to spermine and protons. *Mol. Pharmacol., 49(6),* 1131-1141.

Katayama, S., Ae, N., Nagata, R. (2001) Synthesis of tricyclic indole-2-carboxylic [correction of caboxylic] acids as potent NMDA-glycine antagonists. *J. Org. Chem., 66,* 3474-3483.

Kemp, J.A. & McKernan, R.M. (2002) NMDA receptor pathways as drug targets. *Nature Neurosci. Supp., 5,* 1039-1042.

Kew, J.N., Trube, G., Kemp, J.A. (1998) State-dependent NMDA receptor antagonism by Ro 8-4304, a novel NR2B selective, non-competitive, voltage-independent antagonist. *Br. J. Pharmacol., 123(3),* 463-472.

Khanna, J.M., Morato, G.S., Chau, A., Shah, G. (1995) D-cycloserine enhances rapid tolerance to ethanol motor incoordination. *Pharmacol Biochem Behav., 52(3),* 609-614.

Koek, W., Colpaert, F.C. (1990) Selective blockade of N-methyl-D-aspartate (NMDA)-induced convulsions by NMDA antagonists and putative glycine antagonists: relationship with phencyclidine-like behavioral effects. *J. Pharmacol. Exp. Ther., 252(1),* 349-357.

Kohr, G., Seeburg, P.H. (1996) Subtype-specific regulation of recombinant NMDA receptor-channels by protein tyrosine kinases of the src family. *J. Physiol., 492 (Pt 2),* 445-452.

Koob, G.F. (1992) Drugs of abuse: anatomy, pharmacology and function of reward pathways. *Trends Pharmacol. Sci., 13(5),* 177-184.

Kotlinska, J. & Liljequist, S. (1996) Oral administration of glycine and polyamine receptor antagonists blocks ethanol withdrawal seizures. *Psychopharmacology (Berl), 127(3),* 238-244.

Kotlinska, J. & Liljequist, S. (1997) The NMDA/glycine receptor antagonist, L-701,324, produces discriminative stimuli similar to those of ethanol. *Eur. J. Pharmacol., 332(1),* 1-8.

Kretschmer, B.D. (1999) Modulation of the mesolimbic dopamine system by glutamate: role of NMDA receptors. *J. Neurochem., 73(2),* 839-848.

Kumari, M., Ticku, M.K. (2000) Regulation of NMDA receptors by ethanol. *Prog. Drug Res., 54,* 152-189.

Kuner, T., Schoepfer, R., Korpi, E.R. (1993) Ethanol inhibits glutamate-induced currents in heteromeric NMDA receptor subtypes. *Neuroreport, 5(3),* 297-300.

Lamblin, F., Deuceuninck, D., DeWitte, P. (1993) Modulation of alcohol preference by NMDA antagonists in male rats. *Alcohol Alcohol., 28(6),* 639-647.

Laube, B., Kuhse, J., Betz, H. (1998) Evidence for a tetrameric structure of recombinant NMDA receptors. *J. Neurosci., 18(8),* 2954-2961.

Lerma, J. (1992) Spermine regulates N-methyl-D-aspartate receptor desensitization. *Neuron, 8(2),* 343-352.

Lhuintre, J.P., Daoust, M., Moore, N.D., Chretien, P., Saligaut, C., Tran, G., Boismare, F., Hillemand, B. (1985) Ability of calcium bis acetyl homotaurine, a GABA agonist, to prevent relapse in weaned alcoholics. *Lancet, 1,* 1014-1016.

Lhuintre, J.P., Moore, N., Tran, G., Steru, L., Langrenon, S., Daoust, M., Parot, P., Ladure, P., Libert, C., Boismare, F., et al. (1990) Acamprosate appears to decrease alcohol intake in weaned alcoholics. *Alcohol Alcohol., 25,* 613-622.

Li, C., Peoples, R.W., Weight, F.F. (1994) Alcohol action on a neuronal membrane receptor: evidence for a direct interaction with the receptor protein. *Proc. Natl. Acad. Sci. USA, 91(17),* 8200-8204.

Liljequist, S. (1991) The competitive NMDA receptor antagonist, CGP 39551, inhibits ethanol withdrawal seizures. *Eur. J. Pharmacol., 192(1),* 197-198.

Lovinger, D.M., White G. and Weight, F.F. (1989) Ethanol inhibits NMDA-activated ion current in hippocampal neurons. *Science, 243,* 1721-1724.

Lovinger, D.M., White, G., Weight, F.F. (1990) NMDA receptor-mediated synaptic excitation selectively inhibited by ethanol in hippocampal slice from adult rat. *J. Neurosci., 10,* 41372-41379.

Lovinger, D.M. (1993) Excitotoxicity and alcohol-related brain damage. *Alcohol Clin. Exp. Res., 17(1),* 19-27.

Lovinger, D.M. (1995) Developmental decrease in ethanol inhibition of N-methyl-D-aspartate receptors in rat neocortical neurons: relation to the actions of ifenprodil. *J. Pharmacol. Exp. Ther., 274(1),* 164-172.

Maldve, R.E., Zhang, T.A., Ferrani-Kile, K., Schreiber, S.S., Lippmann, M.J., Snyder, G.L., Fienberg, A.A., Leslie, S.W., Gonzales, R.A., Morrisett, R.A. (2002) DARPP-32 and regulation of the ethanol sensitivity of NMDA receptors in the nucleus accumbens. *Nat. Neurosci., 5(7),* 641-648.

Malinowska, B., Napiorkowska-Pawlak, D., Pawlak, R., Buczko, W., Gothert, M. (1999) Ifenprodil influences changes in mouse behaviour related to acute and chronic ethanol administration. *Eur. J. Pharmacol., 377(1),* 13-19.

Masood, K., Wu, C., Brauneis, U., Weight, F.F. (1994) Differential ethanol sensitivity of recombinant N-methyl-D-aspartate receptor subunits. *Mol. Pharmacol., 45,* 324–329.

Mayer, S., Harris, B., Gibson, D.A., Blanchard, J., Prendergast, M.A., Holley, R.C., Littleton, J. (2002a) Acamprosate has no effect on NMDA-induced toxicity but reduces toxicity induced by spermidine or by changing the medium in organotypic hippocampal slice cultures from rat. *Alcohol. Clin. Exp. Res., 26(5),* 655-662.

Mayer, S., Harris, B.R., Gibson, D.A., Blanchard, J.A., Prendergast, M.A., Holley, R.C., Littleton, J. (2002b) Acamprosate, MK-801, and ifenprodil inhibit neurotoxicity and calcium entry induced by ethanol withdrawal in organotypic slice cultures from neonatal rat hippocampus. *Alcohol. Clin. Exp. Res., 26(10),* 1468-1478.

Meguro, H., Mori, H., Araki, K., Kushiya, E., Kutsuwada, T., Yamazaki, M., Kumanishi, T., Arakawa, M., Sakimura, K., Mishina, M. (1992) Functional characterization of a heteromeric NMDA receptor channel expressed from cloned cDNAs. *Nature, 357(6373),* 70-74.

Meyer, H. (1901) Zur theorie der alkolnarkose der einfluss wechselnder temperatur auf wirkungsstarke und theilungscoefficient der narcotica. *Naunyn-Schmiedeberg's Arch. Exp. Pathol. Pharmacol., 46,* 338–346.

Mihic, S.J., Ye, Q., Wick, M.J., Koltchine, V.V., Krasowski, M.D., Finn, S.E., Mascia, M.P., Valenzuela, C.F., Hanson, K.K., Greenblatt, E.P., Harris, R.A., Harrison, N.L. (1997) Sites of alcohol and volatile anaesthetic action on GABA(A) and glycine receptors. *Nature, 389(6649),* 385-389.

Mirshahi, T., & Woodward, J. (1995) Ethanol sensitivity of heteromeric NMDA receptors: effects of subunit assembly, glycine and NMDAR1 Mg(2+)-insensitive mutants. *J. Neuropharmacology, 34,* 347–355.

Miyakawa, T., Yagi, T., Kitazawa, H., Yasuda, M., Kawai, N., Tsuboi, K., Niki, H. (1997) Fyn-kinase as a determinant of ethanol sensitivity: relation to NMDA-receptor function. *Science, 278(5338),* 698-701.

Monyer, H., Sprengler, R., Schoepfer, R., Herb, A., Higuchi, M., Lomeli, H., Burnashev, N., Sakmann, B., Seeburg. P.H. (1992) Heteromeric NMDA receptors: molecular and functional distinction of subtypes. *Science, 256,* 1217-1221.

Monyer, H., Burnashev, N., Laurie, D.J., Sakmann, B., Seeburg, P.H. (1994) Developmental and regional expression in the rat brain and functional properties of four NMDA receptors. *Neuron, 12(3),* 529-40.

Moraes-Ferreira, V.M., Morato, G.S. (1997) D-cycloserine blocks the effects of ethanol and HA-966 in rats tested in the elevated plus-maze. *Alcohol. Clin. Exp. Res., 21(9),* 1638-1642.

Moriyoshi, K., Masu, M., Ishii, T., Shigemoto, R., Mizuno, N., Nakanishi, S. (1991) Molecular cloning and characterization of the rat NMDA receptor. *Nature, 354(6348),* 31-37.

Morrisett, R.A., Rezvani, A.H., Overstreet, D., Janowsky, D.S., Wilson, W.A., Swartzwelder, H.S. (1990) MK-801 potently inhibits alcohol withdrawal seizures in rats. *Eur. J. Pharmacol., 176(1),* 103-105.

Morrow, A.L., Devaud L.L., Bucci, D., Smith F.D., (1994) GABAA and NMDA receptor subunit mRNA expression in ethanol dependent rats. *Alcohol Alcohol., 2,* 89-95.

Mothet, J.P., Parent, A.T., Wolosker, H., Brady, R.O. Jr,, Linden, D.J., Ferris, C.D., Rogawski, M.A., Snyder, S.H. (2000) D-serine is an endogenous ligand for the glycine site of the N-methyl-D-aspartate receptor. *Proc. Natl. Acad. Sci. USA., 97(9),* 4926-4931.

Murata, S., Kawasaki, K. (1993) Common and uncommon behavioural effects of antagonists for different modulatory sites in the NMDA receptor/channel complex. *Eur. J. Pharmacol., 239(1-3),* 9-15.

Murray, F. Kennedy, J., Hutson, P.H., Elliot, J., Huscroft, I., Mohnen, K., Russell, M.G., Grimwood, S. (2000) Modulation of [3H]MK-801 binding to NMDA receptors in vivo and in vitro. *Eur. J. Pharmacol., 397,* 263–270.

Nagy, J., Müller, F., László L. (2001) Cytotoxic effect of alcohol-withdrawal on primary cultures of cortical neurones. *Drug Alcohol Depend., 61,* 155–162.

Nagy, J. & László L. (2002) Increased sensitivity to NMDA is involved in alcohol-withdrawal induced cytotoxicity observed in primary cultures of cortical neurones chronically pre-treated with ethanol. *Neurochem. Int., 40,* 585–591.

Nagy, J., Kolok, S., Dezső, P., Boros, A. (2003) Szombathelyi, Z. Differential alterations in the expression of NMDA receptor subunits following chronic ethanol treatment in primary cultures of rat cortical and hippocampal neurones. *Neurochem. Int., 42(1),* 35-43.

Nagy J., Boros, A., Dezső, P., Kolok, S., Fodor L. (2003b) Inducible expression and pharmacology of recombinant NMDA receptors, composed of rat NR1a/NR2B subunits. *Neurochemistry International 43,* 19–29.

Nagy, J., Horváth, C., Farkas, S., Kolok, S., Szombathelyi, Z. (2004a) NR2B subunit selective NMDA antagonists inhibit neurotoxic effect of alcohol-withdrawal in primary cultures of rat cortical neurones. *Neurochem. Int., 44(1),* 17-23.

Nagy, J. (2004b) Renaissance of NMDA receptor antagonists: Do they have a role in the pharmacotherapy for alcoholism? *IDrugs: The Investigational Drugs Journal, 7(4),* 339-350.

Nagy, J. (2004c) NR2B type of NMDA receptor subunits: a possible target in treatment for alcohol dependence. *Current Drug Targets CNS Neurol Disord. 3(3),* 169-179.

Narita, M., Soma, M., Narita, M., Mizoguchi, H., Tseng, L F., Suzuki, T. (2000) Implications of the NR2B subunit-containing NMDA receptor localized in mouse limbic forebrain in ethanol dependence. *Eur. J. Pharmacol., 401(2),* 191-195.

Nash, J.E., Hill, M.P., Brotchie, J.M. (1999) Antiparkinsonian actions of blockade of NR2B-containing NMDA receptors in the reserpine-treated rat. *Exp. Neurol., 155(1),* 42-48.

Nash, J.E., Fox, S.H., Henry, B., Hill, M.P., Peggs, D., McGuire, S., Maneuf, Y., Hille, C., Brotchie, J.M., Crossman, A.R. (2000) Antiparkinsonian actions of ifenprodil in the MPTP-lesioned marmoset model of Parkinson's disease. *Exp. Neurol., 165(1),* 136-142.

Nestler, E.J. (1993) Cellular responses to chronic treatment with drugs of abuse. *Crit. Rev. Neurobiol., 7(1),* 23-39.

Nevo, I., Hamon, M. (1995) Neurotransmitter and neuromodulatory mechanisms involved in alcohol abuse and alcoholism. *Neurochem. Int., 26(4),* 305-336.

Nikam, S.S., Meltzer, L.T., (2002) NR2B selective NMDA receptor antagonists. *Current Pharmaceutical Design, 8,* 845-855.

Overton, E. (1896) Uber die osmotischem eigenschaften der zelle in ihrer betdeurtung dur die toxikologie und pharmakolgie. *Z. Physikal Chem., 22,* 189–209.

Parsons, C.G., Danysz, W., Hesselink, M., Hartmann, S., Lorenz, B., Wollenburg, C., Quack, G. (1998) Modulation of NMDA receptors by glycine--introduction to some basic aspects and recent developments. *Amino-Acids., 14(1-3),* 207-216.

Parsons, C.G., Danysz, W., Bartmann, A., Spielmanns, P., Frankiewicz, T., Hesselink, M., Eilbacher, B., Quack, G. (1999) Amino-alkyl-cyclohexanes are novel uncompetitive NMDA receptor antagonists with strong voltage-dependency and fast blocking kinetics: in vitro and in vivo characterization. *Neuropharmacology, 38(1),* 85-108.

Peoples, R.W., Weight, F.F. (1995) Cutoff in potency implicates alcohol inhibition of N-methyl-D-aspartate receptors in alcohol intoxication. *Proc. Natl. Acad. Sci. USA., 92(7),* 2825-2829.

Peoples, R.W., White, G., Lovinger, D.M., Weight, F.F. (1997) Ethanol inhibition of N-methyl-D-aspartate-activated current in mouse hippocampal neurones: whole-cell patch-clamp analysis. *Br. J. Pharmacol., 122(6),* 1035-1042.

Perez-Otano, I., Schulteis, C.T., Contractor, A., Lipton, S.A.., Trimmer, J S., Sucher, N.J., Heinemann, S.F. (2001) Assembly with the NR1 subunit is required for surface expression of NR3A-containing NMDA receptors. *J. Neurosci., 21(4),* 1228-1237.

Piasecki, J., Koros, E., Dyr, W., Kostowski, W., Danysz, W., Bienkowski, P. (1998) Ethanol-reinforced behaviour in the rat: effects of uncompetitive NMDA receptor antagonist, memantine. *Eur. J. Pharmacol., 354(2-3),* 135-143.

Popp, R.L Lickteig, R., Browning, M.D., Lovinger, D.M. (1998) Ethanol sensitivity and subunit composition of NMDA receptors in cultured striatal neurons. *Neuropharmacology, 37(1),* 45-56.

Popp, R.L & Lovinger, D.M. (2000) Interaction of acamprosate with ethanol and spermine on NMDA receptors in primary cultured neurons. *Eur. J. Pharmacol., 394(2-3),* 221-231.

Premkumar, L.S. & Auerbach, A.J. (1997) Subconductance states of a mutant NMDA receptor channel kinetics, calcium, and voltage dependence. *Gen. Physiol., 110(5),* 485-502.

Quartaroli, M., Fasdelli, N., Bettelini, L., Maraia, G., Corsi, M. (2001) GV196771A, an NMDA receptor/glycine site antagonist, attenuates mechanical allodynia in neuropathic rats and reduces tolerance induced by morphine in mice. *Eur. J. Pharmacol., 430(2-3),* 219-227.

alQatari, M.; Bouchenafa, O., Littleton, J. (1998) Mechanism of action of acamprosate. Part II. Ethanol dependence modifies effects of acamprosate on NMDA receptor binding in membranes from rat cerebral cortex. *Alcohol. Clin. Exp. Res. 22(4),* 810-814.

al-Qatari, M., Khan, S., Harris, B., Littleton, J. (2001) Acamprosate is neuroprotective against glutamate-induced excitotoxicity when enhanced by ethanol withdrawal in neocortical cultures of fetal rat brain. *Alcohol. Clin. Exp. Res. 25(9),* 1276-1283.

Rabe, C.S. & Tabakoff, B. (1990) Glycine site-directed agonists reverse the actions of ethanol at the N-methyl-D-aspartate receptor. *Mol. Pharmacol., 38(6),* 753-757.

Rameau, A.G., Akaneya, Y., Chiu, L.Y., Ziff, E.B. (2000) Role of NMDA receptor functional domains in excitatory cell death. *Neuropharmacology, 39,* 2255-2266.

Rammes, G., Mahal, B., Putzke, J., Parsons, C., Spielmanns, P., Pestel, E., Spanagel, R., Zieglgansberger, W., Schadrack, J., (2001) The anti-craving compound acamprosate acts as a weak NMDA-receptor antagonist, but modulates NMDA-receptor subunit expression similar to memantine and MK-801. *Neuropharmacology, 40(6),* 749-760.

Ripley, T.L. & Little, H.J. (1995) Effects on ethanol withdrawal hyperexcitability of chronic treatment with a competitive N-methyl-D-aspartate receptor antagonist. *J. Pharmacol. Exp. Ther., 272(1),* 112-118.

Rock, D.M. & Macdonald, R.L. (1992) The polyamine spermine has multiple actions on N-methyl-D-aspartate receptor single-channel currents in cultured cortical neurons. *Mol. Pharmacol., 41(1),* 83-88.

Ronald, K.M., Mirshahi, T., Woodward J.J. (2001) Ethanol inhibition of N-methyl-D-aspartate receptors is reduced by site-directed mutagenesis of a transmembrane domain phenylalanine residue. *J. Biol. Chem., 276(48),* 44729–44735.

Rossetti, Z.L., Hmaidan, Y., Gessa, G.L. (1992) Marked inhibition of mesolimbic dopamine release: a common feature of ethanol, morphine, cocaine and amphetamine abstinence in rats. *Eur. J. Pharmacol., 221(2-3),* 227-234.

Rossetti, Z.L. & Carboni, S. (1995) Ethanol withdrawal is associated with increased extracellular glutamate in the rat striatum. *Eur. J. Pharmacol., 283(1-3),* 177-183.

Rudolph, J.G., Walker, D.W., Iimuro, Y., Thurman, R.G., Crews, F.T. (1997) NMDA receptor binding in adult rat brain after several chronic ethanol treatment protocols. *Alcohol Clin Exp Res., 21(8),* 1508-1519.

Rumbaugh, G., Prybylowski, K., Wang, J.F., Vicini, S.J. (2000) Exon 5 and spermine regulate deactivation of NMDA receptor subtypes. *Neurophysiol., 83(3),* 1300-1306.

Salter, M.W. & Kalia, L.V. (2004) Src kinases: a hub for NMDA receptor regulation. *Nat. Rev. Neurosci., 5,* 317-328.

Schorge, S. & Colquhoun, D. (2003) Studies of NMDA receptor function and stoichiometry with truncated and tandem subunits. *J. Neurosci., 23(4),* 1151–1158.

Shelton, K.L. & Balster, R.L. (1997) Effects of gamma-aminobutyric acid agonists and N-methyl-D-aspartate antagonists on a multiple schedule of ethanol and saccharin self-administration in rats. *J. Pharmacol. Exp. Ther., 280(3),* 1250-1260.

Smothers, C.T., Mrotek, J.J., Lovinger, D.M. (1997) Chronic ethanol exposure leads to a selective enhancement of N-methyl-D-aspartate receptor function in cultured hippocampal neurons. *J. Pharmacol. Exp. Ther., 283,* 1214-1222.

Smothers, C.T., Clayton, R., Blevins, T., Woodward, J.J. (2001) Ethanol sensitivity of recombinant human N-methyl-D-aspartate receptors. *Neurochem. Int., 38(4),* 333-340.

Snell, L.D., Bhave, S.V., Tabakoff, B., Hoffman, P.L. (2001) Chronic ethanol exposure delays the 'developmental switch' of the NMDA receptor 2A and 2B subunits in cultured cerebellar granule neurons.. *J. Neurochem., 78(2),* 396-405.

Spanagel, R. & Zieglgansberger, W. (1997a) Anti-craving compounds for ethanol: new pharmacological tools to study addictive processes. *Trends Pharmacol. Sci., 18(2),* 54-59.

Spanagel, R., Holter, S., Putzke, J., Pestel, E., Wetzel, C., Zieglgansberger, W., (1997b). Behavioral, molecular and electrophysiological characterization of the action of acamprosate. *Alcohol. Clin. Exp. Res. Suppl. 21,* 637.

Steece-Collier, K., Chambers, L.K., Jaw-Tsai, S.S., Menniti, F.S., Greenamyre, J.T. (2000) Antiparkinsonian actions of CP-101,606, an antagonist of NR2B subunit-containing N-methyl-d-aspartate receptors. *Exp. Neurol., 163(1),* 239-243.

Stork, O., Kojima, N., Stork, S., Kume, N., Obata, K. (2002) Resistance to alcohol withdrawal-induced behaviour in Fyn transgenic mice and its reversal by ifenprodil. *Brain Res. Mol. Brain Res., 105(1-2),* 126-135.

Tang, C.M., Dichter, M., Morad, M. (1990) Modulation of the N-methyl-D-aspartate channel by extracellular H+. *Proc. Natl. Acad. Sci. USA., 87(16),* 6445-6449.

Taniguchi, K., Shinjo, K., Mizutani, M., Shimada, K., Ishikawa, T., Menniti, F.S., Nagahisa, A. (1997) Antinociceptive activity of CP-101,606, an NMDA receptor NR2B subunit antagonist. *Br. J. Pharmacol., 122(5),* 809–812.

The World Health Report (2003) World Health Organization, Geneva, Switzerland.

Thomas, M.P., Davis, M.I., Monaghan, D.T., Morrisett, R.A. (1998) Organotypic brain slice cultures for functional analysis of alcohol-related disorders: novel versus conventional preparations. *Alcohol Clin. Exp. Res., 22(1),* 51-59.

Thomas, M.P. & Morrisett, R.A. (2000) Dynamics of NMDAR-mediated neurotoxicity during chronic ethanol exposure and withdrawal. *Neuropharmacology, 39(2),* 218-226.

Traynelis, S.F. & Cull-Candy, S.G. (1990) Proton inhibition of N-methyl-D-aspartate receptors in cerebellar neurons. *Nature, 345(6273),* 347-350.

Trevisan, L., Fitzgerald, L.W., Brose, N., Gasic, G.P., Heinemann, S.F., Duman, R.S., Nestler, E.J. (1994) Chronic ingestion of ethanol up-regulates NMDAR1 receptor subunit immunoreactivity in rat hippocampus. *J. Neurochem., 62(4),* 1635-1638.

Tsai, G., Gastfriend, D.R., Coyle, J.T. (1995) The glutamatergic basis of human alcoholism. *Am. J. Psychiatry, 152(3),* 332-340.

Tsai, G. & Coyle, J.T. (1998) The role of glutamatergic neurotransmission in the pathophysiology of alcoholism. *Annu. Rev. Med., 49,* 173-184.

Ueno, S., Lin, A., Nikolaeva, N., Trudell, J.R., Mihic, S.J., Harris, R.A., Harrison, N.L. (2000) Tryptophan scanning mutagenesis in TM2 of the GABA(A) receptor alpha subunit: effects on channel gating and regulation by ethanol. *Br. J. Pharmacol., 131(2),* 296-302.

Wang, Y.T., Salter, M.W. (1994) Regulation of NMDA receptors by tyrosine kinases and phosphatases. *Nature, 369(6477),* 233-235.

Whittington, M.A., Lambert, J.D., Little, H.J. (1995) Increased NMDA receptor and calcium channel activity underlying ethanol withdrawal hyperexcitability. *Alcohol Alcohol., 30(1),* 105-114.

Williams, K. (1993) Ifenprodil discriminates subtypes of the N-methyl-D-aspartate receptor: selectivity and mechanisms at recombinant heteromeric receptors. *Mol. Pharmacol., 44(4),* 851-859.

Williams, K., Kashiwagi, K., Fukuchi, J., Igarashi, K. (1995) An acidic amino acid in the N-methyl-D-aspartate receptor that is important for spermine stimulation. *Mol. Pharmacol., 48(6),* 1087-1098.

Williams, K, Pahk, A J, Kashiwagi, K, Masuko, T, Nguyen, N D, Igarashi, K. (1998) The selectivity filter of the N-methyl-D-aspartate receptor: a tryptophan residue controls block and permeation of Mg2+. *Mol. Pharmacol., 53(5),* 933-941.

Wirkner, K., Poelchen, W., Koles, L., Muhlberg, K., Scheibler, P., Allgaier, C., Illes, P. (1999) Ethanol-induced inhibition of NMDA receptor channels. *Neurochem. Int., 35,* 153-162.

Woodward, J.J. & Gonzales, R.A. (1990) Ethanol inhibition of N-methyl-D-aspartate-stimulated endogenous dopamine release from rat striatal slices: reversal by glycine. *J. Neurochem., 54(2),* 712-715.

Wright, J.L., Gregory, T.F., Kesten, S.R., Boxer, P.A., Serpa, K.A., Meltzer, L.T., Wise, L.D., Espitia, S.A., Konkoy, C.S., Whittemore, E.R., Woodward, R.M. (2000) Parallel synthesis of a series of subtype-selective NMDA receptor antagonists. *J. Med. Chem., 43,* 3408-3419.

Yaka, R., Phamluong, K., Ron, D. (2003a) Scaffolding of Fyn kinase to the NMDA receptor determines brain region sensitivity to ethanol. *J. Neurosci. 23(9),* 3623-3632.

Yaka, R., Tang, K.C., Camarini, R., Janak, P.H., Ron, D. (2003b) Fyn kinase and NR2B-containing NMDA receptors regulate acute ethanol sensitivity but not ethanol intake or conditioned reward. *Alcohol Clin Exp Res., 27(11),* 1736-1742.

Yenari, M.A., Bell, T.E., Kotake, A.N., Powell, M., Steinberg, G.K. (1998) Dose escalation safety and tolerance study of the competitive NMDA antagonist selfotel (CGS 19755) in neurosurgery patients. *Clin Neuropharmacol., 21(1),* 28-34.

Zhang, J., Chiodo, L A., Freeman, A S. (1992) Electrophysiological effects of MK-801 on rat nigrostriatal and mesoaccumbal dopaminergic neurons. *Brain Res., 590(1-2),* 153-163.

Zhou, Z.L., Cai, S.X., Whittemore, E.R. (1999) 4-Hydroxy-1-[2-(4-hydroxyphenoxy)ethyl]-4-(4-methylbenzyl)piperidine: a novel, potent, and selective NR1/2B NMDA receptor antagonist. *J. Med. Chem., 42,* 2993-3000.

In: Drug Toxicity: New Research
Editor: Cam E. Vellotis, pp.263-290

ISBN 978-1-60456-320-7

Chapter 8

Antihormonal Agents on the Citotoxicity Increase of Anticancer Drugs in Cervical Cancer

P. García-López*[*] *and R. Jurado
Subdirección de Investigación Básica, Instituto Nacional de Cancerología, Av. San Fernando #22, Tlalpán 14000, Apartado Postal 22026 Mexico, D.F., Mexico.

1. Abstract

Cervical cancer continues to be the major cause of cancer mortality in women in developing countries. Although detection routine screening programs have been implemented since 1975, an increased rate of new cases has also been detected. Some studies have demonstrated a relationship between HPV, cervical intraepithelial neoplasia, and invasive carcinoma of cervix. Additionally, it has been predicted that within 10 years, 66% of all dysplasia -without medical intervention- would progress to carcinoma *in situ*. It is important to bear these data in mind in order to be able to search new alternatives for cervical cancer treatment.

Cisplatin and its derivatives are important drugs in cervical cancer therapy. However, the administration of cisplatin is associated with serious side effects, including nephrotoxic and neurotoxic events. This issue has motivated the search for new agents or new regimens for cisplatin combinations with the purpose of increasing antitumoral activity and decreasing secondary events.

Among the chemosensitizer drugs, antihormonal agents have been used to modulate the cytotoxic activity of antineoplastic agents, principally in hormone-dependent cancers such as breast and prostate cancers. Although the normal cervix is known to respond to steroid sex hormones, hormonal treatments are not frequently employed in cervical carcinoma therapy. In fact, this carcinoma is traditionally considered not to respond to

* Correspondence concerning this article should be addressed to Patricia García-López, Ph.D. Divisiǿn de Investigaciǿn Básica, Instituto Nacional de Cancerología (INCan), Av. San Fernando # 22, Tlalpán 14000, Apartado Postal 22026, México D.F., México. Phone: (52) (55) 5628-0425,26; Fax: (52) (55) 5628-0432; e-mail: garcia_lopez@salud.gob.mx; pgarcia_lopez@yahoo.com.mx.

antihormonal therapy. We hypothesize that exposure to antihormonal agents for sensitizer cervical cancer cells to the antineoplastic treatment can be independent of steroid-receptors. The importance of antihormonal agents used to modulate the cytotoxic activity of anticancer drugs in cervical cancer will be explored in this article.

2. Introduction

Pathogenesis and Epidemiology of Cervical Cancer

Cervical cancer is the third most common cancer in women worldwide and continues to be the major cause of cancer deaths for women in underdeveloped countries, representing approximately 25% of cancer-related deaths in Mexican women. Although routine screening programs for its detection have been implemented since 1975, increase of new cases has been detected (Bosch, 2003; Lorincz, 2003). The epidemiology and molecular biology of cervical cancer are well understood, epidemiologic studies have involved a great variety of risk factors associated with cervical cancer; however, it has been postulated that it is a sexually transmitted disease associated with human papillomavirus (HPV). Cervical condyloma induced by HPV is associated with the development both epidermoide and adenocarcinoma cervical cancer.

Since the DNA isolation of the HPV from cervical cancer cells, many researchers have confirmed the role that has these viruses in the pathogenesis of cervical cancer. HPVs are associated with 99% of cervical cancer (Walboomers et al., 1999). Some studies have demonstrated a relationship between HPV, cervical intraepithelial neoplasia, and invasive carcinoma of the cervix. Additionally, it has been predicted that 66% of all dysplasia -without medical intervention- would progress to carcinoma *in situ* within 10 years. There are >100 types of HPVs, but only a sub-set of high-risk viral types induce cervical carcinogenesis (Wilczynski et al., 1988).

HPVs are small double stranded DNA viruses that infect either cutaneous or mucosal epithelia where they can cause epithelial tumours. Papillomaviruses contain a single molecule of circular double-stranded DNA that is about 8 kilobases in length and encodes eight early genes (E1 to E8) and two late genes (L1 and L2). In addition, there is a non-conding regulatory region called the long control region (LCR). In HPV-infected cells, the HPV genome exists as an extrachromosomal DNA circle. In contrasting in HPV-transformed cells from cervical tumors, the viral genome is often integrated into the host genome (Dürst et al., 1985). Integration commonly takes place within the viral E2 gene and results in the loss of the E2 gene product (Baker et al., 1987; Corden et al., 1999), this suggests that the absence of the E2 protein is an important factor in the development of cervical cancer (Schneider-Maunory et al., 1987). In the HPV-associated cervical cancer, two HPV oncogenes, E6 and E7, are commonly up-regulated in their expression, both multifunctional proteins, display transforming properties in tissue culture, including the ability to contribute to the immortalization process.

The genital HPVs can be divided into low risk types such as HPV-6 and HPV-11, and high-risk types such as HPV-16, 18, 31, 33, and 45. The firsts induce benign genital warts and are very rarely associated with malignancies; and the seconds cause lesions that more frequently progress to cervical carcinoma (Lorincz et al., 1992). However, these HPV types have also been detected in non-malignant cervical tissue, and only a small proportion of women with clinically apparent high–risk HPV infection eventually develop cervical carcinoma, possibly because many of these infections may be transient. Of more than 30 HPV types known to infect human genitalia, HPV-16 is most commonly associated with cervical cancer and is found in 50% of tumors. Women who are not diagnosed through screening usually present with advanced disease and cervical cancer. This the major cause of cancer deaths among young women in some developing countries (Walboomers et al., 1999).

Human papillomavirus infection is not sufficient for tumor development, there are other cofactors associated with cervical cancer –such as cigarette smoking, immunodeficiency, possibly the use of oral contraceptives, recurrent infection, early pregnancy, and hormonal status- may play a role in progression to malignancy (Meanwell, 1991). All HPVs latently infect keratinocyte stem cells in the basal layer of the stratified epithelium; however, while low risk HPVs start to replicate in cells that are still proliferating, the replicate phase of high risk HPVs infection is confined to more differential cells that have already left the cell cycle.

Chemotherapy of Cervical Cancer

Currently, approaches for treating of cancer carcinoma have limited success; consequently, 5 year survival rates for women with this cancer remain low. It is estimated that 500,000 women annually will develop cervical cancer, and 200,000 women die every year from cervical cancer. The prognosis for patients with cervical cancer is dependent of the stage of disease at diagnosis. Cervical cancer is staged using the International Federation of Gynecology & Obstetrics Staging System (FIGO). Routine Pap screening is able to detect precancerous lesions in the cervix (cervical intraepithelial neoplasia) and carcinoma in situ. Preinvasive disease is generally managed through the ablative or excisional procedures such as loop electrosurgical excision procedure, conization, or cryosurgery (Herzog, 2003).

For stages IA to IB disease, radical abdominal hysterectomy and pelvic lymphadenectomy are the standard of care for the surgical treatment of cervical cancer. Early invasive disease (stages IA, IB, and small stage IIA with no parametrial involvement) can be successfully treated with radical hysterectomy or radiotherapy with reported 5-year survival rates in the range of 80–90%. Standard therapy for large locally invasive cervical cancer, including stage Ib2 has been radiotherapy. Radiotherapy has been the standard treatment for patients with advanced cervical cancer and selected patients with early stage disease. However, advanced disease (stages IIB2–IV) is rarely managed surgically because of regional involvement and a high relapse rate. Also, about 50% of advanced disease cases are unresectable. Radiotherapy alone or in combination with chemotherapy, is used to treat these patients. However, current treatment approaches are often ineffective and the 5-year survival rates for patients with stage IIB, III, or IVA tumors are 65, 40, and <20%, respectively (Herzog, 2003; Fiorica 2003; Schilder and Stehman, 2003).

The role of chemotherapy in the treatment of cervical cancer, including the use of new active agents is the actual tendency of therapy because the radiotherapy fails to control the progression of cervical cancer in 35–90% of women with locally advanced disease.

The rationale for combining chemotherapy with radiation is to eradicate systemic micrometastases, which are not eradicated by local radiation. In addition, cisplatin based chemotherapy may synergize with radiation by inhibiting the repair of radiation induced sublethal damage and by sensitizing hypoxic cells to radiation damage (Herzog, 2003).

The concomitant administration of cisplatin based chemotherapy with radiotherapy improves survival rates significantly compared with radiotherapy alone in patients with early stage or locally advanced cervical cancer. For example, the estimated 5-year survival in patients with cervical cancer stages IIB through IVA, with a tumor diameter of at least 5 cm or involvement of pelvic lymph nodes, who were treated with radiotherapy plus cisplatin and 5-fluorouracil was 73%, compared with 58% in patients who received radiotherapy alone. These studies strongly suggest that cisplatin based chemotherapy in cervical cancer patients requiring radiotherapy.

Despite this improvement in the efficacy of treatment, most patients with advanced cervical cancer experience recurrent or persistent disease. Persistent and recurrent cervical cancers are not usually responsive to irradiation therapy. In the other hand, metastases are common in patients with advanced cervical cancer; chemotherapy is an important component of treatment. However, response rates with current chemotherapy regimens are commonly in the range of 20–30% and median survival is approximately 12–14 months (Fiorica, 2003). Several phase II studies have demonstrated that chemotherapy before either radiotherapy or surgery produce a high response rates in patients who had not previously received chemotherapy.

The addition of concurrent chemotherapy to radiotherapy improves the outcome, and is now the standard of care for patients with locally advanced cervical cancer and for those patients with early stage disease and high risk factors (Schilder & Stehman, 2003). The use of concurrent chemoradiation has reduced the overall mortality rate by nearly 50 %. Even in the patients with recurrent cervical cancer or in those women with disseminated disease, recent results with combination chemotherapy suggest major improvement.

The majority of patients considered for combined chemotherapy are those who had failed prior therapy including radiation (Thigpen, 2003).

Although many agents are available, the standard single agent treatment is cisplatin, usually given at a dose of 50 mg/m^2. Response rates of 17–38% have been reported in patients with advanced or recurrent cervical cancer treated with cisplatin; however, these responses are partial and the median overall survival is about 6-7 months (Fiorica, 2003).

The majority of studies of cytotoxic therapy have been realized in squamous cell carcinoma which account for more than 80 % of all cases. Twenty one anticancer agents have been proved in cervical squamous cancer obtaining a response rate of 15 % or grater. The most commonly used are the following:

Three platinum compounds (cisplatin, carboplatin, and iproplatin) have been used in squamous carcinoma of the cervix and produced response rates of 23 %, 15 %, and 11 % respectively. Cisplatin is clearly active against squamous cell carcinoma of the cervix at a dose of 50 mg per m2, given every three weeks. The toxicity of the other two compounds is less than cisplatin but also its citotoxicity.

Ifosfamide acts as a classic alkylating agent. In patients with carcinoma of the cervix and no prior chemotherapy, the response rate is of 31 % to 50 % even if they were prior radiotherapy treated and they have a prolongation of the median progression-free interval (4.6 versus 3.2 months) compared with cisplatin alone. In patients who have received prior chemotherapy, the response rate was only of 8 %. Ifosfamide thus has clear activity in patients with no prior chemotherapy (Fiorica, 2003; Thigpen, 2003).

Dibromodulcitol is a halogenated sugar that acts primarily as an alkylating agent. It has been reported a response rate of 15 % to 29 % in patients with no prior chemotherapy thus showing significant activity in carcinoma of the cervix.

Doxorubicin is an antibiotic who has activity in squamous cell carcinoma of the cervix, showing a 20 % response rate. Doxorubicin is an anthracycline antibiotic which has a wide range of clinical activities. The mechanism of cytotoxicity and the exact intracellular target remains controversial. The target of intracellular drug is intranuclear much of which is intercalated in the DNA. Although DNA intercalation has been felt to be the principle cytotoxic mechanism, more recent evidence suggests that inhibition of topoisomerase-II may play a more important role. Additionally, other cytotoxic actions including helicase inhibition have recently been noted (Rose, et al 2006; Thigpen, 2003).

Taxanes, paclitaxel and docetaxel are important antitumor drugs with a unique mechanism of action: they inhibit microtubule from disassembled. The taxanes bind to a subunit of the tubulin heterodimers that form cellular microtubules; the binding of the taxanes accelerates the polymerization of tubulin, effectively stabilizing and inhibiting the depolymerization of the microtubules. Nocodazole and the vinca alkaloids in contrast inhibit the polymerization of the tubulin heterodimers, in turn preventing the formation of microtubules. The taxanes currently in clinical use are effective against a broad spectrum of human tumors, in particular, ovarian, lung and breast cancers. They have demonstrated a significant activity against many solid tumors as single agent or as an agent combined with other chemotherapeutic agents.

In advanced or recurrent cancer of cervix, Gynecologic Oncology Group conducted phase II trial which demonstrated a moderate activity of paclitaxel with the result of 17% response. In another NCI-supported study, the activity of paclitaxel with the result of 21% partial response was shown in advanced or recurrent cancer of the cervix. Other study report that paclitaxel with previously radiated squamous cell carcinoma produced a 17 % response to 170 mg per m2 once every 3 weeks. After these trials, paclitaxel is widely applied against cervical cancer (Lee et al 2005; Thigpen, 2003).

Gemcitabine (2', 2' -difluorodeoxycytidine) is an antineoplastic agent that inhibits DNA synthesis, resulting in apoptosis. In addition to its established uses in pancreatic and non-small-cell lung cancer, the drug has been shown in clinical trials to be active against a wide variety of solid tumors and, in vitro, is cytotoxic to cervical cancer cell lines at plasma levels similar to those achieved clinically.

As a single agent, gemcitabine has demonstrated little activity as first- or second-line therapy for recurrent or advanced-stage cervical cancer (Mutch & Bloss, 2003).

In view of the limited success of current treatment approaches in patients with advanced disease, the use of a number of new chemotherapy agents has been investigated in clinical trials.

Topotecan has shown promise in a number of clinical trials in cervical cancer patients. This agent, currently licensed for the treatment of recurrent ovarian cancer, inhibits the topoisomerase I enzyme, causing double-stranded DNA breaks during replication which lead to cell death. Topotecan has a significant cytotoxic effect in several squamous cell cancer cell lines of the cervix uteri and vulva, including the C-33, Caski, and CAL-39 cell lines. The cytotoxic activity of topotecan was superior to that of cisplatin in the C-33 and Caski cell lines.

Results of clinical trials with this new agent, in a study who included patients with a measurable cervical cancer lesion received 1.2 mg/m^2 topotecan administered by intravenous (iv) infusion over 30 min for 5 consecutive days, the overall response rate was 18%. The principal toxicity was hematologic; however, all reported incidences of these events were controllable and there were no toxicity related withdrawals. The toxicity levels observed in clinical trials of topotecan in patients with cervical cancer are similar to those observed in patients with relapsed ovarian cancer and are not significantly different from levels observed with other chemotherapy agents (Fiorica, 2003). Also topotecan produces a 19 % response rate with previously radiated squamous cell carcinoma.

Combination treatments with two or more agents can produce higher overall response rates than single agents but are associated with increased toxicity.

Combination chemotherapy improves response rate as it was reported by several studies, also it has been stated that combination chemotherapy is essential if systemic treatment is to have a major impact on survival in patients with squamous cell carcinoma of the cervix.

Platinum based combinations are consistently actives and yield high response rates, particularly in patients with no prior radiation. Response rate in cisplatin combined therapy improves when it is combined from 18 % to 21 % with dibromodulcitol, 31 % with ifosfamide, and 36 % with paclitaxel, and there is a superior progression free survival with no differences in overall survival (Thigpen, 2003).

The combination of cisplatin and ifosfamide has shown a higher response rate, but this was achieved at the cost of considerably greater toxicity and there was no clear impact on overall survival. Concomitant administration of topotecan enhanced the cytotoxic activity of cisplatin, etoposide, and paclitaxel in some cell lines. In addition to its cytotoxic effects, topotecan also has radiation sensitizing activity in vitro in a number of human cancer cell lines. The augmentation of cisplatin activity is thought to occur through inhibition of DNA repair, suggesting that the concomitant administration of these two agents might be advantageous compared with either agent alone. These observations have prompted the instigation of a number of clinical trials of topotecan in cervical cancer patients (Fiorica, 2003).

The combination of cisplatin – doxorubicin results highly toxic when studied in 75 - 100 mg/m^2 in a phase I study, where myelosuppression was dose limiting. There is actually a liposomal doxorubicin (Doxil) preparation which is a polyethylene glycol liposomal encapsulation of doxorubicin. This results in an alteration of the pharmacokinetics in comparison to the parent compound. Specifically, there is minimal hematologic toxicity. Additionally, there is a prolonged circulation time, reduced clearance, a smaller volume of distribution, and limited uptake by the reticulo endothelial system. The liposomal encapsulation of doxorubicin significantly alters the toxicity profile of doxorubicin and in particular the myelotoxicity is considerably reduced. In animals using ovarian xenografts in nude mice, liposomal doxorubicin has resulted in a greater tumor to normal tissue drug uptake and an improved therapeutic index. A report of the pegylated liposomal doxorubicin in combination with carboplatin has demonstrated a 38% response rate among patients with squamous cervix carcinoma cell. Liposomal doxorubicin was well tolerated with minimal myelosuppression and no treatment related deaths (Rose, et al 2006).

In phase II trials, the combination of paclitaxel - cisplatin for metastatic cervical carcinoma has demonstrated response rates as high as 45–50%. A phase III trial by the Gynecologic Oncology Group demonstrated that cisplatin-paclitaxel not only improves response rate over single agent cisplatin, but also progression free survival in patients with FIGO stage IVB, recurrent or persistent squamous cell carcinoma of the cervix. Even in patients previously treated with chemo-radiation, carboplatin-paclitaxel has reasonable activity, is well tolerated, and can be delivered at full dose (Tinker, 2005).

Both in vitro and in vivo studies have shown that gemcitabine and cisplatin act synergistically against cancer cells, suggesting that combining them might lead to greater antitumor activity than would be expected simply by adding the cytotoxic effects of each drug alone. A neoadjuvant regimen based on low doses of gemcitabine combined with cisplatin and followed with definitive surgery or radiotherapy can yield very high overall response rates and prolonged survival. The response rate is higher among patients who had not received radiation therapy previously (57%) than among those who had (30%). Progression-free survival is 1.9 months and overall survival, 4.9 months. The relatively low toxicity of the regimen is very encouraging (Mutch and Bloss, 2003).

Chemotherapy agents are less effective in patients who have already received previous courses of chemotherapy because of relative or absolute drug resistance to the previous treatments. Response rates of >15% can be achieved in chemotherapy naive patients but are lower in previously treated patients. In addition, radical surgery and irradiation both lead to deterioration in the local vasculature, further reducing effects of systemically administered chemotherapy agents.

There is evidence from a number of studies that combination chemotherapy with cisplatin and pelvic irradiation improves progression free survival. This may be due to inhibition of the repair of radiation induced damage, initiation of proliferation, and reduction in the fraction of hypotoxic cells resistant to radiation (Fiorica, 2003).

As with other drugs that have been evaluated in patients with advanced or recurrent cervical cancer, gemcitabine is most active in those who have not had prior chemotherapy or radiation. Concomitant gemcitabine/radiation regimen obtained results with 89% of complete response, and 5% of partial response with a remarkable disease free survival of 84 %, and overall survival of 100% (Mutch and Bloss, 2003).

Other drugs used include at least other 13 agents with a response rate of 15 % or greater, opening the possibility for the development of effective combination chemotherapy.

3. Participating of Steroid Hormones in Cervical Cancer

Hormones can be classified generally into two broad groups: nonsteroidal as amino acids, peptides, and polypeptides, which usually requires cell-membrane localized receptors that regulated second messengers such as cAMP (Adenoside Mono Phosphate cycle) to mediate their action; and steroidal, which bind directly to intracellular receptors to mediate their action. Some examples of steroid hormones include estrogen, androgen, glucocorticoids, mineralocorticoids, and progestin.

Estrogens are endogenous hormones with numerous physiological actions. The most potent naturally estrogen in humans is 17β-estradiol, followed by estrone (E1) and estriol (E3). Estradiol, estrone and estriol are derived from androgenic precursors (androstenedione or testosterone) trough aromatization of the A-ring. Estradiol is oxidized reversibly to estrone, and both estradiol and estrone can be converted to estriol (Birkhauser, 1996). Estradiol is the predominant estrogen during the premenopausal period, and is mainly secreted by the ovaries. After menopause, the main estrogen is estrone. Estrone is synthesized in adipose tissue from adrenal dehydroepiandrosterone.

The biological activity of estrogen is mediated through a specific high-affinity estrogen receptor (ER) located within cell nuclei. The mechanism of action of ER is similar to that of other nuclear receptors. In the absence of hormone, the receptor is sequestered within the nuclei of target cells in a multiprotein inhibitory complex. The binding of ligand induces an activating conformational change within ER, an event that promotes homodimerization and high affinity binding to specific nucleotide sequences termed estrogen response elements (EREs) present in target genes, and these interactions increases, or in some cases decreases, transcription of hormone-regulated genes (Tasai and O`Malley, 1994). In addition to the classic ligand-mediated activation pathway, it has been shown that ER can be activated in the absence of ligand by grow factors or other agents that elevate intracellular cAMP levels (Aronica and Katzenellenbogen, 1993; Ignar-Trowbridge et al., 1993)

In the case of the progesterone, the biological actions are mediated primarily by its progesterone receptor (PR), a member of superfamily of intracellular receptor that mediates the nuclear effects of steroid hormones, thyroid hormone, and the non-nutritional vitamins A and D. The mechanism of action of PR is similar to that of other steroid receptors. In the absence of progesterone, the receptor is transcriptionally inactive and remains sequestered in a large complex of heat shock proteins (HSPs) as HSP-90, HSP-70 (Tsai and O`Malley, 1994). On hormone binding, the receptor undergoes a conformational change, resulting in the dissociation from heat shock proteins, translocations to the nucleus, and dimerization and binding to progesterone responsive elements (PREs) within the promoter regions of target genes (Beato et al., 1995; Mangelsdorf et al., 1995).

Studies reported by Beatson in 1896 were the first that showed that estrogens possess a growth-stimulating effect on breast tumors and that tumor growth could be reduced by removal of the ovaries. There are evidences that involved the association of increased serum estrogens, or estrogen excretion, with postmenopausal breast cancer. Mammary tissues accumulate serum estrogens to concentrations significantly higher than those present in serum (Miller, 1997). Besides, breast tissues also synthesize estrogens trough a pathway similar to that peripheral adipose tissues (Birkhauser, 1996). There are data that show that normal, benign, and malignant breast tissue in postmenopausal women contain concentrations of 17 β-estradiol up to 10-fold higher than those seen in serum (Drafta et al., 1983; Edery et al., 1981). This property of the estrogens, demonstrated by innumerable research studies, has acquired clinical significance in the pharmacological suppression of estrogen production in breast cancer. Estrogen receptor and progesterone receptor status is a well recognized prognostic indicator in women with breast carcinoma, patients with ER-positive tumors have a significantly higher response to antiestrogens than patients with ER-poor or ER-negative tumors. Expression of the progesterone receptor also has been implicated as predictor of response, this likely related to ability of estrogens to induce its expression. Concurrent expression of both ER and PR is often associated with a higher response than in ER-positive, but PR-negative, tumors. So in women with breast carcinoma, hormone receptor status is routinely used as a guide for design therapy.

In the case of the uterine cervix normally responds to stimuli by female sex hormones, which seem to be regulated by mechanisms similar to those proposed for varies target organs. The normal cervix is a hormone-dependent tissue and it has been shown to contain estrogen and progesterone receptors (Terenius et al., 1974; Sanborn et al., 1976; Fujiwara et al., 1997). However, for cervical carcinoma tissues, estrogen and progesterone receptors have also been noted to be present but in a lower percentage than reported for breast and endometrial carcinoma. In fact, there are controversial data suggesting that ER and PR status may be of importance in women with invasive adenocarcinoma of the cervix.

An example showing the importance of steroids on the development of cervical cancer relapse is the fact that not all women infected with HPV develop cervical cancer, HPV infection alone is insufficient for tumor development, and like other cancers, the etiology of cervical neoplasia is a multistep process involving other cofactors. One of these factors can be the sex steroid hormones. The role of estrogens in the development of cervical carcinoma has been widely debated (Piper, 1985). The widespread oral contraceptives use by women in the 1960s and 1970s was associated with an increase in the incidence of cervical dysplasia, however, this idea was abandoned when it was observed that the use of oral contraceptives and the increased risk of HPV exposure was due to a lack of concomitant use of barrier methods. However, some studies have documented that synergism may exist between steroid hormones and HPV in the pathogenesis of cervical cancer; specifically, in vitro studies have demonstrated that the estrogen can enhance the transcription of HPV-16 E6 and E7 oncogenes (Khare et al., 1997; Tewari et al., 2000). In fact, it is know that 17B-estradiol stimulates the proliferation on CaSKi and HeLa cells at the concentration of $1x10^{-6}$ M. Antiestrogens, such as tamoxifen, also showed a similar stimulatory growth effect at low concentrations ($0,1 \times 10^{-6}$M) in Hela cells. However, in HPV-negative cervical cancer such as C33A, the stimulation of cell proliferation by estradiol was not exhibited. These experimental data provide evidence to demonstrate that HPV might play an important role in the hormonal stimulation of cell growth (Kim et al., 2000).

In addition, glucocorticoids have also been shown to enhance the efficiency and frequency of transformation of rodent cell by HPV16 (Brisson et al., 1994; Laga et al., 1992) and together with progestorone can enhance HPV gene expressions through of hormone response elements (Chan et al., 1989; Mittal et al., 1993). Several reports have linked the use of oral contraceptives with a higher risk of being HPV positive and there is an elevated risk of developing cervical cancer with increased duration of oral contraceptives use (Brinton et al., 1986; Hildeshein et al, 1990; Munoz et al., 1994). In addition, pregnant patients had a significantly higher positive rate for HPV infection (Bosch et al., 1995; Fife et al., 1996).

These experimental and clinical studies suggest an important link between steroid homones, high-risk HPV infection, and the development of cervical carcinoma.

Nonetheless, contrasting findings have been reported on the clinical behaviour respect to steroid receptor expression in cervical tumors. Most studies have shown that the content of steroid hormone receptors has not prognostic value for survival (Hunter et al., 1987; Fujiwara et al., 1997; Martin et al., 1986). However, there are data that demonstrate that ER and PR can have prognostic value and might be related to better survival (Gao et al., 1983). Potish et al., (1986) and Twiggs et al., (1987) found that in squamous carcinomas, a higher incidence of ER-positive and PR-positive tumors in comparison with the adenosquamous carcinoma type; while other authors observed no difference between these two types (Gao et al., 1983; Hunter et al., 1987).

Some studies suggest that the number of cervical adenocarcinomas affecting young women in their 20s and 30s may have increased (Parazzini et al., 1990; Peters et al., 1986). In Mexico, it has also been observed that the adenosquamous type is more frequently observed in younger women, while squamous carcinoma predominates in postmenopausal women (Mohar et al., 1993; Ramirez et al., 1987). These data suggest that hormonal profile may participate in histological differentiation and perhaps in the biological behaviour of cervical cancer.

There are experimental data supporting that steroid hormones have the ability to increase the transcription of the oncoproteins E6 and E7 of HPV-16 and HPV-18 (Brake and Lambert, 2005; Kim et al., 2000) the two subtypes most associated with cervical cancer, and part of the therapeutic strategies in the cervical cancer are focused in reducing the transcription of these viral oncoproteins to get the reversion or amelioration of the malignant phenotype even though cervical carcinoma is traditionally considered not to be responsive to antiestrogens (Scambia et al., 1990; Von knebel Doeberitz et al., 1992). However, tamoxifen is only antiestrogen that has been used in this type of cancer, and it is known that this drug has agonist effect in the lower genital tract and it has established an association between the use of tamoxifen in breast cancer and the subsequent development of endometrial carcinoma (Friedrich et al; 1998; Mourits et al., 2002; Tan-Chiu et al., 2003). Indeed, it has been shown that tamoxifen at a low concentration (10^{-9} *M*) causes stimulation of cell proliferation in a cervical cancer cell line (SFR cell line) that does not contain the estrogen receptor (ER) (Hwang et al., 1992). As well, short-term administration of estrogens to cervical carcinoma patients produces an increase in tumor proliferation (Bhattacharya et al., 1997), the potential therapeutic value of pure antiestrogen and antiprogestin on cervical carcinoma justify to be studied on cervical carcinoma.

4. Antihormonal Treatment as Chemosensitizer Drugs

Among the chemosensitizer drugs, antiestrogens such as tamoxifen and ICI 182,780; and antiprogestins as mifepristone have been used to modulate the cytotoxic activity of antineoplastic agents such as doxorubicin, paclitaxel and cisplatin among others.

Role of the Antiestrogen Tamoxifen as a Possible Chemosensitizar

Tamoxifen is a non steroidal estrogen antagonist. In 1985, tamoxifen was approved by the Food and Drug Administration (FDA) as adjuvant therapy with chemotherapy in postmenopausal women with node-positive breast cancer, in 1989 was approved for the use in the treatment of premenopausal women with ER-positive advance breast cancer; and in 1990, approval was obtained for pre- and postmenopausal patients who had node-positive and ER-positive breast cancer. Thus, up to date, it is the most prescribed drug for the treatment of breast cancer and it has been the "gold standard" selective estrogen receptor modulator. However, the use of tamoxifen is limited by the development resistance; the tumors become resistant in metastatic breast cancer after average treatment duration of only 10-12 months.

Some studies have shown that tamoxifen sensitizes the effect of cisplatin in several cell lines. For example, it has been demonstrated that in head and neck squamous cell carcinoma, tamoxifen alone induces a transient G_1 arrest that greatly sensitizes the cells to apoptosis induced by cisplatin (Tavassoli et al., 2002). Recently, it has also been demonstrated that tamoxifen increases the apoptotic effect of cisplatin in primary endometrial cell cultures (Drucker et al., 2003). Following these results, a phase I trial of tamoxifen in combination with cisplatin in patients with lung cancer was done, and it was concluded that a regimen of high-dose tamoxifen in combination with cisplatin can be safety administered, since it did not show any hematological toxicity (Perez et al., 2003).

Tamoxifen has been commonly used for all stages of breast carcinoma. However, several authors have established an association between the use of tamoxifen in breast cancer and the subsequent development of endometrial carcinoma (Friedrich et al, 1998; Mourits et al., 2002; Tan-Chiu et al., 2003), and thromboembolic events (Fisher et al, 1994). Moreover, it has been shown that tamoxifen at a low concentration (10^{-9} M) causes stimulation of cell proliferation in a cervical cancer cell line (SFR cell line) that does not contain estrogen receptor (ER) (Hwang et al., 1992). Therefore, these data suggest the possibility that others antiestrogens may be effective as chemosensitizers in the chemotherapy of cervical carcinoma.

Role of the Antiestrogen ICI 182,780 as a Possible Chemosensitizer

The novel pure antiestrogen, ICI 182,780, is an analogue of estradiol that differs substantially from tamoxifen in terms of the chemical, pharmacologic, and biologic properties. This agent has not intrinsic estrogen–agonist activity and, therefore, is considered a pure antiestrogen. It has advantages over tamoxifen because it is devoid of estrogen agonist activity and its affinity with the ER is approximately 100 times greater than that of tamoxifen (Howell et al., 1994). Studies examining the mode of action have shown that the activity of the ER is completely attenuated by ICI 182,780; there are multiple changes in the ER function as impaired dimerization, increase turnover, and disrupted nuclear localization. Thus, not only is ER blocked functionally, but cellular levels of ER are reduced markedly by ICI 182,780.

It has been used in postmenopausal patients with breast cancer, and clinical results have confirmed that it has useful activity against breast cancer (De Friend et al., 1994), as well as a safety profile that includes reduced adverse effects such as headache and nausea (Thomas et al., 1994). Additionally, there is no evidence of agonist activity in the endometrium of postmenopausal women (Addo et al., 2002). Consequently it has been increasingly used against breast cancer (Cummings, 2002). In accordance with findings of De Vincenzo et al. (1996), in MCF-7 cells and their doxorubicin-resistant variant (MCF-7 ADR), ICI 182,780 increases the effect of doxorubicin, suggesting the participating of the Pgp drug-efflux pump. Also has been reported that this pure steroidal antiestrogen can increase the activity of cisplatin in an estrogen receptor negative ovarian cancer cell line (A2780 WT) and its cisplatin-resistant variant (A2780 CP3). The mechanism involved is not dependent of the cell cycle or apoptosis (Ercoli et al., 2000).

In a work realized by our group (Garcia-Lopez et al., 2004), using in vitro assays, we demonstrated that ICI 182,780 combined with cisplatin was able to enhance cytotoxicity in three cervical cancer cell lines (HeLa, SiHa and CaSki). These cervical carcinoma cells were chosen for the study because they contain the human papillomavirus type 18 (HeLa) and Type 16 (SiHa and CaSki) genotypes, which have been shown in multi-institutional studies to account for >65% of all HPVDNA-positive invasive cervical carcinomas. Moreover, these cells were selected because they represent different histological subtypes; HeLa cells derived from an adenocarcinoma, SiHa cells from a squamous carcinoma, and CaSki cells from an epidermoid cervical carcinoma. The cisplatin was chosen because it is not a substrate for Pgp drug-efflux pump (Nooter and Stoter et al., 1996), and in relation to the studies of De Vincenzo et al. (1996), in MCF-7 cells and their doxorubicin-resistant variant (MCF-7 ADR), ICI 182,780 increases the effect of doxorubicin, suggesting the participation of the P-glycoprotein (Pgp) drug-efflux pump. Therefore, we wanted to study the activity of the drug combination independent of Pgp and in a type of cancer that does not respond to hormonal treatment as cervical carcinoma.

In our studies we found that in the cervical cancer cell lines used, ER and PR gene levels were relatively low compared to those observed in MCF-7 cells. These findings are in accordance with clinical data that show that this type of tumor exhibits low or undetectable level of ER and PR as determined by immunohistochemical and ligand-binding-assays (Hahnel et al., 1979). Although the level of ER and PR gene expression in cervical cancer was low, the levels were enough to demonstrated that ICI 182, 780 effectively down-regulate ER and PR genes in HeLa and SiHa cells, suggesting that these effects were partially responsible for cisplatin sensitization in both cells. It is also important to mention that HeLa cells are considered one of the most sensitive cervical cancer cell lines to cisplatin effect, and SiHa as one of the most resistant cells to this drug. We found a synergistic citotoxic effect more evident in HeLa cells, with approximately 18 times higher potency in comparison to alone cisplastin. However, SiHa and CaSki, resulted in a pontetiation of up to 4.5 fold. These results may be associated to the fact that HeLa cells are adenocarcinoma cells and adenocarcinomas tumors are more likely to hormonally sensitive. It has been reported that estrogens may induce physiological effects at the membrane level, such as synthesis and cyclin expression, indicating that a large amount of cells may respond to estrogenic actions in the absence of its intracellular cognate receptors (Marino et al., 2002). Therefore, chemosensitivity to cisplatin following exposure to ICI 182, 780 in SiHa and CaSki may be related with these mechanisms.

It is known that derivatives of platin such as cisplatin and carboplatin are fixed covalently to DNA forming cisplatin–DNA adducts. This damage is eliminated by the nucleotide excision repair system of the DNA. It has also been demostrated that the high-mobility group (HMG) domain proteins such as HMG1 bind specifically to major cisplatin adducts and that the platinum-DNA-protein complex is involved in mediating cisplatin cytotoxicity by blocking nucleotide excision repair of the damage (Huang et al., 1994). There is an inverse correlation between HMG1 and the ability of cells to repair damage both in vivo and in vitro. Moreover, it has been reported that HMG1 is also able to facilitate the interaction of steroid hormone receptors such as ER and PR with their cognate DNA binding sites (He et al., 2000) In relation to our results, we hypothesize, that exposure to ICI 182,780 could lead to increase in HMG1 expression and therefore to sensitization of ER+ and PR + cells, such as CaSki cells, to the treatment with cisplatin.

In our study we also demonstrated that the combination of ICI 182,780 and cisplatin induced significant increase in G2/M phase of cell cycle in the cervical cancer cells, previous studies have also shown that doxorubicin combined with ICI 82,780 induces G_2/M blockage in MCF-7 breast cancer cells, so this pure antiestrogen is more effective than tamoxifen in inducing G_2/M arrest (De Vincenzo et al., 1996). In the other hand, cervical cancer cell lines in the G_2/M phase of the cell cycle are believed to be more radiosensitive that those in G_0/G_1 phase (Hornback et al., 1994) due to the failure of this checkpoint, genomic instability can be produced resulting in hypersensitivity to radiation. Thus the combination of ICI 182,780 and cisplatin simultaneously with radiotherapy could effectively increase the antiproliferative effect and improve the treatment of cervical cancer.

Other mechanisms that could be involved in the synergistic antiproliferative effect of cisplatin and ICI 182, 780 are those independent of ER, such as decreasing the insulin-like growth factor receptor (IGF-1) (Chan et al, 2001; Huynh et al 1996) and decreasing transforming-growth factor-beta (TGF-beta) (Lackey et al., 2000) or loss of c-fos expression (Hyder et al., 1997). These findings suggest that this pure antiestrogenic compound could be a promising agent to be tested in combination with cisplatin not only in patients with cervical carcinoma, but also in those who are undergoing cisplatin therapy.

ICI 182,780, in addition to be a pure antiestrogen, has also been shown to have antiprogestin activity in human breast cancer cell lines (Rosenberg et al., 2000), as well produces a significant loss in PR expression in tumors and in cell proliferation-related antigen, Ki67 (De Friend et al., 1994). In clinical studies, the effects of three different doses of ICI 182,780 and one dose of tamoxifen on cellular ER and PR levels were examined in postmenoupausal women with primary breast cancer. The doses used were either a single intramuscular injection of ICI 182,780 (50, 125 or 250 mg), or 20 mg of oral tamoxifen, daily for 14-21 days. In this study was demonstrated a dose-dependent reduction in ER ands PR levels; in contrast, tamoxifen treatment produced significant increases in PR levels, possibly due to its estrogen agonist effect (Roberstson et al, 2001).

Role of the Antiprogestin Mifepristone (RU-486) as a Possible Chemosensitizer

As it has mentioned in this chapter, an important event in the malignant progression of cervical intraepithelial neoplasia appears to be the up-regulation of high-risk HPV expression. The steroid hormones have been linked to the progression from malignant in HPV positive lesions. In presence of glucocorticoids and progesterone, the GREs (glucocorticoids response elements) can enhance the transcription of E6-E7 increasing both cell proliferation and tumor growth of cervical tumor cells. According with these studies the glucocorticoid or progesterone antagonists can be used in the treatment of a variety of hormone-dependent tumors (Kettel et al., 1998; Rocereto et al., 2000). These antagonists include compound such as mifepristone, which is a progesterone receptor and glucocorticoid receptor antagonist. In presence of progesterone, mifepristone acts as competitive receptor antagonist, but it is a partial agonist with weak activity when is present alone. It has been widely used as the first-line drug for the termination of early pregnancy (Mahajan et al., 1997).

Biological actions of progesterone are mediated primarily by the progesterone receptor, a member of the nuclear receptor superfamily of transcription factors (Tsai et al 1994; Beato et al., 1995; Mangelsdorf et al.,1995). In the absence of progesterone, the receptor exists in a transcriptional inactive form associated with heat shock proteins (Smith and Toft, 1993). On hormone binding, the receptor undergoes a conformational change, resulting in dissociation from heat shock proteins, translocation to the nucleus, and dimerization and binding to progesterone responsive elements (PREs) within the promoter regions of target genes (Tsai et al., 1994, Beato et al., 1995, Mangelsdorf et al., 1995). When bound to the PRE, the receptor can modulate target gene transcription by directly contacting components of the transcriptional machinery (Ing et al., 1992) or indirectly by means of coactivators, such as steroid receptor coactivator-1 (SRC-1) (Onate et al., 1995) and p300/CBP (CREB-binding protein) (Smith et al., 1996). Progesterone antagonists are synthetic pharmaceutical agents that suppress the transcriptional activity of the natural steroid agonist, progesterone.

Mifepristone acts at the receptor level, binding strongly to progesterone and antiglucocorticoid receptors; its binding affinity for progesterone and glucocorticoid receptors is approximately five times greater than progesterone, and three times greater than dexametasone. Mifepristone, like progesterone, enters to target cell and reaches its receptors; however, it operate differently to progesterone producing conformational changes in the receptor. When the progesterone occupying its receptor in the nucleus may modify the receptor's shape and binding to chromatin, this binding leads to gene transcription and protein synthesis. Mefepristone antagonizes these effects by occupying the receptor without stimulating gene transcription (Spitz et al., 1993; Christian–Maitre et al., 2000). The early metabolism of mifepristone is characterized by rapid demethylation and hydroxylation. The three metabolites as the parental mifepristone retain considerable affinity toward human progesterone and glucocorticoid receptors. Thus, the combined pool of mifepristone plus its metabolites seems to be responsible for the biological actions of mifepristone (Attardi et al., 2004).

Interestingly, recent studies have proved that mifepristone could effectively inhibit the proliferation of PR-positive breast cancer (Liang et al., 2003; El Etreby et al., 1998), ovarian cancer (Rose and Barnea, 1996; Rocereto et al., 2000), endometrial cancer (Schneider et al., 1998), prostate cancer (El Etreby et al., 2000), and gastric cancer (Li et al., 2004).

Despite several reports showing that mifepristone can inhibit human cell growth only limited information is available on the basic mechanism of this effect. Some in vitro and in vivo mechanisms involved in the antiproliferative effects of mifepristone, in the case of the breast cancer, show that mifepristone induces growth arrest and cell death stimulating the activation of caspase-3, -8, and -9 in ER+ PR+, antiestrogen-resistant breast cancer cell (Gaddy et al., 2004). It is known that traditionally, caspase-8 activation is used as an indicator of activation of the extrinsic pathway of apoptosis, whereas caspase-9 activation indicates involved of the intrinsic mitochondrial pathway of apotosis (Kaufmann and Earnshow 2000). The cross-talk between these two death pathways, in part is mediated by caspase-3 activation. Once activated, caspase-3 can amplify apotosis by activating caspase-8 or -9 (Slee et al., 1999; Fujita et al., 2001).

In the case of the endometrial cell proliferation regulation by mifepristone is suggested an antioxidant mechanism by the mifepristone (Murphy et al., 2000). It has been reported an induction of apoptosis through up-regulation of NF-kB (Han and Sidell et al., 2003), one of the early response transcription factors that play a important role in the regulation of genes that are involved in the cascade of events leading to cellular apoptosis (Barkett and Gilmore 1999). The up-regulation of NF-kB in endothelial cells stimulates apotosis by 75% (Matsushita et al., 2000). Simultaneously to a marked increase in NF-kB activity is present an overexpression of Bax oncogen, protein involved in to promote apotosis and down-regulation of Bcl-2, this gene has been shown to rescue cell from apotosis.

It is also known that mifepristone can down-modulate the overexpression of two proteins involved in drug resistance as P-gp and MRP (Multidrug Resistance Protein) in MRP-overexpressing lung tumor GLC4/Sb30 cells (Payen et al., 1999); and induced apoptosis in human LNCaP prostate cancer cells by regulating the expression of apoptosis control gene Bcl-2 and $TGFbeta_1$ proteins (El Etreby et al., 2000); mifepristone has also shown a potent reversal effect on MDR in human gastric adenocarcinoma SGC-7901 cells via inhibiting the function of MRP and P-gp, and modulating the expression of Bcl-2 and Bax proteins (Li et al., 2004).

Other interesting mechanism described for mifepristone is its ability to modulate the activity of antitumor compound such as doxorubicin and vinka alkaloids. There is evidence that some endogenous compounds as steroid hormones also interact with P-gp (Yang et al., 1989). Corticosteroids and mineralocorticoids are substrates for P-gp transport (Ueda el al., 1992). Moreover, some steroid antagonist, such as tamoxifen and toremifen, also interfere with P-gp function, the features that usually describing to these modulators agents are the hydrophobicity and presence of phenyl rings (Hait and Aftab 1992). These properties are also characteristics of antiprogestin mifepristone. Therefore, it has been reported that mifepristone enhance doxorubicin cellular accumulation in resistant human leukaemia cells K562 and RHCL rat hepatoma cells (Lecureur et al., 1994) suggesting a inhibitory effect on P-gp function related to direct interactions with drug binding sites on P-gp, mechanism of action that has already been demonstrated for others chemosensitizers agents, including verapamil and cyclosporine (Ford and Hait 1990).

Recently it has been shown that mifepristone enhances the chemosensitivity of cisplatin in resistant ovarian cancer cell line COC1 (Qin and Wang 2002); finding consistent with the data by Liu et al (2003), showing in a mouse model bearing xenografted cisplatin-resistant ovarian carcinoma, a significantly greater inhibition rates of the tumors in the combined treatment in comparison with alone cisplatin treatment. These effects possibly are due to regulating of Bcl-2 and Bax protein expressions.

5. New Preclinical Advances of the Antiprogestin Mifepristone in the Chemosensitazing of Cisplatin in Cervical Cancer

Cisplatin is one of the most commonly used drugs in cervical carcinoma; however, the side effects as nephrotoxicity, ototoxicity, neuropathy, and mylosuppression; and intrinsic and acquired resistance to cisplatin are major limitations in the use of this drug. The lack of efficacy is generally multifactorial and has been shown to be due to reduced drug accumulation, inactivation by thiol containing species, increased repair/tolerance of platinum-DNA adducts, and alterations in proteins involved in apotosis. It is important to mention that pharmacological agents who are able to modulate any of the above parameters could partially restore the sensitivity to cisplatin; therefore, is important to identify new compound that modulate the cisplatin cytotoxicity in cervical carcinoma, in which cisplatin-based chemotherapy has been the mainstay of treatment since the activity of regimens based on cisplatin was demonstrated.

To date there are not clear data that establishing the participation of mifepristone in the modulation of antineoplastic drug in human cervical carcinoma. In our group we are studying the combination of mifepristone and cisplatin on cervical carcinoma. The aim of the study presented here is to investigate whether mifepristone in combination with cisplatin could act synergistically on the citotoxicity increase in cervical carcinoma; therefore, we propose the analysis of the cisplatin-mifepristone combination as a pharmacological tool to get a synergistic association that permit to potentiate the antiproliferative effect of cisplatin without increasing the serious side effects. Our research, in this chapter, shows the results obtained both *in-vitro* and *in-vivo* using a human cervical cancer cell line HeLa. In an effort to correlate the mechanism of action of this antiprogestin in the modulation of ciplatin activity, we evaluated the intracellular cisplatin accumulation both in the presence and in the absence of mifepristone.

Mifepristone and Cisplatint Treatment *In-Vitro*

We used the HeLa human cervical cell line obtained from ATCC (Rockville, Md.). The effect of mifepristone on proliferation of cell exposed to cisplatin was evaluated using the XTT assay (sodium 3' - [1-(phenylamino-carbonyl) - 3,4 - tetrazolium]–bis (Roche

Molecular Biochemicals) [4]. The assay was based on the cleavage of the yellow tetrazolium salt XTT to form an orange formazan dye by metabolic active cells. The treatment was cisplatin alone or the combination of cisplatin plus mifepristone. Measurement of spectrophotometric absorbance samples was carried out using a microtiter plate ELISA reader at 492 nm.

The cells were conditioned for 4 days with 10 μM mifepristone. Control cells were only exposed to vehicle (final ethanol concentration never exceeded 1% in treated and control samples). At the end of the incubation period, the culture medium was removed and fresh medium with various amounts of cisplatin (0.1-330 μM) was added for 4 h. After simultaneous and individual exposure to the drugs, the cells were cultivated for 24 hours. Cell proliferation was evaluated using the XTT-assay before mentioned. Mean concentration in each set of 3-4 wells was measured by triplicate. The percentage of growth inhibition was calculated and IC_{50} values (concentration of drug to achieve 50% growth inhibition) were obtained graphically from the survival curves distribution.

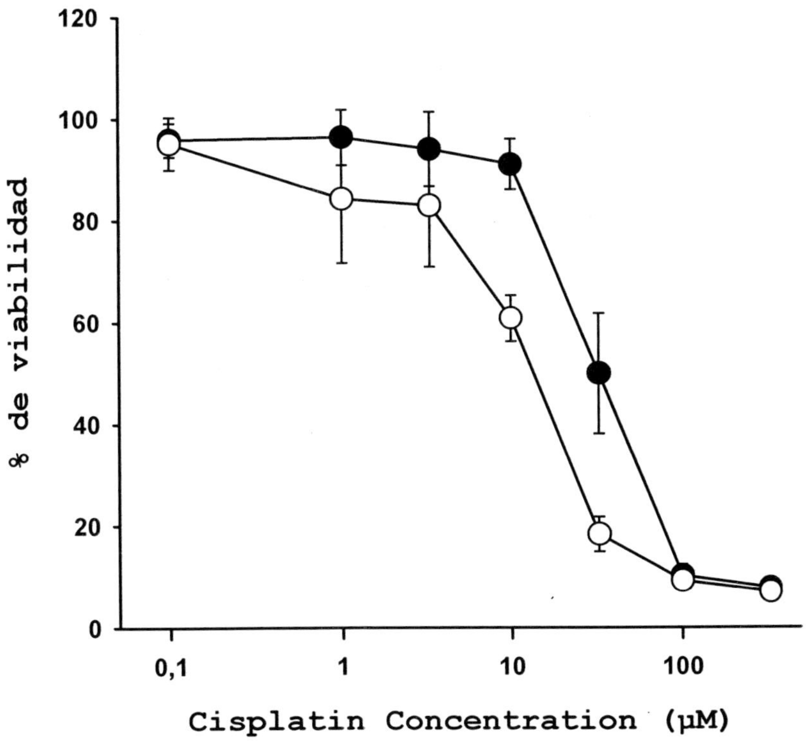

Figure 1. Representative growth inhibition curves of HeLa cells exposed to cisplatin alone (●) and in combination with mifepristone at 10 μM (○). Cells were exposed to mifepristone for 4 days followed by cisplatin for 4 h. After treatment, the effect was evaluated at 24 h. All growth inhibition assays were repeated in triplicate in at least three independent experiments. Values are the means ± SEM.

Synergism or drug additivity can be determined by calculating the combination index (CI) using de equation: $CIx=(D_1/Dx_1)+(D_2/Dx_2)+alfa(D_1)(D_2)/(Dx_1)(Dx_2)$. CIx represents the CI value for X% effect. Dx_1 and Dx_2 are the doses of agents 1 and 2 required to exert X% effect alone, whereas D_1 and D_2 represent the doses of agents 1 and 2 that elicit the same x%

effect in combination with the other agent respectively. Alfa describes the type of interaction: alfa=0 for mutually exclusive drugs (similar mechanisms of action), alfa=1 for mutually non-exclusive drugs (independent modes of action), the equation was resolved for alfa=1. CI=1 indicates additivity, CI<1 synergism and CI>1 antagonism.

Growth inhibition experiments Citotoxicity is expressed as percentage growth inhibition of HeLa cells treated with cisplatin for 4 h, or cisplatin in combination with mifepristone pre-treatment (Fig. 1). The antiproliferative effect of cisplatin (0.1-330 μM) was potentiated in combination with mifepristone (10 μM). The IC_{50} of cisplatin in combination with mifepristone was lower (14.2 μg/mL) than that of cisplatin alone (34.2 μg/mL). To determine whether the combination effect of mifepristone and cisplatin was synergistic or additive, the CI was determined using the equation before mentioned. The CI obtained showed that the interaction of mifepristone and cisplatin was synergistic throughout of the dose of 10 and 33 μg/mL.

Intracellular Cisplatin Accumulation

In the preparation of the cell samples, HeLa cervix cancer cell line were plated at 1×10^5 cells /mL in specific medium supplemented as above was described. After 24 h the medium was replaced with fresh medium containing cisplatin alone for 4 h to a final concentration of 33μg/m or in combination with mifepristone (10 μM). As control non-exposed cells were treated with vehicle and cultured for the same period. The cells were harvested after 24 h and washed twice with PBS. After that they were counted with a haemocytometer and lysed with buffer (Tris 100 mM, EDTA 5 mM, NaCl 200 mM, SDS 0.2%, at pH 8) by 3 h at 55°C. The intracellular concentration of cisplatin was estimated by High Performance Liquid Chromatograpic method previously reported (Lopez-Flores et al., 2004). Briefly, the homogenate was ultrafiltrated, derivatized with DDTC in 0.1 N NaOH, samples were incubated in a 37°C water bath for 15 min, and extracted with 80 μl chloroform by vortexing at maximal speed for 1 min. The two layers were separated by centrifugation at 10,000 rpm for 5 min. Finally, 20 μl of chloroform layer was injected into the chromatographic system.

The results of intracellular levels of cisplatin indicated that mifepristone increased cellular cisplatin retention. The concentration used of mifepristone of 10 μM was able to enhance cisplatin accumulation by approximately 2-fold, this dose of mifepristone is in the range of plasma concentration usually observed in humans after oral administration of the drug (Kartner et al., 1985).

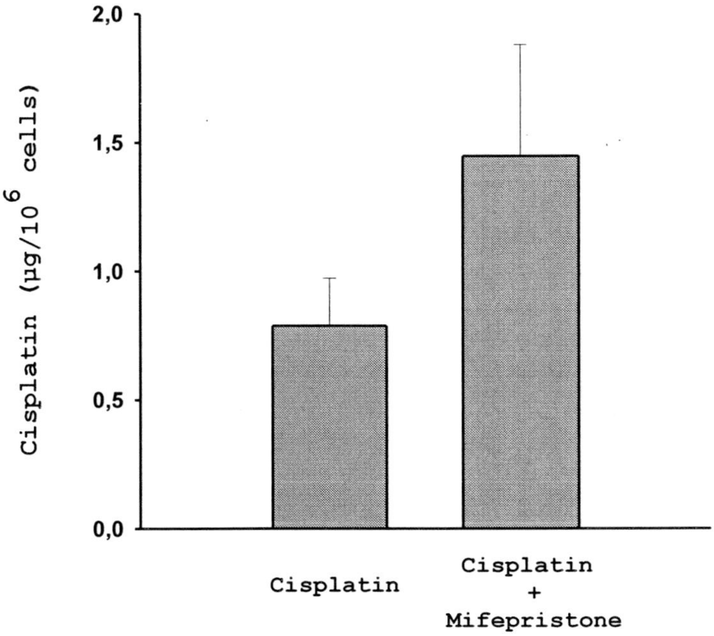

Figure 2. Effect of mifepristone on cisplatin accumulation in HeLa cells. The cells were incubated with 33 µg/mL of cisplatin for 4 h either alone or in presence of 10 µM of mifepristone. The intracellular cisplatin levels were then determined using the HPLC method. The values are the mean ± SEM of three independent experiments.

Mifepristone and Cisplatin Treatment *In-Vivo*

For xenograft model in nude mice we used female *nu/nu* mice (National Institute of Nutrition, Mexico City) between 6-8 weeks of age, they were kept in a pathogen-free environment and fed *ad lib.* The protocol for animal experiments was approved by the ethic committee of National Institute of Cancerology (Mexico, City). The *nu/nu* mice were subcutaneously injected with $6x10^6$ HeLa cells in a flank. Once tumors were approximately 5 mm x 5 mm, the animals were treated with a subcutaneous injection of mifepristone 2 mg/kg/day for 3 dáy previously to the administration of cisplatin (3 mg/kg daily on days 1 through 3). The control animals received only the vehicle. The tumor volumes were measured with a caliper and calculated using the following formule: $\pi[width^2 (mm) x length (mm)]/4$. The tumor growth was followed by 8 weeks.

The measurement of the tumor volume revealed a reduction of tumor growth in cisplatin-treatment alone and mifepristone-treatment alone with regarding to control animals; however, the tumor growth-inhibiting effect was more evident when the mice were treated with the combination of cisplatin and mifepristone (Fig. 3), revealing an effect modulator of mifepristone on cisplatin activity *in-vivo.* These findings are consisted with previous reports that show an improvement of antitumor effect of cisplatin against human ovarian carcinoma cells by mifepristone *in-vivo* (Liu Y et al., 2003).

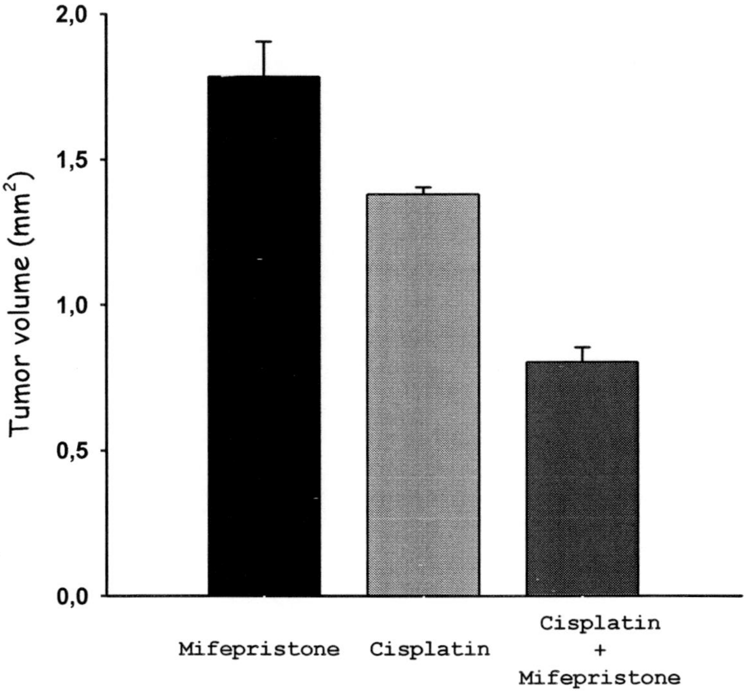

Figure 3. Effects of mifepristone, cisplatin, and mifepristone plus cisplatin on growth of HeLa tumor in nude mice after 8 weeks, the drug-treatments were indicated in the text. Data are expressed as the mean of 8 animals ± S.E.M.

6. Conclusion

Even when there are many antihormonal agents used in the treatment of patients with cancer, the primary use of these agents is in hormonally responsive cancer such as breast, prostate or ovarian cancer. However, due to the structural properties, they become attractive drugs as modulator agents of chemotherapeutic drugs in several carcinomas. Aside from the action mechanism of antihormonal agents described in this chapter, there is evidence that not all effects of steroid hormones are mediated via the regulation of genomic or transcriptional events, the importance of these nontranscriptional actions in cervical carcinoma is not known; in fact, it is important to mention that these nontranscriptional mechanisms could be involved in the action of antihormonal agents as chemosensitizers of chemotherapeutics drugs in cervical carcinoma. Taking into account that this carcinoma is traditionally considered to not respond to antihormonal therapy, the understanding of the mode of action of antihormonal compounds will allow the development of new treatment strategies to improve patients outcome with cervical carcinoma.

Acknowledgment

This work was support by CONACYT (México), grants I35551-M and P44176-M .

7. References

Addo, S; Yates, RA; Laight A. A phase 1 trials to assess the pharmacology of the new oestrogen receptor antagonist fulvestran on the endometrium in healthy postmenopausal volunteers. *Br J Cancer*, 2002 87:1354-1359.

Attardi, BJ; Burgenson, J; Hild, SA; Reel, JR. In vitro antiprogestational/ antiglucocorticoid activity and progestin and glucocorticoid receptor binding of the putative metabolites and syntetic derivatives of CDB-2914, CDB-4124, and mifepristone. *J Steroid Biochem Mol Biol*, 2004 88:277-288.

Aronica, SM; Katzenellenbogen, BS. Stimulation of estrogen receptor-mediated transcription and alteration in the phosphorylation state of the rat uterine estrogen receptor by estrogen, cyclic adenosine monophosphate, and insulin-like growth factor-I. *Mol Endocrinol*, 1993 7:743-52

Barket, M; Gilmore, TD. Control of apoptosis by Rel/NF-KB transcription factors. *Oncogene*, 1999 18:6910-6924

Baker, CC; Phelps, WC; Lindgren, V; Braun, MJ; Gonda, MA; Howley, PM. Structural and transcriptional analysis of human papillomavirus type 16 sequences in cervical carcinoma cell lines. *J Virol*, 1987 61:962-97.

Beato, M; Herrlich, P; Schutz, G. Steroid hormone receptors: many actors in search of a plot. *Cell*, 1995 83:851-857

Beatson, GT. On the treatment of inoperable cases of carcinoma of the mamma: Suggestion from a new method of treatment, with illustrative cases. *Lancet*, 1896 ii:104-107

Bhattacharya, D; Redkar, A; Mitra, I; Sutuaria, U; MacRae, KD. Oestrogen increase S-phase fraction and estrogen and progesterone receptors in human cervical cancer in vivo. *Br J Cancer*, 19975 7:554-558

Bosch, FX; Manos, MM; Muñoz, N; Sherman, M; Jansen, AM; Peto, J; Schiffman, MH; Moreno, V; Kurman, R; Shah, KV. Prevalence of human papillomavirus in cervical cancer, a worldwide perspective: International biological study on cervical cancer (IBSCC) study group. *J Natl Cancer Inst*, 1995 81:796-802

Bosch, FX. Epidemiology of human papillomavirus infections: new option for cervical cancer prevention. *Salud Publica Mex*, 2003 45:S326-S329

Birkhauser, MH. Chemistry, Physiology, and Pharmacology of sex steroids. *J Cardiovasc Pharmacol*, 1996 28:S1-S13

Brake, T; Lambert, P. Estrogen contributes to the onset, persistence, and malignant progression of cervical cancer in a human papillomavirus-transgenic mouse model. *Proc Natl Acad Sci USA*, 2005 102:2490-2495.

Brinton, LA; Huggins, GR; Lehman, HF;, Mallin, K; Savitz, DA; Trapid, E; Rosenthal, J; Hoover, R. Long-term use of oral contraceptives and risk of invasive cervical cancer. *Int J Cancer*, 1986 38:339-344.

Chan, TW; Pollak, M; Huynh, H Inhibition of insulin-like growth factor signaling pathways in mammary gland by pure antiestrogen ICI 182,780. *Clin Cancer Res*, 2001 7:2545-2554

Chan, WK; Klock, G; Bernhardt, HU. Progesterone and glucocorticoid response elements occur in the long control regions of several human papillomaviruses involved in anogenital neoplasia. *J Virol*, 1989 63:3261-3269.

Christin-Maitre, S; Bouchard, P; Spitz, IM. Drug Therapy: medical termination of pregnancy. *N Engl J Med*, 2000 342:946-56

Corden, SA; Sant-Cassia, LJ; Easton, AJ; Morris, AG. The integration of HPV-18 DNA on cervical carcinoma. *Mol Pathol*, 1999 52:275-278.

Cummings, FJ. Envolving uses of hormonal agents for breast cancer therapy. *Clin Ther*, 2002 24:C3-C25

DeFriend, DJ; Howell, A; Nicholson, RI; Anderson, E; Dowsett, M; Mansell, RE. Investigation of a new pure cancer. *Cancer Res*, 1994 54:408-414

De Vincenzo, R; Scambia, G; Benedetti, PP; Fattorasi, A; Bonanno, G; Ferlinic, C; Isola, G; Pernisco, S; Mancuso, S. Modulatory effects of tamoxifen and ICI 182, 780 on Adriamycin resistance in MCF-7 human breast cancer cells. *Int J Cancer*, 1996 68:340-348.

Drafta, D; Priscu, A; Neacsu, E; Gangura, M; Schindler, AE; Stroe, E; Anghel, C; Panaitescu, G. Estradiol and progesterone receptor levels in human breast cancer in relation to cytosol and plasma estrogen level. *J Steroid Biochem* 1983, 8:459-63.

Drucker, L; Stackieviez, R; Radnay, J; Shapiro, H; Cohen, I; Yarkoni, S. Tamoxifen enhances apoptotic effect of cisplatin on primary endometrial cell cultives. *Anticancer Res*, 2003 23:1549-1554.

Durst, M; Kleinheinz, A; Hotz, M; Gissmann, L. The physical state of human papillomavirus type 16 DNA in benign and malignant genital tumours. *J Gen Virol* 1985 66:1515-22.

Edery, M; Goussard, J; Dehennin, L; Scholler, R; Reiffsteck, J; Drosdowsky, MA. Endogenous oestradiol-17beta concentration in breast tumours determined by mass fragmentography and by radioimmunoassay: relationship to receptor content. *Eur J Cancer*, 1981 17:115-20.

El Etreby, MF; Liang, Y; Wrenn, RW; Schoenlein, PV. Additive effect of mifepristone and tamoxifen on apoptotic pathways in MCF-7 human breast cancer cells. *Breast Cancer Res Treat*, 1998 51: 149-168

El Etreby, MF; Liang, Y; Johnson, MH; Lewis, RW. Antitumor activity of mifepristone in the human LNCaP, LNCaP-C4, and LNCaP-C4-2 prostate cancer models in nude mice. *Prostate*, 2000 42: 99-106

Ercoli, A; Battaglia, A; Raspaglio, G; Fattorossi, A; Alimonti, A; Petrucci, F; Carola, S; Mancoso, S; Scambia, G. Activity of cisplatin and ICI 182,780 on estrogen receptor negative ovarian cancer cells: cell cycle and cell replication rate perturbation, Chromatin texture alteration and apoptosis induction. *Int J Cancer*, 2000 85:98-103

Fife, KH; Katz, BP; Roush, J; Handy, VD; Brown, DR;, Hansell, R. Cancer associated Human papillomavirus types are selectively increased in the cervix of women in the first trimester of pregnancy. *Am J Obstet Gynecol*, 1996 174:1487-1493.

Fiorica, JV. The role of topotecan in the treatment of advanced cervical cancer. *Gynecol Oncol*, 2003 90:S16-21.

Fisher, B; Constantino, JP; Redmond, CK; Fisher, ER; Wickerham, DL; Cronin, WM; Endometrial cancer in tamoxifen-treated breast cancer patients: findings from the National Surgical Adjuvant Breast and breast Project (NSA BP) B-14. *J Natl Cancer Inst*, 1994 86:527-537.

Ford, JM; Hait, WN. Pharmacology of drugs that alter multidrug resistance in cancer. *Pharmacol Rev*, 1990 42:155-99.

Friedrich, M; Mink, D; Villena-Heinsen, C; Woll-Hermann, A; Schmidt, W. Tamoxifen and proliferation of vaginal and cervical epithelium in postmenopausal women with breast cancer. *Eur J Obstet Gynecol Reprod Biol*, 1998 80:221-225.

Fujita, E; Egashira, J; Urase, K; Kuitda, K; Mommi, T. Caspase-9 processing by caspase-3 via feedback amplification loop in vivo. *Cell Death*, 2001 8:335-344

Fujiwara, H; Tortoledo-Luna, G; Mitchell, MF; Koulos, JP; Wright, TC Jr.. Adenocarcinoma of the cervix. Expression and clinical significance of estrogen and progesterone receptors. *Cancer*, 1997 79:505-512.

Gaddy, VT; Barrett, JT; Delk, JN; Kallab, AM; Porter, AG; Schoenlein, PV. Mifepristone induces growth arrest, caspase activation, and apoptosis of estrogen receptor-expressing, antiestroogen-resistant breast cancer cell. *Clin Cancer Res*, 2004 10:5215-5225.

Gao, YL; Twiggs, LB; Leung, BS; Yu, WC; Potish, R; Okagaki, T; Adcock, L; Prem KA. Cytoplasmic estrogen and progesterone receptors in primary cervical carcinoma: clinical and histopatologic correlates. *Am J Obstet Gynecol*, 1983 146:299-306.

Garcia-Lopez, P; Rodriguez-Dorantes, M; Perez-Cardenas, E; Cerbon, M; Mohar-Betancourt, A. Synergistic effects of ICI 182,780 on the cytotoxicity of cisplatin in cervical carcinoma cell lines. *Cancer Chemother Pharmacol*, 2004 53:533-540.

Hait, WN; Aftab, DT. Rational design and pre-clinical pharmacology of drugs for reversing multidrug resistance. *Biochem Pharmacol*, 1992 43:103-107

Hahnel, R; Martin, JD; Masters, AM; Ratajezak, KT; Twaddle, E. Oestrogen receptors and blood hormone levels in cervical carcinoma and other gynecological tumors. *Gynecol Onco*l, 1979 8:226-233

Hand, S; Sidell, N. RU486-induced growth inhibition of human endometrial cells involves the nuclear factor-kappa B signaling pathway. *J Clin Endocrinol Metab*, 2003 88:713-719.

He, Q; Liang, CH; Lippard, SJ. Steroid hormones induce HMG1 overexpression and sensitize breast cancer cells to cisplatin and carboplatin. *Proc Natl Acad Sci*, 2000 97:5768-5772

Herzog, TJ. New approaches for the management of cervical cancer. *Gynecol Oncol*, 2003 90: S22–S27.

Hildeshein, A; Reeves, WC; Brinton, L; Lavery, C; Brenes, M; DeLa Guardia, ME; Godoy, J; Rawls, WE. Association of oral contraceptive use and human papillomaviruses in invasive cancers. *Int. J Cancer*, 1990 45:860-864.

Hornback, NB; Shen, RN; Sutton, GP; Shidnia, H; Kaiser, HE. Synergistic cytotoxic and antitumor effects of irradiation and taxol on human HeLa cervix carcinoma and mouse B16 melanoma cells. *In vivo*, 1994 8:819-823.

Howell, A; Osborne, CK; Morris, CH; Wakeling, AE. ICI 182 780 (Faslodex), Development of a novel, "pure" antiestrogen. *Cancer,* 2000 89:817-825

Huang, JC; Zamble, DB; Reardon, JT; Lippard, ST; Sancar, A. HMG-domain proteins specifically inhibit the repair of the major DNA adduct of the anticancer drug cisplatin by human excision nuclease. *Proc Natl Acad Sci,* 1994 91:10394-10398.

Hunter, R; Longcope, C; Keough, P. Steroid hormone receptors in carcinoma of the cervix. *Cancer*, 1987 60:392-396.

Huynh, H; Nickerson, T; Pollak, M; Yang X. Regulation of insulin-like growth factor I receptor expression by the pure Antiestrogen ICI 182,780. *Clin Cancer Res*, 1996 2:2037-2042.

Hwang, JY; Lin, BY; Tang, FM; Yu, WC. Tamoxifen stimulates human papillomavirus type 16 gene expression and cell proliferation in a cervical cancer cell line. *Cancer Res*, 1992 52:6848-6852.

Hyder, S; Chiappetta, C; Murthy, L; Stancel, G. Selective inhibition of estrogen–regulated gene expression in vivo by the pure antiestrogen ICI 182,780. *Cancer Res*, 1997 57:2547-2549.

Ignar-Trowbridge, DM; Teng, CT; Ross, KA; Parker, MG; Korach, KS; McLachlan, JA. Peptide growth factors elicit estrogen receptor-dependent transcriptional activation of an estrogen-responsive element. *Mol Endocrinol*, 1993 7:922-8.

Ing, NH; Beekman, JM; Tsai, SY; Tsai, MJ; O'Malley, BW. Members of the steroid hormone receptor superfamily interact with TFIIB (S300-II). J Biol Chem, 1992 267: 17617-17623.

Kaufmann, SH; Earnshaw, WC. Induction of apoptosis by cancer chemotherapy. *Exp Cell Res*, 2000 256:42-9.

Kartner, N; Evernden-Porelle, D; Bradley, G; Ling, V. Detection of P-glycoprotein in multidrug-resistant cell lines by monoclonal antibodies. *Nature*, 1985 316:820-823.

Ketter, LM; Murphy, AA ; Morales, AJ; Yen, SS. Preliminary reports on the treatment of endometriosis with low-dose mifeprostone (RU486) *Am J Obstet Gynecol* 1998 178:1151-1156.

Khare, S; Pater, MM; Tang, SC; Pater, A. Effect of glucocorticoid hormones on viral gene expression, growth, and dysplastic differentiation in HPV16-immortalized ectocervical cells. *Exp Cell Res*, 1997 232:353-360.

Kim, CJ; Um, S; Kim, TY; Kim, E; Park, TC; Kim, SJ; Namkoong, SE; Park, JS. Regulation of cell growth and HPV genes by exogenous estrogen in cervical cancer cells. *Int J Gynecol Cancer*, 2000 10:157-164.

Lackey, BR; Gray, SL; Henricks, DM. Synergistic approach to cancer therapy: exploiting interactions between anti-estrogens, retinoids, monoterpenes and tyrosine kinase inhibitors. *Med Hypotheses*, 2000 54:832-836

Laga, M; Icenogle, JP; Marsella, R; Manoka, AT; Nzila, N; Ryder, RW; Vermund, SH; Heyward, WL; Nelson, A; Reeves; WC. Genital papillomavirus infection and cervical dysplasia –opportunistic complications of HIV infection. *Int J Cancer*, 1992 50:45-48.

Lecureur, V; Fardel, O; Guillouzo, A. The antiprogestatin drug RU 486 potentiates doxorubicin cytotoxicity in multidrug resistant cells through inhibition of P-glycoprotein function. *FEBS Lett*, 1994 355:187-91.

Lee, KH; Yim, EK; Kim, CJ; Namkoong, SE; Um, SJ; Park, JS.. Proteomic analysis of anti-cancer effects by paclitaxel treatment in cervical cancer cells. *Gynecol Oncol* 2005. 98:45-53.

Li DQ, Wang ZB, Bai J, Zhao J, Wang Y, Hu K, Du YH. Effects of mifepristone on proliferation of human gastric adenocarcinoma cell line SGC-7901 in vitro. *World J Gastroenterol*, 2004 10:2628-2631.

Liang, Y; Hou, M; Kallab, AM; Barrett, JT; El Etreby, F; Schoenlein, PV. Induction of antiproliferation and apoptosis in estrogen receptor negative MDA-231 human breast cancer cells by mifepristone and 4-hydroxytamoxifen combination therapy: a role for TGFbeta1. *Int J Oncol*, 2003 23: 369-380.

Liu, Y; Wang, LL; Deng, Y. Enhancement of antitumor effect of cisplatin against human ovarian carcinoma cells by mifepristone in vivo. *Di Yi Jun Yi Da Xue Xue Bao*, 2003 23:242-4.

Lopez-Flores, A; Jurado, R; Garcia-Lopez, P. A high-performance liquid chromatographic assay for determination of cisplatin in plasma, cancer cell, and tumor samples. *J pharmacol Toxicol Methods*, 2005 52:366-372.

Lorincz, AT. Screening for cervical cancer: new alternatives and research. *Salud Publica Mex*, 2003,45:S376-387.

Lorincz, AL; Reid, R; Jonson, AB; Greenberg, MD; Lancaster, W; Kurman, RJ. Human papillomavirus infection of the cervix: relative risk associations of 15 common anogenital types. *Obstet Gynecol*, 1992 79:328,

Mahajan, DK; London, SN. Mifepristone (RU486): a review. Fertil Steril, 1997 68: 967-976

Mangelsdorf, DJ; Thummel, C; Beato, M; Herrlich, P; Schutz, G; Umesono K; Blumberg, B; Kastner, P; Mark, M; Chambon, P; Evans, RM. The nuclear receptor superfamily: the second decade Cell, 1995 83:835-839.

Marino M, Acconcia F, Bresciani F, Weisz A, Trentalance A (2002) Distinct nongenomic signal transduction pathways controlled by 17B-estradiol regulate DNA synthesis and cyclin D1 gene transcription in HepG2 cells. *Mol Biol Cell* 13:3720-3729.

Martin, JD; Hahnel, R; Mc Cartney, AJ; DeKlerk, N. The influence of estrogen and progesterone receptors on survival in patients with carcinoma of the uterine cervix. *Gynecol Oncol*, 1986 23:329-335.

Matsushita, H; Morishita, R; Nata, T; Aoki, M; Nakagami, H; Taniyama, Y; Yamamoto, K; Higaki, J; Yasufumi, K; Ogihara, T. Hypoxia-induced endothelial apoptosis through nuclear factor-kappaB (NF-kappaB)-mediated bcl-2 suppression: in vivo evidence of the importance of NF-kappaB in endothelial cell regulation. *Cir Res*, 2000 86:974-81.

Meanwell, CA. The epidemiology and etiology of cervical cancer. In:Blackledge GRP, Jordan JA, Shingleton HM, eds. *Textbook of gynecologic oncology*. Philadelphia: WB Saunders, 1991:250.

Miller, WR. Uptake and synthesis of steroid hormones by the breast. *Endocr Related Cancer*, 1997 4:307-311.

Mittal, R; Tsutsumi, K; Pater, A; Pater, MM. Human papillomavirus type 16 expression in cervical keratinocytes: role of progesterone and glucocorticoid hormones. *Obstet Gynecol*, 1993 81:5-12.

Mohar, A; Frias, M; Beltran, A; Mora, T; Solorza, G; Herrera, A; Ramírez, J. Epidemiología descriptiva del cancer cervico uterino. Instituto Nacional de Cancerología 1985-1991. *Rev Inst Nal Cancerol (Mex)*, 1993 39:1849-1854.

Mourits, MJ; Hollema, H; De Vries, EG; Ten-Hoor, KA; Willemse, PH; VanDer Zee, AG.) Apoptosis and apoptosis-associated parameters in relation to tamoxifen exposure in postmenopausal endometrium. *Hum Pathol*, 2002 33:341-346.

Muñoz, N; Bosch, FX; de Sanjose, S; Shah, KV. The role of HPV is the etiology of cervical cancer. *Mutat. Res*, 1994 305:293-301.

Murphy, AA; Zhou, MH; Malkapuram, S; Santanam, N; Parthasarathy, S; Sidell, N. RU486-induced growth inhibition of human endometrial cells. *Fertil Steril*, 2000,74:1014-9.

Mutch, DG; Bloss, JD. Gemcitabine in cervical cancer. *Gynecol Oncol* 2003 90:S8-15.

Nooter, K; Stoter, G. Molecular mechanisms of multidrug resistance in cancer chemotherapy. *Pathol Res Pract*, 1996 192:768-780.

Onate, SA; Tsai, SY; Tsai, MJ; O'Malley, BW. Sequence and characterization of a coactivator for the steroid hormone receptor superfamily. *Science*, 1995 270: 1354-1357

Parazzini, F; LaVecchia, C. Epidemiology of adenocarcinoma of the cervix. *Gynecol Oncol*, 1990 39:40-46.

Payen, L; Delugin, L; Courtois, A; Trinquart, Y; Guillouzo, A; Fardel, O. Reversal of MRP-mediated multidrug resistance in human lung cancer cells by the antiprogestatin drug RU486. *Biochem Biophys Res Commun*, 1999 258: 513-518.

Perez, EA; Gandara, DR; Edelman, MJ; O'Donnell, R; Lauder, IJ; DeGregorio, M. Phase I trial of high-dose tamoxifen in combination with cisplatin in patients with lung cancer and other advanced malignancies. *Cancer Invest*, 2003 21:1-6.

Peters, RK; Chao, A; Mack, TM; Thomas, D; Bernstein, L; Henderson, BE. Increased frequency of adenocarcinoma of the uterine cervix in young women in Los Angeles Country. *J Natl Cancer Inst*, 1986 1986:423-8.

Piper, JM. Oral contraceptives and cervical cancer. *Gynecol Oncol*, 1985 22:1-14.

Potish, RA; Twiggs, LB; Adcock, LL; Prem, K; Savage, JE; Leung, BS. Prognostic importance of progesterone and estrogen receptors in cancer of the uterine cervix. *Cancer*, 1986 58:1709-1713.

Qin, TN; Wang, LL. Enhanced sensitivity of ovarian cell line to cisplatin induced by mifepristone and its mechanism. *Di Yi Jun Yi Da Xue Xue Bao*, 2002 22:344-6.

Ramirez, J; Luévano, E; Mora, A; Solorza, G; Alcal, J; Verduzco, L; Guadarama, R; Beltran, A. Carcinoma cervico uterino: Análisis epidemiológico de 140 casos. *Rev Inst Nal Cancerol (Mex)*, 1983 3:417-442.

Roberstson, JF; Nicholson, RI; Bundred, NJ; Anderson, E; Rayter, Z; Dowsett, M; Fox, JN; Gee, JM; Webster, A; Wakeling, AE; Morris, C; Dixon, M. Comparison of the short-term biological effects of 7ά-[9-(4,4,5,5,5-pentafluoropenthylsulfinyl)-nonyl]estra-1,3,5,(10)-triene-3,17 beta-diol (faslodex) versus tamoxifen in postmenopausal women with primary breast cancer. *Cancer Res*, 2001 61: 6739-6746.

Rocereto, TF; Saul, HM; Aikins, JA Jr; Paulson, J. Phase II study of mifepristone (RU486) in refractory ovarian cancer. *Gynecol Oncol*, 2000 77: 429-432.

Rose, FV; Barnea, ER. Response of human ovarian carcinoma cell lines to antiprogestin mifepristone. *Oncogene*, 1996 12: 999-1003.

Rose, PG; Blessing, JA; Lele, S; Abulafia, O. Evaluation of pegylated liposomal doxorubicin (Doxil) as second-line chemotherapy of squamous cell carcinoma of the cervix: A phase II study of the Gynecologic Oncology Group. *Gynecol Oncol*, 2006 [Epub ahead of print].

Rosenberg-Zand, RS; Grass, L; Magklara, A; Jenkins, DJ; Diamandis, EP.) Is ICI 182,780 an antiprogestin in addition to being an antiestrogen?. Breast Cancer Res Treat, 2000 60:1-8.

Sanborn, BM; Held, B; Kuo, HS. Hormonal action in human cervix-II. Specific progestogen binding proteins in human cervix. *J Steroid Biochem*, 1976 7:665-672.

Scambia, G; Panici, B; Baiochi, G; Battaglia, F; Ferrandina, G; Greggi, S; Mancuso, S. Steroid hormone receptors in carcinoma of the cervix: look of response to an antiestrogen. *Gynecol Oncol*, 1990, 37:323-326.

Schilder, JM; Stehman, FB. Stage Ia - IIa cancer of the cervix. *Cancer J*, 2003 9:395-403.

Schneider, CC; Gibb, RK; Taylor, D; Wan, T; Gercel-Taylor, C. Inhibition of endometrial cancer cell lines by mifepristone (RU 486*). J Soc Gynecol Investig*, 1998 5: 334-338.

Schneider-Maunory, S; Croissant, O; Orth, G. Integration of human papillomavirus type 16 DNA sequences: a possible early event in the progression of genital tumors. *J Virol*, 1987 61:3295-3298.

Slee, EA; Harte, MT; Kluck, RM; Wolf, BB; Casiano, CA; Newmeyer, DD; Wang, HG; Reed, JC; Nicholson, DW; Alnemnri, ES; Green, DR; Martin, SJ. Ordering the cytocrome c-eliminated caspase cascade: hierarchial activation of caspase -2,-3,-6,-7,-8, and 10 in caspase -9-dependent manner. *J Cell Biol*, 1999 144:281-292.

Smith, CL; Onate, SA; Tsai, MJ, O'Malley, BW. *Proc. Natl. Acad. Sci. USA*, 1996 93: 8884-8888.

Smith, DF; Toft, DO. Steroid receptors and their associated proteins. *Mol Endocrinol*, 1993 7:4-11.

Spitz, IM; Bardin, CW. Mifepristone (RU486), a modulator of progestin and glucocorticoid action. *N Engl J Med*, 1993 329:404-12.

Tan-Chiu, E; Wang, J; Costantino, JP; Paik, S; Butch, C; Wickerham, DL; Fisher, B; Wolmark, N. Effects of tamoxifen on benign breast disease in women at high risk for breast cancer. *J Natl Cancer Inst*, 2003 95:302-307.

Tavassoli, M; Soltaninia, J; Rudnicka, J; Mashanyare, D; Johnson, N; Gaken, J. Tamoxifen inhibits the growth of head and neck cancer cells and sensitizes these cells to cisplatin induced apoptosis: role of TGF-beta1. *Carcinogenesis*, 2002 23:1569-1575.

Terenius, L; Lindell, A; Persson, BH. Binding of estradiol-17-beta to human cancer tissue of the female genital tract. *Cancer Res*, 1971 31:1895-1898.

Tewari, KS; Taylor, JA; Liao, SY; DiSaia, PJ; Burger, R; Monk, B; Hughes, CC; Villarreal, LP. Development and assessment of a general theory of cervical carcinogenesis utilizing a severe combined immunodeficiency murine-human xenograft model. *Gynecol Oncol*, 2000 77:137-148.

Thigpen, T. The role of chemotherapy in the management of carcinoma of the cervix. *Cancer J*, 2003 9:425-432.

Thomas, EJ; Walton, P; Thomas, NM; Dowsett, M. The effects of ICI 182,780, a pure anti-estrogen, on the hypothalamic-pituitary-gonadal axis and on endometrial proliferation in pre-menopausal women. *Hum Reproduction*, 1994 9:1991-1996.

Tinker, AV; Bhagat, K; Swenerton, K; Hoskins, PJ. Carboplatin and paclitaxel for advanced and recurrent cervical carcinoma: the British Columbia Cancer Agency experience. *Gynecol Oncol*, 2005 98:54-58.

Tsai, MJ; O'Malley, BW. Molecular mechanism of action of steroid/thyroid receptor superfamily members. *Ann Rev Biochem*, 1994 63:451-486.

Twiggs, S; Potish, R; Leung, B; Carson, L; Adcock, L; Savage, J; Prem, K. Cytosolic estrogen and progesterone receptors as prognostic parameters in stage IB cervical carcinoma. *Gynecol Oncol,* 1987 28:156-160.

Ueda, K; Okamura, N; Hirai, M; Tanigawara, Y; Saeki, T; Kioka, N; Komano, T; Hori, R. Human P-glycoprotein transports cortisol, aldosterone, and dexamethasone, but not progesterone. *J Biol Chem*, 1992 267:24248-52.

Von Knebel Doeberitz, M; Bauknecht, T; Bartsch, D; ZurHausen, H. Influence of chromosomal integration on glucocorticoid regulated transcription of growth -stimulating papillomavirus genes E6/E7 in cervical carcinoma cells. *Proc Natl Acad Sci USA*, 1991 88:1411-1415.

Von Knebel Doeberitz, M; Rittmuller; Zur Hausen, H; Durst, M. Inhibition of tumorigenicity of cervical cancer cells in nude mice by HPV E6/E7 anti-sense RNA. *Int J Cancer*, 1992 51:831-834.

Walboomers, JM; Jacobs, MV; Manos, MM; Bosch, FX; Kummer, JA; Shah, KV, Snijders, PJ; Peto, J; Meijer CJ; Munoz, N. Human papillomavirus is a necessary cause of invasive cervical cancer worldwide. *J Pathol*, 1999 189:12-19.

Wilczynski, SP; Bergen, S; Walker, J; Liao, SY; Pearlman, LF. Human papillomaviruses and cervical cancer: analysis of histopathologic features associated with different viral types. *Hum Pathol*, 1988 19:697-704.

Yang, CP; DePinho, SG; Greenberger, LM; Arceci, RJ; Horwitz, SB. Progesterone interacts with P-glycoprotein in multidrug-resistant cells and in the endometrium of gravid uterus. *J Biol Chem*, 1989 264:782-8.

In: Drug Toxicity: New Research
Editor: Cam E. Vellotis, pp.291-299
ISBN 978-1-60456-320-7

Chapter 9

Influence of Low-Toxicity Chemical Agents at Low Doses on Oxidative Processes in the Liver of Mice

M.V. Kozlov, V.V. Urnysheva and L.N. Shishkina
N.M. Emanuel Institute of Biochemical Physics, Russian Academy of Sciences,
ul. Kosygin 4, Moscow, 119991 Russia

Abstract

It was shown that the scale or direction of correlations between both the several parameters of the lipid composition and the generalized parameters of the phospholipids composition of the murine liver depend on the kinetic characteristics of their lipids (the lipid peroxides content, the capacity of lipids to decompose peroxides). In was found that the combined intraperitoneal administration of the low- toxicity surfactant (Tween 80) and acetone at low doses causes disturbances in the lipid peroxidation regulatory system which manifest themselves in 1 month after the action.

Key words: lipid peroxidation, low doses, liver of mice, Tween 80, acetone, combined effect

Aims and Background

The hematopoietic system and hepatocytes of liver play a important role in the maintenance of the homeostasis in organism. In [1, 2] it was shown that hepatocytes are also having high sensitive to technogenic contamination of the environment. The detoxification which consists in the removal of various chemical substances that are products of the vitally important processes in organism and alien compounds is one of the main function of liver [3].

The investigation of the state of lipid peroxidation (LPO) is one of the perspective lead in the search for tests for the estimation of biological consequences of damaging effects because of a high sensitivity of the LPO regulatory system parameters in tissues of wild rodents and laboratory animals to the action of unfourable factors [1, 2, 4, 5].

Polyoxyethylensorbitanmonooleate (Tween 80) which is one of the common technogenic unfourable factors – surfactant and acetone were chosen as chemical agents. The surfactant's role in the development of biological consequences of the combined effect of different agents enhances due to their properties to facilitate the penetration of hydrophobic compounds into cells. In practice, this distinction of surfactants is used for the prophylactic or therapeutic administration of lipid soluble substances into organism [6, 7]. Acetone is also one of the chemical agents which is widely used as a solvent and intermediate in the chemical, pharmaceutic and food industry.

It is well known that liver is the main organ of accumulation and metabolism of chemical agents in organism. This organ was chosen as an object for investigating of the remote consequences of the action of the chemical agents on organism.

The aim of this work is to study the combined effect of the surfactant and acetone at low doses on the parameters of the LPO regulatory system in the murine liver.

Experimental

The experiments were carried out on Balb/c mice (males, weight 16 – 20 g before the experiments, n = 13). The mice were divided into two groups. The first group (8 mice) was used as the intact biological control. The Tween 80 (Ferak Berlin, FRG) at the dose of 30 mg/kg as 0.3% solution in 10% mixture of acetone in water was administration intraperitoneally at the second group of mice (5 mice). The solution of 0.3% Tween 80 in the 10% aqueous solution of acetone (special purity grade) was prepared immediately before the experiment. Decapitation of mice was performed in 1 month after administration of chemical agents. Decapitation of intact mice was performed simultaneously with the experimental group. The murine liver was placed in ice-cooled weighting bottles immediately after the decapitation. The parameters to be studied were determined for each mouse.

Lipids of the liver were isolated by the method of Blay and Dyer in the Kates modification [8]. The qualitative and quantitative composition of phospholipids (PL) was determined by thin-layer chromatography as it was described in [9]. We used type G silica gel (Sigma, USA), glass plates 9 × 12 cm and the mixture of solvents - chloroform: methanol: glacial acetic acid: water (25:15:4:1) as a mobile phase. All the solvents were of special or chemical purity grade. The development of chromatograms was performed by iodine vapour. For the colour reaction for phosphorus, we used ammonium molybdate and ascorbic acid (Serva, FRG) and chemical purity perchloric acid. The amount of inorganic phosphorus was determined from the optic density of the solutions at the wavelength $\lambda = 800$ nm with KFK-3 (Russia) instrument. In addition to the quantitative analysis of different fractions of PL, the following generalized parameters of the lipid composition were also evaluated: the PL proportion in the total lipid composition (% PL); the ratio of phosphatidyl choline to phosphatidyl ethanolamine (PC/PE) content in PL; the ratio of the sums of the more easily to the more poorly oxidizable fractions of PL (ΣEOPLΣPOPL). The ΣEOPLΣPOPL value was calculated by the formula: ΣEOPLΣPOPL = (PI + PS + PE + CL + PA)/(LPC + SM + PC), where PI is phosphatidyl inositol, PS is phosphatidyl serine, CL is cardiolipin, PA is phosphatidic acid, LPC are PL lysoforms and SM is sphingomielin.

The content of LPO products, which have reacted with 2-thiobarbituric acid (TBA-reactive substances, TBA-RS) was determined spectrophotometrically by the method described in [10] with adding 10 μl of the 0.01% 4-methyl-2,6–ditert.butylphenol solution in ethanol. Protein was determined according to [11]. The peroxides concentration in lipids was determined iodometrically.

The data were processed by a commonly used variational statistic method [12] and by the KINS program given in [13].

Results and Discussion

One of the primary significance in the development of both the early and remote biological consequences of those effects have changes in the hematopoietic system induced by damaging effects. The inevitable changes in the organ weight observed under different experimental conditions made it possible to use these parameters as a criterion for the organ activity [14]. In larger animals, the organ weight is larger. As expected there is a direct correlation between the weight of liver and that of a mouse for the age control group with the correlation coefficient $R = 0.91 \pm 0.06$. However, in 1 month after the administration of surfactant and acetone the correlation between these parameters is absent for this group of mice ($R = 0.32$). This is evidence for a long-term persistence of the disturbances in the liver activity on the physiological level after the combined effect of chemical agents at the low doses. It should be noted that the variability of the liver weight in the experimental group decreased drastically as compared with that for the control group. Visually the murine liver in the experimental group was dark and the size of the gallbladder is smaller than in the control group.

The influence of the unfourable low-toxicity ecological factors of the chemical nature at low doses on the LPO process in Balb/c mice liver was assessed.

From our experiments we found that the liver lipids of mice in the control age group exhibit different kinetic characteristics. Liver lipids of one subgroup of the intact animals contain peroxides ($[ROOH]_0$), liver lipids of another control subgroup had a capacity of decomposing peroxides, i.e. exhibit an antiperoxide activity (APA). In these cases the concentration of peroxide in liver lipids is equal to zero. It was found that depending on the kinetic characteristics of lipids there are differences in values of the several generalized parameters of the lipid composition and the scale and direction of correlation between these parameters in these groups of control mice. Thus, when lipids exhibit the property of the peroxide decomposition, the average values of the PL fraction in the total lipid content and the ratio of the sums of the more easily to the more poorly oxidizable PL fractions are significantly lower as compared with the control animals whose lipids contain peroxides (figure 1). The average value of the PC/PE ratio in the group of mice with APA of their liver lipids also tends to decrease as compared with that for the another control animals. On the contrary, the concentration of the oxidation products ([TBA-RS]) in the subgroup of mice with APA of their liver lipids tends to increase as compared with that for the another control animals (figure 1).

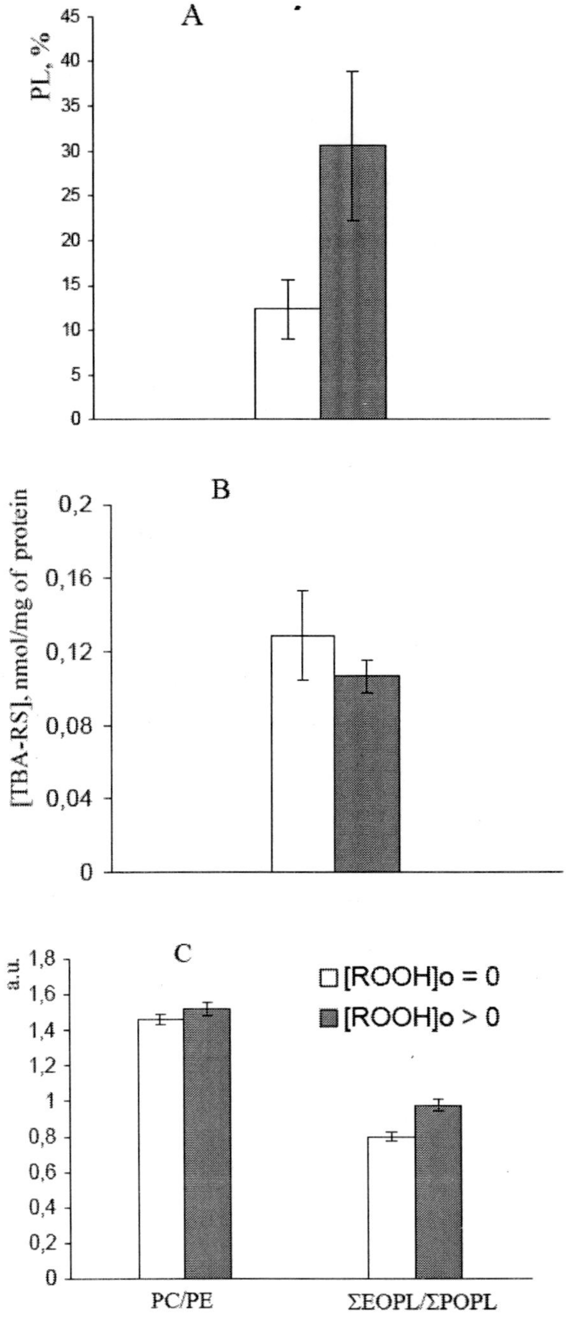

Figure 1. Parameters of the lipid peroxidation in liver of the control mice: □ - the liver lipids exhibit an antiperoxide activity; ■ - the liver lipids contain peroxides; A – the phospholipids proportion in the total lipid composition; B – the amount of the TBA-reactive substances; C – the ratio of phosphatidyl choline to phosphatidyl ethanolamine and the ratio of the sums of the more easily to the more poorly oxidizable fractions in phospholipids.

The dependence of the scale and/or direction of correlations on the lipid kinetic characteristics was revealed in the study on the interrelations between lysoforms of PL and PC amounts and the ratio of the more easily and the more poorly oxidizable fractions and the PC/PE ratio in PL liver in the control group of mice. Thus, the interrelation between the lysoform relative content and the PC proportion in the murine liver PL whose lipids have the APA properties is practically linear (R = 0.999) with the linear regression coefficient 1.53 ± 0.03 (figure 2,A). In mice, whose liver lipids contain peroxides, the similar correlation is reciprocal (R = – 0.90 ± 0.08) with the linear regression coefficient 1.1 ± 0.2 (figure 2,A).

Regardless of the presence or absence of peroxides in their liver lipids the reciprocal linear correlations between the ratio of the more easily and the more poorly oxidizable fractions and the PC/PE ratio in PL liver in the control age group of Balb/c mice were revealed. However, because of the significant decrease in the proportion of the more easily oxidizable fractions in the murine liver PL when lipids exhibit the APA properties (figure 1) the experimental data are positioned on different correlation lines (figure 2,B) Furthermore, the certain differences are determined for the coefficients of the linear regression of the correlation between the lipid ability to oxidation and the structural state of the membrane system of liver. For the control age groups of mice the coefficient of the linear regression of the reciprocal correlation between the parameters of ΣEOPL/ΣPOPL and PC/PE is equal to 0.516 ± 0.065 (R = – 0.98 ± 0.02) for lipids with APA properties and to 0.324 ± 0.075 (R = – 87 ± 0.11) for lipids containing peroxides.

In the experimental group of mice the liver lipids as rule contain peroxides. APA lipids was found only in liver of one mouse. The analysis of consequences of the single administration of the surfactant and acetone at the low doses to Balb/c mice was performed relative to the same parameters of LPO process for the control group of mice whose liver lipids also contained peroxides.

It should be noted that the extent of changes in the various average parameters of LPO in liver of mice is different in 1 month after administration of the 0.3 % Tween 80 in the 10 % aqueous acetone solution. The average values of the content of the TBA-reactive substances in liver homogenate, the amounts of the peroxides in lipids and the PL proportion in the total lipid composition do not differ significantly in the experimental and control groups due to the high individual variability of these parameters (figure 3,A; 3,B). The average magnitude of the ratio of the sums of the more easily to the ore poorly oxidizable fraction is the significantly lower and the PC/PE ratio tends to increase for the liver PL in the experimental group as compared with that in the control group (figure 3,C).

The administration of the solution of the 0.3 % Tween 80 in the 10 % aqueous acetone to Balb/c mice causes the disturbance of biochemical and biophysical parameters in tissues that is revealed in a change in the scale and direction of interrelations between the LPO regulatory system parameters. The absence of the correlation (R = – 0.10) between the content of lysoforms and the relative content of PC in the murine liver PL in 1 month after the action of the chemical agents was shown (figure 2,A). The reciprocal correlation between the lipid oxidizability and the PC/PE ratio retains (R = – 0.998 ± 0.002) in the experimental group of mice, however, coefficient of the linear regression (0.864 ± 0.025) is 2.7 times higher than that for the control group (figure 2,B).

The analysis of the interrelation between the primary and secondary products of oxidation in the murine liver in the experimental and control groups showed great changes in the function of the murine liver after injection of the surfactant and acetone at low doses (figure 4). While the direct correlation (R = 0.96 ± 0.03) between the content of the TBA-reactive substances in the homogenate and the amount of peroxides in liver lipids was revealed for the control group, the correlation was reciprocal in the murine liver for the experimental group (R = – 0.77 ± 0.21).

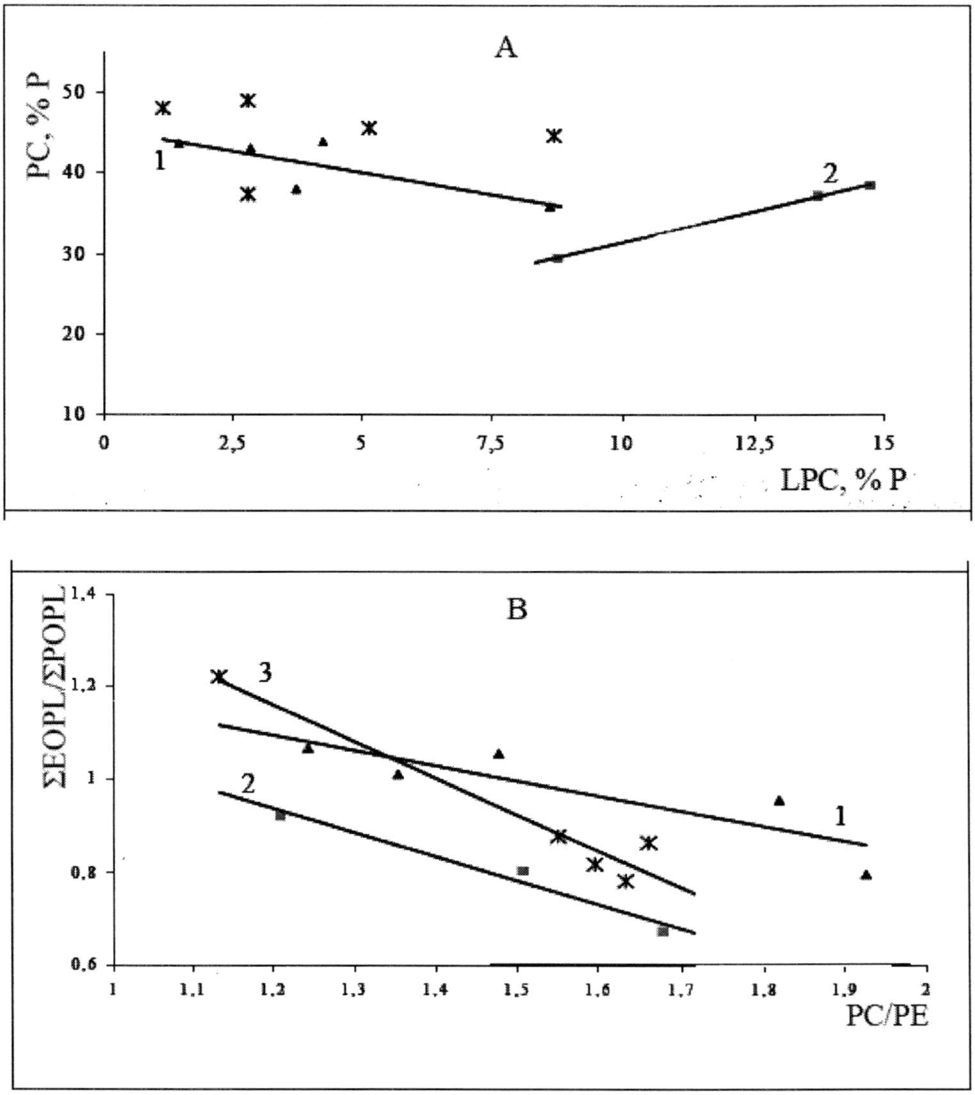

Figure 2. Interrelation between the proportion of phosphatidyl choline and the relative content of lysoforms of phospholipids (A) and between the ratio of the sums of the more easily to more poorly oxidizable fractions and the ratio of phosphatidyl choline to phosphatidyl ethanolamine (B) in the liver phospholipids.: 1 – the liver lipids contain peroxides (the control group of mice); 2 – the liver lipids exhibit an antiperoxide activity (the control group of mice); 3 (*) – the liver lipids contain peroxides (the experimental group of mice, i.e. in 1 month after the Tween 80 and acetone administration.

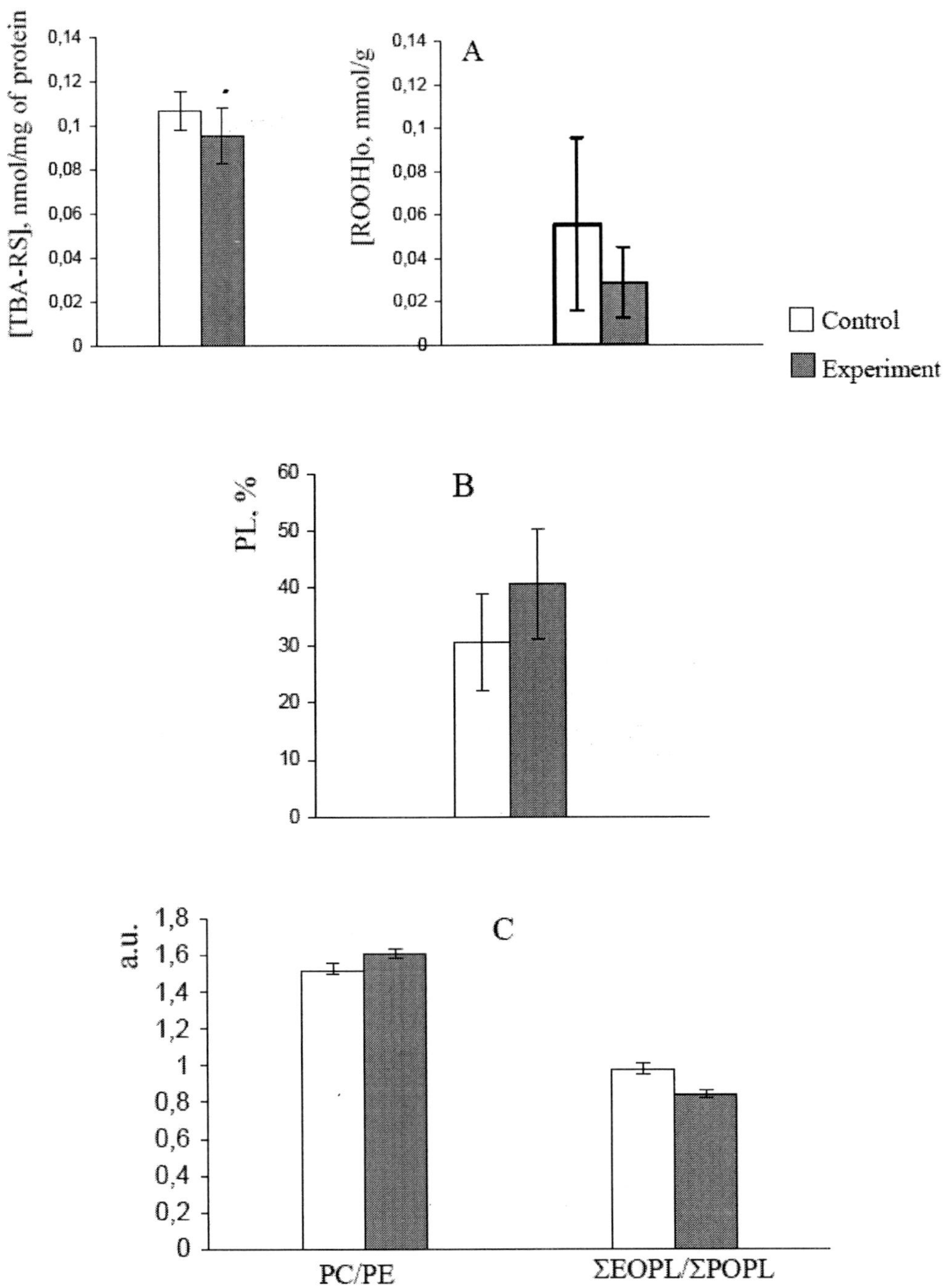

Figure 3. Various parameters of the lipid peroxidation in liver of mice in the control and experimental groups: A – the content of the TBA-reactive substances and the amount of peroxides in lipids; B – the phospholipid proportion in the total lipid composition; C – the ratio of phosphatidyl choline to phosphatidyl ethanolamine and the ratio of the sums of the more easily to the more poorly oxidizable fractions in phospholipids.

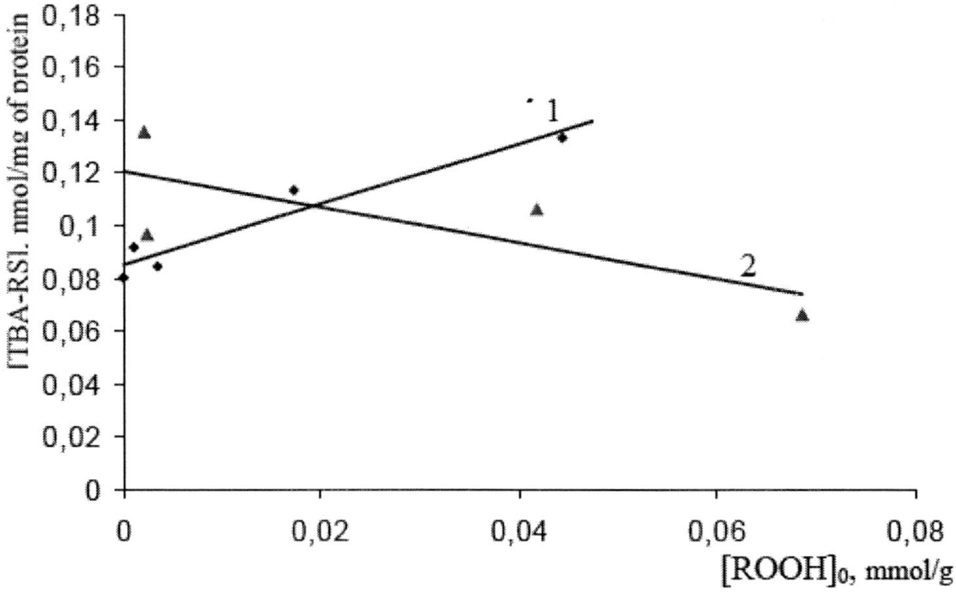

Figure 4. The influence of the intraperitoneal administration of Tween 80 and acetone on the interrelation between the content of the TBA – reactive substances in the homogenate and the amount of peroxides in the liver lipids of the control mice (1) and in 1 month after the action (2).

The data obtained lead us to conclusion about the substantial role of the kinetic characteristic of lipids for the function activity of the murine liver and the persistence of the disturbances in the intensity of the oxidative process and the disbalance in processes of the biosynthesis and degradation of PL a long time after the action of the low-toxicity chemical agents at the low doses on the animal organism.

This work was support by the Foundation of the Program of Presidium of Russian Academy of Sciences "Basic sciences – for medicine".

References

[1] A.G. Kudyasheva, L.N. Shishkina, N.G. Zagorskaya, A.I. Taskaev, "Biochemical mechanisms of the radiation damage of the natural rodent population", St.-Petersburg, *Nauka,* 1997, 156 pp. (In Russian)

[2] E.V. Shtamm, L.N. Shishkina, N.B. Kozlova et al. *"Vodosnab. and sanitar. tekhnika",* N 10, pp. 18 – 21, 1997 (in Russain).

[3] T.I. Bonashevskaya, N.N. Belyaeva, "Morphofunctional evaluation of the genotoxic action of the chemical environment factors", pp. 20 – 25, in the book *"Structural – functional and biochemical mechanisms of effect of the environmental factors on humans and experimental animals",* Moscow, 1986 (in Russian).

[4] V.V. Urnisheva, L.N. Shishkina, *Biophysics* Vol. 48., N 4., pp. 744 – 753, 2003.

[5] V.V. Urnisheva, L.N. Shishkina, *Bull. RAS, Ser. Biology,* N 2, pp. 163 – 168, 2004.

[6] Frankfurt, Voprosy onkol., Vol. 21, N 10, pp. 63 – 67, 1975 (in Russian).

[7] E.B. Burlakova, A.V. Alesenko, E.M. Molochkina, N.P. Pal'mina, N.G. Khrapova, "Bioantioxidants in the Radiation Damage and the Tumor Growth", Moscow, *Nauka,* 1975, pp. 214 (in Russian).

[8] M. Kates. The technique of lipidology. Moscow: *Mir,* -1975. 322. pp. (Russian version).

[9] 9. "Biological membranes. A practice approach." / Eds J. B.C. Findlay, W.H. Evans – Moscow: *Mir,*-1990. 424 pp. (Russian version).

[10] T. Asakawa, S. Matsushita. *Lipids.* - 1980. - V. 15. - No. 3. pp. 137-140.

[11] R. Itzhaki, D.M. Gill. A*nal.Biochem.*- 1964.- V. 9. pp. 401 - 409.

[12] G.F. Lakin. Biometry. 3rd publication. Moscow: Higher school, 1990. 293 pp. (in Russian).

[13] E.F. Brin, S.O. Travin, *Chem. Phys. Reports,* Vol. 10, N 6, pp. 830 – 837, 1990.

[14] O.K. Khmel'nitskii, V.L. Bykov, *Arkhiv patolog.,* Vol. XIII, N 6, pp. 3 – 9, 1986 (in Russian).

In: Drug Toxicity: New Research
Editor: Cam E. Vellotis, pp.301-304

ISBN 978-1-60456-320-7

Chapter 10

Nephrotoxicity of D-serine in Rats

Ryuichi Konno*
Department of Microbiology, Dokkyo Medical University, Japan.

Keywords: D-serine, nephrotoxicity, rat, D-amino-acid oxidase, glucosuria

1. Introduction

D-Serine is nephrotoxic in rats. Intraperitoneal injection of d-serine causes necrosis of the cells in the proximal tubules, resulting in glucosuria, aminoaciduria, proteinuria, and polyuria [1,2]. However, the precise mechanism by which D-serine induces nephrotoxicity is not well understood. D-Amino-acid oxidase (EC 1.4.3.3) is suspected to be involved in the D-serine-induced nephrotoxicity because (a) D-serine is reabsorbed in the straight part (pars recta) of the proximal tubules, where cell damage is observed [1-3], (b) D-amino-acid oxidase is localized in this region [4,5], (c) D-serine is a good substrate for this enzyme [6], and (d) one of the products of the D-amino-acid oxidase reaction, hydrogen peroxide, is a cytotoxin.

However, there are perplexing problems: (a) D-serine is not nephrotoxic in mice, guinea pigs, rabbits, dogs, hamsters, or gerbils that have D-amino-acid oxidase activity comparable to rats [7,8]; (b) D-alanine, which is also a good substrate for D-amino-acid oxidase, is not nephrotoxic in rats [8]. These facts cast doubt on the involvement of this enzyme in d-serine-induced nephrotoxicity.

Thus, D-serine-induced nephrotoxicity is a challenging problem. One example of the induction of the kidney damage by D-serine is described here.

* Correspondence concerning this article should be addressed to Ryuichi Konno, E-mail: konno@dokkyomed.ac.jp, FAX: +81-282-86-5616.

2. Materials

1. Male Fischer 344 rats (F344 rats, 6-10 weeks old, 100-250 g).
2. D-Serine (Sigma Chemical Co., St. Louis, MO, USA).
3. Metabolic cages (Model SN-781, Shinano Manufacturing Co., Ltd., Tokyo, Japan, or an equivalent).
4. Glucose assay kit (Wako Pure Chemicals, Osaka, Japan)

3. Methods

1. Male F344 rats are housed in individual metabolic cages. They are allowed free access to the commercial diet and tap water.
2. Urine is collected for 24 h prior to D-serine administration.
3. D-Serine is dissolved in 0.85% NaCl at 80 mg/ml and is injected intraperitoneally into the rats at a dose of 0.8 g/kg.
4. Urine is collected daily at 24-h intervals for a week.
5. The volume of the urine is measured and the glucose content is measured.

4. Results

Male adult F344 rats excreted approximately 6.0 ml of urine during 24 h (Day -1) and their urine contained approximately 0.2 mg of glucose/ml. Intraperitoneal injection of D-serine into the F344 rats caused glucosuria (Figure 1A). Urine collected for the first 24 h (Day 1) after the D-serine injection contained about seven times more glucose than that collected for the 24 h (Day -1) before the injection. However, the urinary glucose level dropped significantly on Day 2 and returned to the normal level on Day 4.

The high level of glucose in the urine was accompanied by an increase in the urinary volume (Figure 1B). The urinary volume after the D-serine injection was increased about three times on Day 1. In contrast to urinary glucose, the high level of the urine volume continued until Day 7.

5. Notes

1. Inbred F344 rats are more sensitive to D-serine than Sprague-Dawley rats.
2. D-Serine doses of 0.5-1.0 g/kg are used to induce the obvious damage in the kidney.
3. Amino acid concentration in the urine is determined as follows [9]. Sulfosalicylic acid (20%) is added to the urine at a final concentration of 5% and vortexed. The mixture was centrifuged at 14,000 g for 10 min and the supernatant solution is filtered through a 0.22-µm membrane (Ultra-free C3GV, Nihon Millipore, Tokyo, Japan). The filtrate is applied to an automated amino acid analyzer (Model L-8500A, Hitachi, Tokyo, Japan). The amino acid concentration in the urine is usually expressed on the basis of the creatinine content in the urine. The creatinine content is determined using an assay kit (Wako Pure Chemicals).

4. The protein content in the urine is determined using a Non-Interfering Protein Assay kit (Geno Technology, St. Louis, Mo., USA) [9].
5. For histopathological examination, the kidney is fixed in 10% formalin and embedded in parfifin. Thin tissue sections are cut on a microtome and are stained with hematoxylin and eosin [9].
6. It has become clear that D-amino-acid oxidase is involved in D-serine-induced nephrotoxicity because D-serine injection did not cause glucosuria or polyuria in mutant rats lacking D-amino-acid oxidase [10]. The results that pretreatment of rats with sodium benzoate, a competitive inhibitor of D-amino-acid oxidase, resulted in a dose-dependent reduction of D-serine-induced nephrotoxicity [11] are consistent with this conclusion.

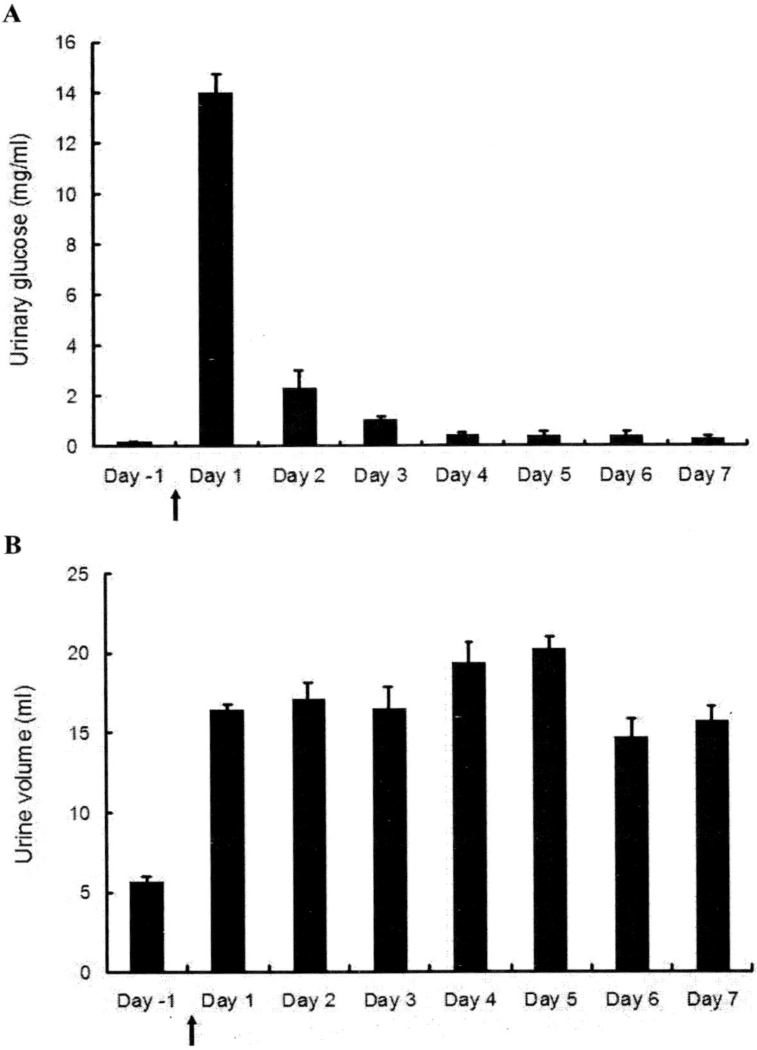

Figure 1. Glucosuria and polyuria induced by the administration of D-serine. D-Serine was injected intraperitoneally into adult male F344 rats at a dose of 0.8 g/kg (arrow). Their urine was collected daily at 24-h intervals for seven days. The glucose content in the urine (A) and the volume of the urine (B) were measured. The values represent the mean ± SEM in five rats. (Reprinted with permission from Maekawa *et al.*, *Chem Res Toxicol*, *18*, 1678-1682, Copyright (2005) American Chemical Society.)

Acknowledgement

This work was supported in part by Research Grant from Asahi Glass Foundation.

References

[1] Ganote, C. E., Peterson, D. R. and Carone, F. A. (1974). The nature of D-serine-induced nephrotoxicity. *Am J Pathol 77*, 269-282.

[2] Carone, F. A. and Ganote, C. E. (1975). D-Serine nephrotoxicity. *Arch Pathol 99*, 658-662.

[3] Silbernagl, S., Völker, K. and Dantzler, W. H. (1999). D-Serine is reabsorbed in rat renal pars recta. *Am J Physiol 276*, F857-F863.

[4] Usuda, N., Yokota, S., Hashimoto, T. et al. (1986). Immunocytochemical localization of D-amino acid oxidase in the central clear matrix of rat kidney peroxisomes. *J Histochem Cytochem 34*, 1709-1718.

[5] Perotti, M. E., Gavazzi, E., Trussardo, L. et al. (1987). Immunoelectron microscopic localization of D-amino acid oxidase in rat kidney and liver. *Histochem J 19*, 157-169.

[6] Dixon, M. and Kleppe, K. (1965). D-Amino acid oxidase. II. Specificity, competitive inhibition and reaction sequence. *Biochim Biophys Acta 96*, 368-382.

[7] Morehead, R. P., Poe, W. D., Williams, J. O. et al. (1946). The influence of age and species on the nephrotoxic action of DL-serine. *Am J Pathol 22*, 658.

[8] Kaltenbach, J. P., Ganote, C. E. and Carone, F. A. (1979). Renal tubular necrosis induced by compounds structurally related to D-serine. *Exp Mol Pathol 30*, 209-214.

[9] Konno, R., Ikeda, M., Yamaguchi, K. et al. (2000). Nephrotoxicity of D-propargylglycine in mice. *Arch Toxicol 74*, 473-479.

[10] Maekawa, M., Okamura, T., Kasai, N. et al. (2005). D-Amino-acid oxidase is involved in D-serine-induced nephrotoxicity. *Chem Res Toxicol, 18,* 1678-1682.

[11] Williams, R. E. and Lock, E. A. (2005). Sodium benzoate attenuates D-serine induced nephrotoxicity in the rat. *Toxicology 207*, 35-48.

Index

A

B

C

D

E

F

G

H

I

J

K

L

M

N

O

P

Q

R

S

U

V

W

X

Y

Z